Socializing Medicine

Crossings: Asian Cinema and Media Culture

Series Editor: Man-Fung Yip (University of Oklahoma)

The series "Crossings" publishes books in English and Chinese that investigate Asian cinema and media from cross-disciplinary and cross-methodological perspectives. It situates Asian cinema and media within a global or regional framework and explores different dimensions of transnationality in relation to production, distribution, and reception. It also entails trans-medial interrogations of past and present media culture, looking into the complex interactions of media forms and how they have shaped aesthetic and social practices. Wide-ranging in scope and method, the series places special emphasis on cutting-edge scholarship that draws on careful archival research or that derives from vigorous, insightful theoretical study.

Also in the series:

Chinese Cinema: Identity, Power, and Globalization
Edited by Jeff Kyong-McClain, Russell Meeuf, and Jing Jing Chang

Malaysian Cinema in the New Millennium: Transcendence beyond Multiculturalism
Adrian Yuen Beng Lee

Remapping the Sinophone: The Cultural Production of Chinese-Language Cinema in Singapore and Malaya before and during the Cold War
Wai-Siam Hee

Screening Communities: Negotiating Narratives of Empire, Nation, and the Cold War in Hong Kong Cinema
Jing Jing Chang

Working the System: Motion Picture, Filmmakers, and Subjectivities in Mao-Era China, 1949–1966
Qiliang He

《重繪華語語系版圖：冷戰前後新馬華語電影的文化生產》
許維賢

《市井香港：戰前香港的粵語電影、宣傳電影和文化空間》
趙傑鋒

Socializing Medicine

Health Humanities and East Asian Media

Edited by Pao-chen Tang, Yuqian Yan, and
Ling Zhang

HKU PRESS
香港大學出版社

Hong Kong University Press
The University of Hong Kong
Pok Fu Lam Road
Hong Kong
https://hkupress.hku.hk

ISBN 978-988-8876-81-5 (*Hardback*)

British Library Cataloguing-in-Publication Data
A catalogue record for this book is available from the British Library.

Digitally printed

Contents

Illustrations

Acknowledgments

The editors wish to extend their deepest appreciation to friends and colleagues for their invaluable assistance throughout the creation of this volume. Our heartfelt thanks go to Paula Halperin, Kristine Harris, Paola Iovene, and Agustin Zarzosa for their support in facilitating an online workshop that allowed our contributors to present and discuss their drafts. We are equally grateful to the members of the "Dare to Win" interdisciplinary writing group for their insightful feedback on an early draft of our introduction. Our contributors deserve special recognition for their patience, diligence, and the originality of their chapters, which have been instrumental in bringing this volume to fruition. We owe a debt of gratitude to Kenneth Yung from Hong Kong University Press for his unwavering trust and guidance throughout this journey, and to the Press's copyediting and production team for the support during the editing process. We are also thankful for the perceptive and elaborate comments provided by two anonymous reviewers on the book manuscript.

Pao-chen Tang thanks the University of Manchester and the University of Sydney for various research supports, and Max Bledstein and Mei Yen Chua for their editing work. Yuqian Yan expresses gratitude toward Zhejiang University, Shanghai Film Studio, and Shi Chuan for helping to make connections. Ling Zhang is thankful to the State University of New York at Purchase College for their support. The editors also wish to acknowledge Wang Yujue, Wu Xueshan, Yuke Ma, Jeehey Kim, Jin Xu, Stephanie Su, Yuhang Li, Mia Yinxing Liu, Liang Luo, André Stufkens, National Sanatorium Nagashima Aiseien, Toho, Ke Chin-yuan, and Shengze Zhu for kindly assisting or permitting us to reprint the images on the book cover and in several chapters.

Contributors

Max Balhorn is an independent researcher who studies the intersections of media culture and Korean environmental history. He is also a Korean–English translator specializing in film studies and critical theory.

Jeehey Kim is an assistant professor of the art history program at the University of Arizona. Her first book, *Photography and Korea* (2023), is the first book on the history of Korean photography in English. She is currently working on a book project: *Photography and Death: Funerary Photo-Portraiture in East Asia*. She has also been writing articles on vernacular photographic practices, documentary films, and visual culture concerning the Cold War and gender politics in East Asia.

Lilian Kong is a PhD candidate at the University of Chicago, enrolled in the East Asian Languages and Civilizations and Cinema and Media Studies joint program. She studies contemporary Chinese film and media, with interests in genre, media atmosphere, transmedial and transnational methodologies, and digital media aesthetics.

Lu Liu is an assistant professor of Chinese at the Georgia Institute of Technology. Her research broadly examines the interplay of subject formation, science and technology, and visual and media cultures. Her book manuscript examines how the figuration of the pest from the 1930s to contemporary China produces socialist subjectivities. She is also working on a second book project about the conceptual exchange of microbiology, Cold War politics, and popular culture in China's socialist period.

Yuki Obayashi is a lecturer in Asian American studies at San Francisco State University. She received her doctoral degree in Literature at the University of California, Santa Cruz with designated emphases in Critical Race and Ethnic Studies and Feminist Studies. An introduction for Etsu Inagaki Sugimoto's *A Daughter of the Samurai* was coauthored with Karen Tei Yamashita for Penguin Random House's edition in 2021. Her research interests include Cold War and post–Cold War historiography in Asia and the Pacific, transnational Asian American Studies, comparative empire studies, nuclear militarism, and environmental racism.

Kathryn M. Tanaka is an associate professor at the University of Hyogo. Her research focuses on Hansen's disease literature and gender. Articles that focus on gender and Hansen's disease include "For the Purity of the Nation: Ogawa Masako and the Gendered Ethics of *Spring on the Small Island* (*Kojima no haru*)" in *U.S.-Japan Women's Journal* and "The Abject Woman and the Meaning of Illness in Kōda Rohan's 'Tai dokuro' (Encounter with a Skull)" in *Japanese Studies*. She is currently completing a book manuscript focused on Hansen's disease in Japan: *The Gendered Experience of Hansen's Disease in Literature and Public Discourse*.

Pao-chen Tang is a lecturer in film studies at the University of Sydney. He is currently writing his first book, which thinks about broadscale themes of environment and contemporary East Asian cinema through the logic and language of animism. Among other venues, his writings have appeared in *Screen, Journal of Cinema and Media Studies, Screen Bodies, Interdisciplinary Studies in Literature and Environment, Journal of Chinese Cinemas,* and *Early Popular Visual Culture*.

Chang-Min Yu is an assistant professor in the Department of Foreign Languages and Literatures at National Taiwan University. He received his PhD in Film Studies from the University of Iowa. His articles have appeared in *Film Criticism, Quarterly Review of Film and Video, NECSUS: European Journal of Media Studies,* and *The Cine-Files*. His current research interests lie in corporeal cinema, contemporary digital cinema, and Sinophone film historiographies.

Ban Wang is William Haas Professor in Chinese Studies at Stanford University. His publications include *The Sublime Figure of History* (Stanford University Press, 1997), *Illuminations from the Past* (Stanford UP, 2004), *History and Memory* (*Lishi yu jiyi*) (Oxford, 2004), *China in the World: Culture, Politics, and World Vision* (Duke University Press, 2022) and *At Home in Nature: Technology, Labor, and Critical Ecology* (Duke University Press, 2023). His edited volumes include *Chinese Visions of World Order: Tianxia, Culture, and Word Politics* (2017), *Words and Their Stories* (2011), *Debating Socialist Legacy* (2014), *China and Left Visions* (2012), and *Trauma and Cinema* (2004).

Chao Wang is a lecturer at The Chinese University of Hong Kong, Shenzhen. He is a historian of modern China specializing in disability studies and the social studies of medicine. He is writing his first book on the social history of blindness in modern China, which rethinks bodily difference as distributed capacity and the making of "disabled but not useless" persons at the intersections of the family, community, and the welfare state.

Yuqian Yan is an associate researcher at Zhejiang University in China. She received her PhD from the Department of Cinema and Media Studies and East Asian Languages and Civilizations at the University of Chicago. Her research interests include early Chinese cinema, historical representation, film and material culture, documentary, and contemporary media culture. She has published articles and book chapters on Chinese documentary as well as cinematic and theatrical representations of history. She is currently working on her book manuscript entitled *Assembling the Past: Ancient Costume Films in Republican China.*

Ling Zhang is an associate professor of cinema studies at the State University of New York at Purchase. She is completing her book manuscript entitled *Unruly Sounds: Chinese Cinema and Transnational Acoustic Culture, 1929–1949*. Zhang received her PhD from the Department of Cinema and Media Studies at the University of Chicago and specializes in film sound, Chinese-language cinema, documentary, women and cinema, Third World cultural exchange, and the cultural Cold War. She has published in both English and Chinese journals and anthologies including *Journal of Cinema and Media Studies, Film Quarterly, Journal of Chinese Cinemas, Comparative Cinema, The Journal of Popular Culture,* and *Asian Cinema,* among others.

Introduction

Pao-chen Tang, Yuqian Yan, and Ling Zhang

On July 23, 2021, fifteen minutes into the opening ceremony of the Tokyo Olympics, Japanese dancer Moriyama Mirai took the stage alone in a nearly empty stadium. Draped in white and illuminated by a spotlight, Moriyama's body gracefully unfolded from a crouched position, moving with a deliberate and forceful elegance before settling into a posture reminiscent of *Balasana* (child's pose)—a symbolic stance encapsulating both life and death. Throughout the performance, Moriyama's pale and expressionless face conveyed a palpable sense of unease and even terror, heightened by the eerie and unsettling music that accompanied the dance. Indeed, the performance was followed by a reminder of the social tenebrosity that the venue's strong spotlight could not dispel: a silent tribute to those who perished during the global COVID-19 pandemic. It was therefore fitting that Moriyama performed the *ankoku butō* (often abbreviated to *butō*)—literally the "dance of darkness"—developed by avant-garde choreographer Hijikata Tatsumi (1928–1986) in post–World War II Japan, when the disintegrating empire was reordered and reconstructed under American occupation. Drawing on the raw features, unpolished behaviors, and overtly sexualized expressions of marginalized individuals such as criminals, prostitutes, the ill, and the impoverished, Hijikata endeavored to acknowledge these subaltern subjects, who are often invisible or intentionally excluded from Japan's aesthetic canons.[1] By referencing such postwar extremism, Moriyama's performance channeled the spirits of those whose lives were lost due to the questionable public health policies of many governments during the ongoing pandemic in 2021.

The richness of Moriyama's dance gains additional depth when contextualized within the framework of the pandemic-influenced Olympics. The 2021 event, necessitated by global circumstances, was purposefully crafted for televisual broadcast.

1. Vicki Sanders, "Dancing and the Dark Soul of Japan: An Aesthetic Analysis of 'Butō'," *Asian Theatre Journal* 5, no. 2 (1988): 148–63.

Despite the longstanding global broadcast of the Olympics through communication satellites since the 1964 Tokyo Summer Games, the 2021 edition took on a new dimension as a technologically mediated spectacle, tailored exclusively for television and online streaming. The imposition of an emergency state, leading to the exclusion of live audiences except a few, transformed the Tokyo venues into spaces primarily for virtual engagement by both domestic and international viewers. Moriyama's dance, therefore, was not merely a live performance but was conceived as a media spectacle from the outset, reflecting themes of illness and mortality in a time of pervasive unease, indignation, and collective mourning.

Moriyama's dance and its subsequent media dissemination highlight the intersection of corporeality, well-being, and the regional and national hierarchies embodied in medical and ecological practices at the center of this volume. As of 2022 and 2023, when we worked on this book amid the unremitting surge of COVID-19 and other respiratory infectious diseases, there was a renewed emphasis on the interplay among public health, structural inequity, and mass media. The so-called new normal of the everyday saw continuous media updates on infection statistics, health guidelines, and preventative strategies, which have created or reinforced the boundaries of various imagined communities. Despite proclamations of the pandemic's conclusion by several political leaders, racially motivated violence against (East) Asian communities in Europe and North America remained unabated. Although the pandemic was undeniably a global phenomenon, the complex cultural and geopolitical region of East Asia had been thrust into the limelight of Western media scrutiny. This focus led to the propagation of essentialist cultural perceptions, particularly regarding collectivism and conformity, stereotypes about hygiene practices, racialized discourse about East Asian bodies, and techno-orientalist narratives concerning East Asian approaches to digital surveillance and epidemic disease management.

Individual and public health were thus entangled with the mechanisms of representation and (re)mediation, with the pandemic itself metamorphosing into a media spectacle inseparable from myriad audiovisual forms and platforms. A plethora of cultural and media productions—documentary and fictional films, television programs, photographs, songs, vlogs, and digital diagrams, among others—has since proliferated across platforms in response to the pandemic.[2] They often position the COVID-19 emergency within an extended discourse on medical and public health history. These works of popular science not only convey medical knowledge to the public but also foster a collective awareness regarding how the production of

2. Some examples from China and the United States include documentaries such as *The Lost Spring* (Fan Jian, 2020), *76 Days* (Wu Hao and Chen Weixi, 2020), and Ryo Takeuchi's *Nanjing Anti-epidemic Scene* (2020), *Long Time No See, Wuhan* (2021), and *China's Post-Pandemic Era: Winning Against All Odds* (2021).

this knowledge and public health protocols can be historicized. Between 2020 and 2022, for instance, a host of Chinese documentaries and videos revisited the 1911 Manchurian pneumonic plague.[3] This media wave offered a multifaceted exploration of the epidemic by exploring the scientific and political dynamics of the era and examining the audiovisual methods employed in recounting this historical event. Central to this media examination is the role of Dr. Wu Lien-teh, a Cambridge-educated physician of Malaysian Chinese descent. Appointed by the Qing court as the director of the anti-plague campaign, Wu implemented crucial quarantine and disinfection measures, including the development of layered surgical masks, framed as the precursor of the current N95 mask in contemporary media. To execute their agenda, Wu's team had to negotiate with various political and military powers in Manchuria, including Russian and Japanese colonial forces. The contemporary portrayal of Wu as a heroic medical figure is thus often imbued with nationalistic overtones, not least because the political backdrop of the 1911 plague invites comparisons with present-day China, facing contention with the West on ideological, political, technological and military fronts.

In addition to repurposing historical materials to comment on present circumstances, this corpus of works self-reflexively engages with the material foundation of media technologies. The abundance of audiovisual media detailing Wu's contribution to public health is made possible due to Wu's own meticulous documentation and orchestration of his team's endeavors through photography and textual narratives, such as a bilingual (English and Chinese) photo album that chronicles the crisis through the lens of Wu's epistemic and epidemiological knowledge.[4] This album, alongside Wu's autobiography that details the anti-plague initiatives, have shaped the commemoration of his legacy. It is upon the foundation of such archival materials that contemporary media productions reinterpret a tumultuous past with the aim of bridging past and present narratives.

Just as Moriyama's dance summoned the ghosts of the subaltern from postwar Japan, and contemporary Chinese media reinterpreted the 1911 Manchurian plague, *Socializing Medicine: Health Humanities and East Asian Media* explores the intersection of public health and popular media within the historical and geopolitical frameworks of East Asia. Organized both chronologically and thematically, the

3. On March 30, 2020, for instance, China Central Television's primary channel serving Chinese-speaking audiences overseas (CCTV-4) screened a documentary on the Great Manchurian Plague of 1911. On May 28, 2022, another documentary on the historical event was aired on the science and education channel of the CCTV (CCTV-10). Numerous short videos on the event and other relevant topics by individual content creators appeared on video sharing platforms such as Youku and Bilibili.
4. For an analysis of the photo album, see Christos Lynteris, "Photography, Zoonosis and Epistemic Suspension After the End of Epidemics," in *The Anthropology of Epidemics*, ed. Ann H. Kelly, Frédéric Keck, and Christos Lynteris (London: Routledge, 2019), 84–101.

ten chapters of this volume offer a transregional, multimedia, and interdisciplinary exploration that encompasses a diverse range of locales, including Japan, South Korea, mainland China, and Taiwan. The title *Socializing Medicine* carries a twofold significance. First, it underscores a commitment to social justice in media productions that envision accessible and equitable medical and health care practices. Second, it challenges the reductive view of medicine and health as merely "scientific" and "objective" by accentuating their sociopolitical aspects and institutional infrastructures. In anchoring these emphases in the East Asian context, the volume further challenges the Western-centric tendencies prevalent in the fields of medical and health humanities, as well as their intersection with media.

Incorporating a non-Western perspective is crucial for the diversification and decolonization of knowledge production and intellectual discourse. This approach not only expands the geographical and cultural horizons of existing literature but also reshapes the dominant paradigms through which the intersections among medicine, public welfare, political economy, and audiovisual media have been discussed. By focusing on East Asia, this volume underscores the necessity for the interdisciplinary confluence of these fields to be attuned to cultural and geopolitical specificities. Indeed, some contributors elucidate the complex relations of medicine and media against the backdrop of imperialism and (neo)colonialism, including Japan's colonization of Korea and the postwar Pax Americana that profoundly shaped the developments of Japan, South Korea, and Taiwan. By clarifying the hierarchical social structures within these historical and global-regional frameworks, their shared goal is to locate alternative approaches to health care and media practices that are anti-imperial and anti-colonial in nature. Some other contributors highlight the tension between capitalist and socialist systems during the Cold War. By critically examining the ideologies of medicine and media productions in the "high socialist" period in the People's Republic of China (spanning the early 1950s to the late 1970s), they complicate the entrenched Cold War narratives that tend to depict socialist medicine and media as mere myths and propagandistic tools. Building on the foundation of these inquiries regarding early to mid-twentieth century history, the volume further addresses pertinent and urgent concerns in the neoliberal capitalist East Asia today, including environmentalism, ableism, and the culture of mental health and healing—not least articulated through digital media.

Facilitating a dialogue among health humanities, media studies, and East Asian studies, the following pages will first define the concepts of medical humanities and health humanities and then delineate how this volume engages with and diversifies these fields by introducing an East Asian, media-sensitive perspective. Subsequently, we will explore the entanglements of medicine, health humanities, and media in modern and contemporary East Asian history and geopolitics before providing an overview of the book's four sections that host ten chapters.

Health Humanities: An Interdisciplinary Approach to Medicine, People, and Environments

Heeding the recent appeals from scholars in the medical humanities to transcend the conventional "humanistic perspective on medicine" and foster "*a cross-disciplinary and cross-cultural space for a bidirectional critical interrogation of both biomedicine (simplistic reductions of life to biology) and the humanities (simplistic reductions of suffering and health injustice to cultural relativism)*,"[5] *Socializing Medicine* understands medicine as a biocultural paradigm. This perspective acknowledges the integration of scientific inquiry and practice with culturally contingent realms, including aesthetics, ethics, biopolitics, and public policy. Exploring these junctures entails an investigation into the discursive underpinning of medicine as a sociocultural construct. In the context of media analysis, this approach recognizes that discussions of media products about medicine and public health must move beyond the one-dimensional theoretical sphere of representation. Indeed, texts, images, and sounds are intrinsically interwoven with, and reflective of, the tangible physical and institutional realities they engage with and, concurrently, interpret, mediate, and mold.

Socializing Medicine aims to engage the academic realms of medical and health humanities by exploring how diverse media forms and curative practices are mutually constitutive and firmly entrenched in sociopolitical contexts and collective human well-being. The conceptual framework of "medical humanities" emerged in the 1970s to investigate the ethical dimensions of medicine by integrating disparate disciplinary fields. It gained prominence in academic and clinical discourse, particularly in the late twentieth century.[6] Medical humanities scholars employ methodologies from various humanities and social sciences disciplines, including history of medicine, anthropology, and sociology.[7] As Anne Whitehead and Angela Woods point out, the field's foundation rests on three "E"s: ethics (including both medical ethics and bioethics), education, and experience (focusing on the qualitative aspects of illness).[8] Generally speaking, the field seeks to enhance the patient-clinician

---

5. Julia Kristeva, Marie Rose Moro, John Ødemark, and Eivind Engebretsen, "Cultural Crossings of Care: An Appeal to the Medical Humanities," *Medical Humanities* 44, no. 1 (2018): 56, emphasis original.
6. Sander L. Gilman, *Illness and Image: Case Studies in the Medical Humanities* (London: Routledge, 2015), xi; Lisa M. DeTora, and Stephanie M. Hilger, "Introduction: Bodies and Transitions in the Health Humanities," in *Bodies in Transition in The Health Humanities: Representation of Corporeality*, ed. Lisa M. DeTora and Stephanie M. Hilger (London: Routledge, 2020), 3; and Cole, Carlin, and Carson, *Medical Humanities*, 7.
7. Gilman, *Illness and Image*, xi.
8. Anne Whitehead and Angela Woods, "Introduction," in *The Edinburgh Companion to the Critical Medical Humanities*, ed. Anne Whitehead, Angela Woods, Sarah Atkinson, Jane Macnaughton, and Jennifer Richards (Edinburgh: Edinburgh University Press, 2016), 3.

relationship and foster empathy in medical practitioners by immersing them in diverse cultural perspectives on health and illness.[9] Moreover, the field of medical humanities aims to address the increasing imbalance between the technological advancements of health care and the intrinsically human aspects of care provision. This divide has been exacerbated by the commodification of health care systems and the pervasive reliance on costly medical technologies and biomedicine, deepening depersonalization within clinical environments. Such trends are symptomatic of institutional shifts toward profit maximization, often at the detriment of patient welfare and the well-being of physicians and medical trainees. These negative developments highlight the importance of recentering human experience in medical practice and health care systems.

The medical humanities paradigm, while invaluable, has encountered critiques for its limitations, as suggested by scholars such as Lisa M. DeTora and Stephanie M. Hilger. They argue that this approach, without a critique of the larger social forces behind the medicalization of illness and disability, may inadvertently reinforce existing hierarchical structures instead of deconstructing them to establish more equitable power and expertise dynamics.[10] In response, the concept of "health humanities" has gained prominence, either complementing or partially supplanting medical humanities. This approach expands the purview of medical humanities' inquiry to encompass the broader impacts of medicine beyond the patient-medical professional relationship. In other words, it seeks to transcend the confines of clinical settings as well as the emphasis on empathy and patient narratives by integrating a wider array of critical concerns, such as social justice, systemic inequalities in health care, the sociological aspects of medicine, and the role of various institutions from hospitals to advertising agencies. The primary objective of health humanities is to articulate alternative perspectives to the prevailing norms, thereby fostering a more comprehensive and socially conscious understanding of health and medicine.[11]

The health humanities framework not only expands the field of medicine but also advocates for a more politically engaged interpretation of "humanities." Sari Alschuler notes a divergence in how the term has been conceptualized within medical contexts versus humanities scholarship. In medical spheres, "humanities" is often perceived as a means to infuse humaneness into the scientific rigidity of

9. Therese Jones, Delese Wear, and Lester D. Friedman, "Introduction: The Why, the What, and the How of the Medical/Health Humanities" in *Health Humanities Reader*, ed. Therese Jones, Delese Wear, and Lester D. Friedman (New Brunswick, NJ: Rutgers University Press, 2014), 1–9.

10. DeTora and Hilger, Foreword to *Bodies in Transition in The Health Humanities: Representation of Corporeality*, xix.

11. Gilman, *Illness and Image*, xxvi; Rishi Goyal and Arden Hegele, "Introduction," in *Culture and Medicine: Critical Readings in the Health and Medical Humanities*, ed. Rishi Goyal and Arden Hegele (London: Bloomsbury Academic, 2023), 1–8.

medicine. Conversely, in humanities scholarship, it signifies "the ability to navigate the complexities of interpersonal interaction and their ethical implications, to relate the individual to the structural, to historicize encounters, to communicate accurately and effectively across a variety of media, and to engage in creative analytical thinking about health care."[12] Health humanities scholars, dedicated to establishing the field's legitimacy, emphasize the shared core values and a commitment to social justice that unite practitioners from various disciplines.[13]

Socializing Medicine aligns with such objectives, stressing the importance of understanding humanity beyond mere notions of humaneness and humanism. As Samuel Dubal argues, liberal humanism frequently overlooks the problematic terms and conditions upon which its fulfillment is built.[14] It is these foundational aspects of humanity, along with their underlying assumptions and implications, that our volume seeks to critically interrogate. Health humanities compel us to acknowledge that medicine is not a purely neutral, objective science as per post-Enlightenment ideologies. Rather, it is deeply influenced and shaped by cultural-economic forces, social privileges, and ingrained biases pertaining to class, gender, sexuality, race, ethnicity, age, and disability, among other factors.[15] Health humanities scholars have thus critiqued the evidence-based approach of biomedical sciences and the ideology of scientific objectivity, demonstrating how these concepts have been utilized to justify the marginalization, discrimination, and even genocide of disadvantaged and oppressed people. Notorious historical instances include the abhorrent Nazi medical experiments,[16] the egregious biological warfare perpetrated by Japanese Military Medical Unit 731 in Manchuria,[17] and the covert, nonconsensual sterilizations of Indigenous American women of childbearing age undertaken by the

12. Sari Alschuler, "Humanities" in *Keywords for Health Humanities*, ed. Sari Alschuler, Jonathan M. Metzl, and Priscilla Wald (New York: New York University Press, 2023), 109.
13. Thomas R. Cole, Nathan S. Carlin, and Roald A. Carson, *Medical Humanities: An Introduction* (Cambridge: Cambridge University Press, 2015); Craig Klugman and Erin Gentry Lamb, eds., *Research Methods in Health Humanities* (Oxford: Oxford University Press, 2019).
14. Samuel Dubal, "Humanity," in *Keywords for Health Humanities*, 115.
15. Lesa Scholl, "Introduction: Medicine and Modernity," in *Medicine, Health and Being Human*, ed. Lesa Scholl (London: Routledge, 2018), 10.
16. Scholl, "Introduction: Medicine and Modernity," 8.
17. Ruth Rogaski, "Vampires in Plagueland: The Multiple Meanings of *Weisheng* in Manchuria," in *Health and Hygiene in Chinese East Asia: Policies and Publics in the Long Twentieth Century*, ed. Angela Ki Che Leung and Charlotte Furth (Durham, NC: Duke University Press, 2010), 132–59; Tsuneishi Keiichi, "Unit 731 and the Japanese Imperial Army's Biological Warfare Program," in *Japan's Wartime Medical Atrocities: Comparative Inquiries in Science, History, and Ethics*, ed. Jing-Bao Nie, Nanyan Guo, Mark Selden, and Arthur Kleinman (London: Routledge, 2010), 23–31.

government across the United States from the 1930s to the 1970s.[18] Echoing this critical perspective, Sander L. Gilman argues that medical imagery is more than a transparent conveyor of information; rather, it is imbued with a history of scientific racism.[19] This concept is explored in this volume, particularly in Jeehey Kim's "Contagious Disease and Visual Media in Colonial Korea" and Yuki Obayashi's "Deformed Bodies in Nuclear Family Rhetoric: The Hiroshima Maidens Project in the Early Cold War." Both emphasize that medical renditions in media are intertwined with broader sociocultural and historical narratives of, respectively, colonialism and neocolonialism.

Furthermore, *Socializing Medicine* utilizes methodologies from health humanities to explore three interconnected realms. First, the volume redresses the prevalent North American and Euro-centric tendencies in health humanities. It critiques dominant Western ideological paradigms and highlights regional health disparities and discriminatory practices through an anti-colonial and geopolitical perspective, especially in the first section, "Medical and Media Imperialism." Second, it foregrounds alternative frameworks for understanding capitalist medicine, health, and political economy that are often overshadowed by various social, political, ecological, and historical influences of the Cold War. One such framework is the "cooperative medical service" model in socialist China, discussed in the second section, "Socialist Medicine in Revolution." Third, the book delves into the complex relationship between historical and contemporary media and health through a transmedial and interdisciplinary approach. This aspect is explored in the volume's third and fourth sections, "Precarious Ecology and Body" and "Digital Embodiment and Neoliberalism," respectively.

As these three focal areas demonstrate, the volume positions health as a phenomenon beyond the narrow confines of individual or public concerns traditionally associated with the medical profession. Within neoliberal capitalist societies, health care has been transformed into a profit-driven enterprise, characterized by the commodification and corporatization of medicine. This practice reflects deep-seated structural inequalities—historical and emergent alike—that are often exacerbated by minimal government intervention. This trend is starkly evident in the monopolization of medical resources by biomedical pharmaceutical complexes, medical insurance corporations, hospital conglomerates, and the escalating costs of medical education. These entities collectively exert excruciating financial, physical, and emotional strain on patients, health care professionals, and the general populace. In a

18. Brianna Theobald, *Reproduction on the Reservation: Pregnancy, Childbirth, and Colonialism in the Long Twentieth Century* (Chapel Hill, NC: The University of North Carolina Press, 2019); Sophia Shepherd, "The Enemy is the Knife: Native Americans, Medical Genocide, and the Prohibition of Nonconsensual Sterilizations," *Michigan Journal of Race and Law* 27 (2021): 89–106.

19. Gilman, *Illness and Image*, xxvi.

highly developed capitalist country like the United States, this situation is acutely visible: nearly 7–8 percent of the population, amounting to approximately thirty million individuals, are unable to afford medical insurance. Additionally, a significant portion of the population incurs debilitating debt due to exorbitant health care costs. These burdens disproportionately affect ethnic minorities and working class people, epitomizing the structural inequalities inherent in the current health care system.[20]

Norman Bethune (1890–1939), a prominent Canadian thoracic surgeon renowned for his staunch advocacy of socialized medicine and his internationalist medical contributions during pivotal historical events such as the Spanish Civil War and China's War of Resistance against Japanese, incisively critiqued the state of health care in his era. He poignantly observed, "Medicine, as we are practicing it, is a luxury trade. We are selling bread at the price of jewels."[21] His reflections—articulated in the 1930s amid a capitalist crisis marked by economic depression, rampant infectious diseases such as tuberculosis among the working class, and global warfare—resonate with even greater urgency today. In his "Speech on Socialized Medicine," Bethune argues that health is not solely a technical or scientific concern but is deeply intertwined with political, ethical, and economic factors, necessitating consideration within a broader social framework. He critiques the capitalist model founded on individualism, competition, and private profit, highlighting the paradox of "poverty of health in the midst of scientific abundance of knowledge of disease."[22] Annually, countless people, both in advanced capitalist and developing nations, suffer premature deaths due to the inaccessibility of adequate, albeit available, health care. This predicament, according to Bethune, is not a transient ailment of the body but rather a systematic malady requiring comprehensive treatment. Advocating for a thorough transformation, Bethune called for a restructuring of the economic system and the eradication of ignorance, poverty, and unemployment. He emphatically asserted that in a modern industrial society, health cannot be regarded as a private matter. He asserted that all health is public, underscoring the shared responsibility and interconnectedness of health outcomes across societal strata.

Drawing inspiration from Bethune's insights, *Socializing Medicine* calls for a reevaluation of the relationship between medical ethics and audiovisual media. We perceive this relationship not simply as a set of professional etiquette among physicians, but as a broader framework of justice and morality that interconnects medicine, humanity, the environments, and media. This perspective posits health as a

20. Brian Tsai, "U.S. Uninsured Rate Hits Record Low in First Quarter of 2023," accessed November 15, 2023: https://blogs.cdc.gov/nchs/2023/08/03/7434/#:~:text=Highlights%20from%20the%20report%3A,the%20same%20period%20in%202022.
21. Norman Bethune, *The Wounds* (Ontario: Alive Press, 1939), 5.
22. Bethune, *The Wounds*, 4–6.

fundamental human right, rather than a privilege, advocating for its recognition as a core responsibility of the state to its citizens. It suggests that socialized medicine and the limitation of private medical practice are practical means to actualize this right. However, some pivotal questions arise in the era of globalized neoliberal capitalism: How can the primary aim of medicine shift from maximizing profit to serving the public? How might a just public medical and health system be established to ensure equitable distribution of health care resources, irrespective of class, race, and gender, while also addressing the exploitation of "imported" medical workers from the developing world?

Delving deeper into these critical inquiries, *Socializing Medicine* tackles two interrelated domains: the geopolitical context of East Asia and the realm of audio-visual media. The volume scrutinizes the interaction between local, national, and transnational dynamics of health socialization and media cultures across East Asia. Spanning sundry periods and sites in modern East Asian history, the book investigates the role of mass media in mediating and disseminating the socialization of health. It assesses how media has supported or contested an array of ideologies, including imperialism, colonialism, socialism, internationalism, neoliberal capitalism, developmentalism, and environmentalism. The aim of this exploration is to uncover the complex ways in which media has historically influenced, and continues to shape, public understanding and policies concerning health within the dynamic sociopolitical landscape of East Asia.

Health and Media in East Asian Geopolitics

The formation of public health discourse in Europe generally took place in the context of capitalist industrialization and urbanization in the early nineteenth century, as social reformers and civic leaders saw the prevention of disease as part of a broader humanitarian campaign against poverty. In contrast, the trajectory in East Asia, as Susan L. Burns suggests, predated industrialization. In Japan, for instance, public health consciousness "took form in response to concerns about imperialism" in the mid-nineteenth century. This is exemplified in the treatments of cholera outbreaks in Nagasaki, a treaty port that Western imperialist powers forced the Bakufu government to open, following the locals' interactions with infected foreign seamen and tradesmen.[23] To discuss public health discourse in the East Asian context, we must therefore take into account the entanglements between health and cultural-political

23. Susan L. Burns, "Constructing the National Body: Public Health and Nation in Meiji Japan," in *Nation Work: Asian Elites and National Identities*, ed. Timothy Brooks and Andre Schmid (Ann Arbor, MI: University of Michigan Press, 2000), 21.

ideologies that have long been pivotal in shaping national and regional identities, sovereignty, and resistance against colonialism and imperialism.

From the late nineteenth century onward, public health discourse in East Asia was further associated with the region's political identity and degree of modernization, as the epistemological framing of health shifted from personal well-being to national strength. A salient example is the evolving interpretation of the classical Chinese phrase *weisheng* (*eisei* in Japanese), which historically denoted personal well-being but gradually came to be associated with public health institutions. As Ruth Rogaski argues, the notion of hygienic modernity emerged when *weisheng* gained a public connotation, initially as part of Japan's Meiji-era sanitary movement, and later across the broader East Asian cultural sphere. Over time, *weisheng* began to symbolize not only the ideal of public health as a civic right but also the legitimization of modern state authority and the bureaucratic apparatus for the implementation of public health policies.[24] A problematic outcome of this tendency was the convergence of medical and political narratives, as exemplified by the racially charged and derogatory term "the Sick Man of East Asia." Coined by Western imperialists to denigrate the declining Qing empire following its debilitating defeats in wars against Western and Japanese colonial forces since the mid-nineteenth century, this label referred not only to public health crises, such as rampant opium addiction and escalating epidemics exacerbated by poverty and colonial exploitation, but also to the Qing leaders' ineffective governance amid political and social upheaval. Consequently, the term encapsulated both the literal public health crises and the metaphorical political and social "sickness" of the empire. It reflected the pervasive themes of social Darwinism, the power dynamics in colonial domination, and racial discrimination.

The association of health with national strength and global hierarchies has historically been manipulated by Western imperialists as a justification for their military incursion and colonial aggression. However, this perception of health has also been strategically leveraged by East Asian politicians and intellectuals as an impetus for social reform or a revolutionary movement. In the wake of Japan's forced opening to Western powers, for instance, the Meiji government, inspired by the German medical system, embarked on domestic medical reforms beginning in 1868. These reforms instigated pivotal changes in Japan's sociopolitical system, propelling the nation toward a self-transformation into an imperialist power itself. Indeed, the valorization of the German system (rather than the Dutch or the French one) was due to the perceived positive image of Prussia as "a monarchic state with

24. Charlotte Furth, "Introduction: Hygienic Modernity in Chinese East Asia," in *Health and Hygiene in Chinese East Asia*, 7; Ruth Rogaski, *Hygienic Modernity: Meanings of Health and Disease in Treaty-Port China* (Berkeley, CA: University of California Press, 2004).

a strong military that had succeeded in industrializing rapidly"—a model of power and wealth that the Meiji leaders sought to learn from for improving the health of their own empire.[25] This sociopolitical transformation precipitated Japan's subsequent colonization of regions such as Taiwan (1895), Korea (1910), and Manchuria (1931) in the late nineteenth and early twentieth centuries.

The urgency to discard the racially disparaging label of "Sick Man of East Asia" likewise galvanized Chinese reformers at the turn of the twentieth century to pursue social transformations. As Rogaski points out, the Qing government perceived the 1911 Manchurian Plague as an opportunity to demonstrate that its response to the pandemic was superior to those of neighboring Russia and Japan. The stigma associated with the "Sick Man" was thus inverted into a symbol that fostered "national solidarity around the well-being of all citizens."[26] Consequently, the rhetoric of national illness was repurposed to motivate defiant changes and imbricated into revolutionary discourses, which persisted in China throughout the twentieth century, including the uprisings against the Qing government, leftist critiques of the Republican regime in the first half of the century, and the various revolutions and confrontations in socialist China during the Cold War.

Resonating with existing narratives in health humanities and modern East Asian history, this volume explores the dialectical tension between health and politics as a pivotal lens through which we can understand the socialization of medicine in the specific historical and geopolitical milieu of modern and contemporary East Asia. Indeed, the past two decades have witnessed an increasing academic interest in the history of medicine and health care in East Asia, as evidenced by the publication of over a dozen high-caliber monographs and anthologies.[27] Our volume contributes

---

25. Susan L. Burns, "Constructing the National Body: Public Health and Nation in Meiji Japan," 24.
26. Ruth Rogaski, "The Manchurian Plague and COVID-19: China, the United States, and the 'Sick Man,' Then and Now," *American Journal of Public Health* 111, no. 3 (2021): 428.
27. Some recent works include Volker Scheid, *Chinese Medicine in Contemporary China* (Durham, NC: Duke University Press, 2007); Angela Ki Che Leung and Charlotte Furth, eds., *Health and Hygiene in Chinese East Asia* (Durham, NC: Duke University Press, 2010); Ann Jannetta, *The Vaccinators: Smallpox, Medical Knowledge, and the Opening of Japan* (Stanford, CA: Stanford University Press, 2012); Xiaoping Fang, *Barefoot Doctors and Western Medicine in China* (Rochester, NY: University of Rochester Press, 2012); Bridie Andrews, *The Making of Modern Chinese Medicine* (Honolulu, HI: University of Hawai'i Press, 2014); Hoi-eun Kim, *Doctors of Empire: Medical and Cultural Encounters in Between Imperial Germany and Meiji Japan* (Toronto: University of Toronto Press, 2014); Sean Hsiang-lin Lei, *Neither Donkey nor Horse: Medicine in the Struggle over China's Modernity* (Chicago: The University of Chicago Press, 2014); Miriam Gross, *Farewell to the God of Plague: Chairman Mao's Campaign to Deworm China* (Oakland, CA: University of California Press, 2016); Sun-yang Kim, *Health Politics in Korea: The Political Dynamics of Healthcare Reform* (Seoul: Seoul National University Press, 2016); Lincoln C. Chen, Michael R. Reich, and Jennifer Ryan, ed., *Medical Education in East Asia Past and Future* (Bloomington, IA: Indiana University Press, 2017); Mary Augusta Brazelton, *Mass Vaccination: Citizen's Bodies and State Power in Modern China* (Ithaca, NY: Cornell University Press, 2019); Sonja M. Kim, *Imperatives of Care: Women and Medicine in Colonial*

to the growing inquiries into the sociopolitical histories of medicine in East Asia by emphasizing the influential role of mass media in constructing and mediating these historical narratives. Adopting an interdisciplinary approach that spans a broad historical-geopolitical spectrum, our analysis explores the potential production and reinforcement of racist medical discourses through (neo)colonial media in East Asia. We also examine how practices of socialized medicine—in a broad sense, promoted by photography, films, and other audiovisual media—may act as countering forces to these hegemonic discourses. Additionally, *Socializing Medicine* investigates how audiovisual media afford the documentation of historical transformations in public health policies through facilitating collaboration and mutual comprehension across local, national, and transregional grounds, and enhancing contemporary understandings of public health emergencies.

By investigating the media ecology of medicine and health, and by diversifying the burgeoning field of medical media studies—which has, until now, predominantly focused on Western texts and contexts—this volume aims to develop innovative methodologies. Over the past two decades, academic works on medical media have mainly embraced a thematic approach, focusing on the portrayal of specific themes related to health, well-being, and medical practices. Examples include Brian Glasser's *Medicinema: Doctors in Films,* which provides a comprehensive analysis of the titular medical professional in Western cinema; and *Diseased Cinema: Plagues, Pandemics and Zombies in American Movies,* by Robert Alpert, Merle Eisenberg, and Lee Mordechai, which traces the evolution of the disease film genre in relation to the development of capitalism in the United States.[28] Similarly, *The Silvering Screen: Old Age and Disability in Cinema* by Sally Chivers and *Cultures of Representation: Disability in World Cinema Contexts* edited by Benjamin Fraser address the cinematic representation of aging as well as physical and neurological disabilities by engaging with theoretical frameworks from disabilities studies, critical gerontology, and cultural studies.[29] The anthology *Medicine's Moving Pictures: Medicine, Health, and Bodies in American Film and Television* likewise examines media's power in molding public perceptions, practices, and policies related to health. This collection constitutes a rich cultural and historical archive, encompassing fictional features, educational

---

Korea (Honolulu, HI: University of Hawai'i Press, 2019), and Wayne Soon, *Global Medicine in China: A Diasporic History* (Stanford, CA: Stanford University Press, 2020).

28. Brian Glasser, *Medicinema: Doctors in Films* (Oxon: Radcliffe, 2010); Robert Alpert, Merle Eisenberg, and Lee Mordechai, *Diseased Cinema: Plagues, Pandemics and Zombies in American Movies* (Edinburgh: Edinburgh University Press, 2023).
29. Sally Chivers, *The Silvering Screen: Old Age and Disability in Cinema* (Toronto: University of Toronto Press, 2011); Benjamin Fraser, ed., *Cultures of Representation: Disability in World Cinema Contexts* (New York: Columbia University Press, 2016).

films, and television programs.[30] Collectively, these works lay bare the importance of media in reflecting and shaping societal attitudes and understandings of health and medicine, paving the way for further scholarly inquiry in this interdisciplinary domain.

Socializing Medicine aligns with the pivotal concerns of these seminal works but distinguishes itself in terms of scope, source materials, and theoretical interventions. Our objective is to think beyond the analysis of individual experiences or medical symptoms as represented in media, aiming instead to forge a more comprehensive understanding of how mass media facilitates the interaction between health, illness, and a broader assemblage that comprises diverse social actors, environments, and institutions. The commitment to rethinking existing epistemological divisions also motivates our decision to extend our focus beyond cinema to encompass a wider array of mass media forms. Contrasting with existing scholarship that predominantly centers on filmic representations, our anthology situates socialized medicine within a larger media ecology, which includes fiction films, documentaries, educational films, television programs, poetry, photography, lantern slides, vlogs, and online streaming. By moving beyond a representational perspective, we adopt approaches rooted in (re)mediation and materiality, which enables us to perceive physical and mental health at the textual level as inextricably interwoven with paratextual elements and conditions spanning individual, institutional, social, and environmental dimensions. The analyses of various media objects within this volume thus aim to reveal how conventional aesthetic inquiries, such as content, form, style, and genre, cannot be disentangled from a broader social history of media. Conversely, employing close audiovisual analysis as a methodological approach in media studies allows us elucidate the hierarchical operation of power and ideology embedded in the realm of aesthetics.

The volume's emphasis on East Asia indicates another crucial methodological departure from prevailing narratives in medical media studies. While the above scholarly works have substantially enriched our knowledge of media production in relation to health, medicine, and the human body, they have mainly engaged with European and North American cases, contexts, and frameworks. For example, in *Medicinema*, the only non-Western director explored in depth is Akira Kurosawa; similarly, in *Cultures of Representation*, only four of the seventeen chapters address non-Western films. The Western-centric inclination is also evident in other anthologies, such as the lack of engagement with non-Western cinema in *Signs of life: Cinema*

30. Leslie J Reagan, Nancy Tomes, and Paula A. Treichler, eds., *Medicine's Moving Pictures: Medicine, Health, and Bodies in American Film and Television* (Rochester, NY: University of Rochester Press, 2007).

and Medicine.[31] In recognition of the critical need for non-Western perspectives and case studies, particularly those with historical, conceptual, and geopolitical attributes, *Socializing Medicine* seeks to enrich scholarly discourse at the intersection of media studies and health humanities by offering an East Asian perspective.

Film and the Chinese Medical Humanities, an anthology in parallel with our thematic interests, offers critical insights into the portrayal of Chinese medical and health narratives in cinema across both historical and contemporary contexts.[32] While resonating with this anthology, *Socializing Medicine* nevertheless expands its scope to encompass transregional interactions in medical and media cultures. Moving beyond a sole focus on mainland China, our anthology fosters a dialogue among East Asian regions (such as Japan, South Korea, and Taiwan) and acknowledges the global forces that have operated within or out of East Asia at different historical junctures. Although a considerable portion of our anthology addresses Chinese media, we endeavor to complicate the notion of "China" by situating it within diverse temporal and spatial frameworks. This includes examining Chinese-language media produced beyond the Mainland and offering a thorough historical analysis of the interplay between public health and media from the Republican era through the Maoist period to the present. In our exploration of Japan, the inquiries also extend beyond the main islands to address its impact on other regions in East Asia, particularly colonial Korea. We also examine the aftermath of Japanese imperialism, focusing on how Japan itself became a subject of medicalization under the racialized and gendered gaze of the West.

By transcending the conventional national framework, *Socializing Medicine* unravels the sociopolitical ramifications and historical pertinence of transregional interactions. This viewpoint not only highlights the distinctive aspects of East Asian localities but also interrogates the constructed nature of "East Asia" as a conceptual category. Collectively, the ten chapters challenge the reduction of East Asia to a monolithic, homogenized entity. Instead, they explore the myriad media narratives that have constituted the region's diverse histories and experiences from a health humanities perspective.

Chapter Breakdown

The structure of *Socializing Medicine* is designed to guide readers through a comprehensive exploration of the multifaceted aspects of East Asian medical and media

---

31. Graeme Harper and Andrew Moor, eds., *Signs of life: Cinema and Medicine* (New York: Wallflower Press, 2005).
32. Vivienne Lo, Chris Berry, and Guo Liping, eds., *Film and the Chinese Medical Humanities* (London: Routledge, 2020).

cultures. It commences with a section on the influence of early twentieth-century imperialism and post–World War II neo-imperialism on East Asian medical culture, then moves chronologically to the second section devoted to anti-imperialist medical theories and practices, featuring socialist medical service in the PRC during the Cold War. The final two sections of the book then examine the diverse ramifications of ideological conflicts in areas such as gender and sexuality, human-environment relations, the experiences of differently abled bodies, and digital media in the age of neoliberal global capitalism.

By emphasizing the dominant social ideologies in different historical moments of modern East Asia, the structure of this book demonstrates our attempt to trace various transregional networks and exchanges among key social actors, institutes, and discourses related to health humanities. As noted by Charlotte Furth, public health is commonly analyzed within the context of state- and nation-building projects.[33] However, our volume illuminates the extensive transnational influences and interventions that shape local situations and power structures. The audiovisual media formats, materials, and platforms discussed herein further broaden the conventional focus on literature, cinema, and visual arts in health humanities scholarship.

Section I: Medical and Media Imperialism

The first section of *Socializing Medicine*, comprising three chapters, delineates the role of print and audiovisual media in shaping and complicating Japanese colonial and American neocolonial medical discourses on race, gender, and humanism during the first half of the twentieth century. Japanese imperialist expansion was intricately linked to its colonial medical culture, serving as a multifaceted tool for domination and control. The expansionist agenda of Japan in the late nineteenth and early twentieth centuries utilized medical practices as a means of asserting authority over colonized territories and their inhabitants. The establishment of hospitals, public health centers, and medical schools in these regions aimed to transplant Japanese medical standards and systems into conquered areas. Health care initiatives, including disease control and vaccination campaigns, not only served public health purposes but also bolstered Japanese cultural hegemony and promoted immigration to colonized territories. In a comprehensive study of Japanese colonial medicine, Michael Shiyung Liu argues that "medicine" and "civilization" were two major themes employed by the Japanese government to justify their rule in Taiwan,

33. Furth, "Introduction: Hygienic Modernity in Chinese East Asia," 2, 5–6.

which was considered a "model colony."[34] Influenced by the prevailing racial and eugenic ideologies of the time, Japan used medical justifications to solidify the notion of racial superiority and to legitimize discrimination and differential treatment based on race and ethnicity.

Jeehey Kim's chapter, "Contagious Disease and Visual Media in Colonial Korea," examines the pivotal role of media in constructing and reinforcing the image of the colonized people as inferior and in need of Japanese guidance and control for their purported benefit. The chapter investigates the strategic use of lantern slides, photo albums, postcards, and films by the Japanese imperial authority in Korea to form a culture of ostracization, thereby normalizing the racialization and segregation of those with contagious diseases. Kim's thorough analysis of photographs from the official records of cholera outbreaks in colonial Korea reveals the administration's tactic of blaming disease spread on the noncompliance of Korean subjects. The deployment of magic lantern shows and hygiene films also became an instrumental part of this control mechanism, instilling fear and justifying the segregation of leprosy patients on Sorok Island. The ironic promotion of the island as a tourist destination erased the physical presence of the patients from visual representations, reducing these permanent residents to mere statistical figures in news reports or bearers of social stigma.

Back in Japan, societal attitudes toward leprosy were deeply stigmatized and profoundly influenced by the policies of the imperial health system. The 1930s marked a period during which Japan's social and medical responses to leprosy emphasized the isolation and segregation of those afflicted. Kathryn M. Tanaka's chapter, "Ink on the Silver Screen: Medical Culture and Poetic Voices in *Spring on the Small Island*," unpacks the experiences of leprosy patients through a nuanced examination of Toyoda Shirō's film *Spring on the Small Island* (*Kojima no haru,* 1940). Adapted from Dr. Ogawa Masako's popular travel diary, the film adheres to the episodic structure of the original text, accentuated by the inclusion of written or chanted tanka poems. Challenging the common perception of the film as either propagandistic or humanistic, Tanaka engages with Bakhtin's concept of heteroglossia to demonstrate how the film incorporates complex layers of voices, especially poems by the patients, to convey subtle forms of resistance against dominant narratives. Furthermore, the portrayal of discriminatory treatment based on the patients' gender and class affords a critical distance to reflect upon these issues.

34. As Liu argues, the reduction in mortality rate and the improvement of general health in colonial Taiwan was mainly due to the increase of income from economic development rather than benefiting directly from Japan's medical measures. Michael Shiyung Liu, *Prescribing Colonization: The Role of Medical Practices and Policies in Japan-Ruled Taiwan, 1895–1945* (Ann Arbor, MI: Association for Asian Studies, 2009).

Parallel to the plight of leprosy patients, the disfigurement of nuclear war survivors presented challenges to mainstream media narratives and representational policies. The American atomic bombings of Hiroshima and Nagasaki altered Japan's history and reshaped global perceptions, transitioning the country's image from a militaristic aggressor during World War II to that of a victimized nation grappling with catastrophic aftermaths and radiation effects. Yuki Obayashi's chapter, "Deformed Bodies in Nuclear Family Rhetoric: The Hiroshima Maidens Project in the Early Cold War," explores US television's portrayal of disfigured female survivors from Hiroshima, recasting Japan as a deserving recipient of humanitarian aid. Since World War II, the United States, as a dominant political, military, economic, and cultural force in East Asia, has wielded substantial influence over regional dynamics and national image construction and dissemination. The Hiroshima Maidens Project on television, initially intended to transform anti-Japanese sentiments and national guilt into "benevolence," marked a pivotal shift in American attitudes towards Japan, which significantly impacted East Asian geopolitics. Focusing on the discourses surrounding the so-called American generosity and humanitarianism during the Cold War, Obayashi investigates the ways in which US media outlets and project contributors perpetuated racialized images of Japanese women's bodies for political purposes.

From the early 1950s to the 1970s, the global Cold War rivalry between the capitalist camp led by the United States and the socialist bloc led by the Soviet Union, was acutely felt in East Asia. This period was characterized by the prominent presence of numerous US military bases in Japan and South Korea, surrounding the nascent People's Republic of China (PRC). The Korea War (1950–1953), involving multiple international forces, stood as a stark manifestation of American anti-communist policies in the region. Amid this geopolitical turmoil, the PRC, emerging as a newly independent and impoverished third world nation, adopted a policy of self-reliance across economic, political, cultural, and medical sectors. Although there were collaborations and exchanges with the Soviet Union, the relationship diverged in the early 1960s. In this context, concepts of health and medical sovereignty, alongside socialist medicine and mass participation, became central to the PRC's national agenda: the promotion of anti-colonial, anti-imperialist, and anti-interventionist sentiments under socialism. The renditions and mediations of these themes in popular media, set against the backdrop of intense global and regional Cold War politics, will be explored in the subsequent section.

Section II: Socialist Medicine in Revolution

This section provides an expansive and nuanced view of the interaction between socialist medical services and mass media in the PRC from the 1950s to the late

1970s. British surgeon Joshua Horn (1914–1975), who worked in China from 1954 to 1969, noted that the PRC's socialist medical services, established on the "mass line," transformed health care by providing the masses with medical care previously unavailable before 1949. This system dismantled hierarchical and profit-driven health care structures, focusing on demystifying the medical profession through state-led initiatives.[35] A key strategy was the dispatch of mobile medical teams from urban hospitals to rural areas. These teams were instrumental in serving rural populations and training paramedical workers, or "barefoot doctors," who were recruited from local peasant communities.[36] This strategy, initiated in the 1950s, gained momentum for expansion following Chairman Mao Zedong's June 26, 1965 directive, which stated that the main emphasis in medical and health work was to be on rural areas where the majority of population resides.[37] Between 1966 and 1969, approximately one million peasant paramedical workers were trained and supported by larger medical facilities and mobile teams comprising physicians, nurses, and other health professionals. These barefoot doctors were central in providing essential medical services in rural communities, often free or at minimal cost. They represented a crucial transformation in China's health care system that emphasized universal care and preventive measures.[38]

After 1949, China developed new medical treatments and techniques. Commencing in 1954, Traditional Chinese Medicine (TCM), including acupuncture and herbal medicine, underwent a resurgence. Previously suppressed by some Republican elites as unscientific, TCM was integrated into medical school curricula in the 1950s and practiced alongside Western medicine in hospitals and clinics following Mao's June 26 directive.[39] This revival signified an ideological reassessment of Chinese medicine. TCM's cost-effective local production and alignment with the principle of self-sufficiency particularly enhanced its appeal.[40] During the 1960s and 1970s, the community-operated socialist health care system gained acclaim from Western observers, who viewed it as a potential model for global health care due to its emphasis on preventive care, cooperative health plans, mass participation, and

35. Joshua Horn, "The Mass Line," in *Health Care in China* (London: Anglo-Chinese Educational Institute, 1976), 11.
36. Horn, "The Mass Line," 2; Xiaoping Fang, *Barefoot Doctors and Western Medicine in China* (University of Rochester Press, 2015).
37. Peter Kong-ming New, "Barefoot Doctors and Health Care in the People's Republic of China," *Ekistics* 38, no. 226 (1974): 220.
38. Horn, "The Mass Line," 4; New, "Barefoot Doctors and Health Care in the People's Republic of China," 223.
39. New, "Barefoot Doctors and Health Care in the People's Republic of China," 220–21.
40. New, "Barefoot Doctors and Health Care in the People's Republic of China," 221.

public accountability.[41] Notable achievements by socialist medical workers in this period include controlling epidemic diseases such as syphilis, leprosy, and schistosomiasis, advancing treatments for severe burns and limb reimplantation, promoting planned parenthood among peasants, and becoming the first in the world to create synthetic protein (insulin).[42]

This section's three chapters explore how various media forms from the 1950s to the 1970s were mobilized to promote and envision the progression of the Chinese socialist medical program. Lu Liu's chapter, "A Battle for Life: Bacteriophage Therapy and Socialist Medicine in the Great Leap Forward," traces the transnational and transmedial trajectory of phage therapy. Despite initial skepticism in the Soviet Union, the therapy gained prominence in the PRC during the Great Leap Forward (1958–1962) and subsequent years. By comparing diverse media formats such as news reports, reportage literature, and adaptations in stage and film, Liu analyzes the consistent tension between medical knowledge and its media portrayal. This tension often resolves in favor of dramatic elements over medical accuracy, notably in fiction films such as *Spring Reigns Everywhere* (*Chunman renjian* 春滿人間, dir. Sang Hu, 1959), and in various literary, theatrical, and cinematic works, including science and education films.

In their chapter, "From Curing to Revolutionizing: The Politics of Disability in Chinese Socialist Medicine and Media," Chao Wang and Yuqian Yan reassess the portrayal of curing deaf-mute people through acupuncture in PRC media and films from the 1950s to the 1970s. Focusing on the dual transformation of acupuncture into a state-sponsored scientific therapy and the disabled into revolutionary subjects, they argue that treating people with disabilities was a form of political inclusion. The cure of deaf-muteness advanced the politics of disability in socialist media, in which the socialist goal of "giving voice to the people" was aligned with an aspiration to unleash the revolutionary potential for vulnerable members of society.

Ban Wang's chapter, "The Mass Biopolitics of Medicine in Socialist Chinese Films," provides an in-depth analysis of the Chinese socialist films *Spring Comes to a Withered Tree* (*Kumu fengchun* 枯木逢春, 1961) and *Spring Sprouts* (*Chunmiao* 春苗, 1975). Wang explores how these films depict the political mobilization of the rural peasantry, emphasizing their education, political consciousness, and participation in curing diseases and combatting epidemics. The films illuminate a vision of health care dedicated to serving the masses, while critiquing the increasing inequalities in the health care system that favors urban elites to the detriment of workers, peasants,

41. The Committee of Concerned Asian Scholars, *China! Inside the People's Republic* (Toronto: Bantam, 1972), 240.
42. Joshua S. Horn, *Away with All Pests: An English Surgeon in People's China, 1954–1969* (New York: Monthly Review Press, 1971); Gross, *Farewell to the God of Plague*.

and soldiers. The chapter reveals how these films promote a "mass-line" approach to medicine, challenging elitist and professional biases in health care and addressing the inequities between urban and rural health care provision.

While not covered in this anthology, an important facet of Chinese socialist medicine and media is medical internationalism. Since the 1960s, the Chinese government has sent medical teams to African countries to help with the construction of medical infrastructure, manufacture supplies, work alongside local medical workers, and integrate TCM methods such as acupuncture into patient care.[43] These medical aid initiatives, founded on principles of third world solidarity and used as diplomatic leverages, merit further scholarly exploration.

Another significant transnational trend since the 1970s is the rise of global capitalism and labor division, exemplified by the economic surge of the so-called Four Asian Tigers (Hong Kong, Singapore, South Korea, and Taiwan). With their developmentalist and export-oriented policies, South Korea and Taiwan experienced rapid industrialization and sustained high-growth rates for several decades. While these developments generally improved living standards, they also led to physical and psychological health issues, ecological degradation, and environmental crises. Both fictional films and documentaries have addressed these challenges, a topic that will be explored in the next section.

Section III: Precarious Ecology and the Body

The first two sections of the book examine the influence of imperialism, colonialism, and socialism on the development of medical culture, along with the corresponding responses through audiovisual media in the early to mid-twentieth century. The subsequent sections shift focus to the late twentieth and early twenty-first centuries by analyzing the formation and mediation of medical culture in relation to the prevailing ideologies of this later period: state developmentalism and neoliberal capitalism. As South Korea and Taiwan transitioned from political dictatorship or military governance to market economies in the 1970s and 1980s—a period characterized by rapid industrialization, urbanization, and globalized capitalism—they grappled with the tension between state-led industrialization and market-oriented principles. To varying degrees, they were influenced by substantial changes in industrial conditions and social relations, which have significantly reshaped the culture of public health concerning media production, distribution, and consumption. New social

43. Dongxin Zou, "Socialist Medicine and Maoist Humanitarianism: Chinese Medical Missions to Algeria, 1963–1984," Dissertation, Columbia University, 2019; *Yi Bai Qiuen wei guanghui bangyang: zhongguo yisheng he gongcheng jishu renyuan zai guowai* (Shanghai: Shanghai renmin chubanshe, 1970).

dynamics emerged between the individual and the collective, and between humans and the environment, leading to novel conceptualizations of public health: health began to be perceived not only as the wellness of the individual and collective body but also as a political allegory for the body of the imagined state undergoing rapid economic growth.

The third section examines the effects of industrial development on public health in South Korea and Taiwan during the 1970s and 1980s. This focus marks an exchange between the health humanities and environmental humanities. As scholars in this interdisciplinary field have reminded us: "we must learn to understand the mental health implications of climate change, the anxiety caused by increasingly toxic environmental conditions, and the overarching challenges of facing vast, slow processes that jeopardize not only the more-than-human world but also our own safety."[44] The two chapters trace the historical shaping of public medical-environmental consciousness in South Korea and Taiwan, mediated by various social actors through mass media, including government-endorsed "culture films" and public television documentaries. They demonstrate how mass media can either align audience perception of environmental pollution with official narratives or serve as a conduit for civic participation, stimulating public policy debates and eco-activist counter-discourses against collusion between governments and major corporations.

Max Balhorn's chapter, "Ecological Crisis and Pathologies of Modernity in the South Korean Films *Crowded* and *Zero Woman*," analyzes how two South Korean films, *Crowded* (*Manwŏn*, 1977) and *Zero Woman* (*Yŏngnyŏ*, 1979), suggest public anxieties over birth defects, chronic illnesses, and neuroses due to industrial expansion around Seoul and excessive pesticide use. Balhorn examines how these state-endorsed films frame environmental issues as individual moral failings rather than the repercussions of state-led developmentalism, echoing the neo-Malthusian theories prevalent in 1970s South Korea. These theories linked biological and social reproduction with human-environment interactions. As South Korea transitioned to a regime prioritizing capital accumulation through pollution-intensive industrialization, concerns over urban air and noise pollution, and rural chemical pollution, intensified. The films portray these issues as imminent threats to reproductive health and the social reproduction of the nation, blaming ecological devastation on the so-called irresponsible sexual behaviors of the urbanized populace. Against this backdrop, environmental changes are framed as consequences of individual consciousness, deflecting discussions of pollution away from criticism of the intrinsic

44. Scott Slovic, Swarnalatha Rangarajan, and Vidya Sarveswaran, "Introduction: Toward a Medical-Environmental Humanities. Why Now?" in *The Bloomsbury Handbook to The Medical-Environmental Humanities*, ed. Scott Slovic, Swarnalatha Rangarajan, and Vidya Sarveswaran (London: Bloomsbury Academic, 2022), 2.

damages of unregulated capitalist development. The two films reveal the apprehensions held by government officials and medical experts about the long-term consequences of marginalizing environmental considerations as "externalities" in the name of capitalist growth, which they feared could undermine national identity and the reproduction of the Korean capitalist system itself.

With a similar concern, Pao-chen Tang's chapter, "Beyond Locality: Ke Chin-yuan's Environmentalist Documentary and Cultural Nativism," illustrates how Taiwanese filmmaker Ke Chin-yuan's recent television documentaries address environmental pollution and public health hazards by presenting diverse eco-activist strategies to confront the prevalent neoliberal capitalist regime in contemporary Taiwan. Ke's documentaries explore the profound connection between citizens and the land, spanning from the regional to the national and even the post-national levels. By tracing Ke's creative trajectory and examining how these documentaries investigate various aspects of community formation, the chapter argues that Ke's films employ discourses about the human-environment relationship for distinct ideological and activist purposes. They consistently avoid the dominance of any single narrative but, rather, promote the necessity of dialectical reflection on the advantages and conceptual blind spots of these imagined communities. This approach enables us to chart a path to collective flourishing. Particularly, Ke's films challenge a specific type of environmentalist discourse that emphasizes the importance of nativist culture, tradition, and prestige for environmental protection and public health. They instead propose that the key to an effective model for eco-politics and ethics lies in the capacity of audiovisual media to cultivate collective empathy that transcends locality and even extends to cross-species understanding.

Section IV: Digital Embodiment in Neoliberal Capitalism

In the current digital platform economy, characterized by excitement, anxiety, and often frenzy, the concept of health and illness transcends traditional measures. Health monitoring apps and devices not only collect data for corporate profits or governmental records, they also shape medical culture in its digital form, influencing both our physical and affective well-being through constant interactions with screen-based devices. This transformation extends beyond practical telemedicine applications, popularized during the COVID-19 pandemic, or the quest for online health care information, which can vary in accuracy. Digital media's materiality and the aesthetic proliferation of these platforms engender specific experiences related to health and medical culture. Consider, for instance, how virtual reality and live streaming filters can create "flawless" faces or bodies, while ASMR (autonomous sensory meridian response) videos may induce "soothing" or "healing" sensations. As though the image now assumes a tangible presence, stylistic devices are more than mere audiovisual features; they serve as conduits of well-being. This paradigm shift reflects the intricate ways in which digital platforms have become integral to molding and defining our contemporary engagements with health and medical aesthetics.

The nuanced interplay between contemporary digital media and neoliberal capitalism warrants thorough analysis, especially in the aftermath of the recent global pandemic and health crises that have exposed severe deficiencies of capitalist systems. The volume earlier articulates that the foundation of Chinese socialist health care was predicated on a mass-oriented approach. However, this system has deteriorated since the 1980s, succumbing to the overwhelming forces of a market-driven economy and the commodification inherent in transnational capitalism. Neoliberalism has become hegemonic in China, as it embraced an American mode of political-economic discourse, which proposes that human well-being can be advanced by enhancing individual entrepreneurial freedoms within a system of strong private property rights, free markets, and free trade. However, this purported freedom disproportionately favors the powerful and privileged, within or beyond national borders, at the expense of labor rights, social justice, welfare provisions, and reproductive activities, seeking to bring all human activity under market transactions. In China, while a state-supervised market economy has delivered economic growth and improved living standards since the early 1990s, it has also led to privatization of public assets, labor exploitation, social inequality, rampant consumerism and individualism, environmental degradation, and the reconstitution of capitalist class power.[45] The chapters in this section address China's post-socialist era by investigating how digital media, from live streaming to vlogging, has reshaped healthcare practices and perceptions of physical and psychic well-being in a capitalist framework. Atomized individuals, whether online or offline, navigate diverse experiences. Some seek solace and healing in digital media, while others grapple with challenges due to disabilities and gender hierarchies.

Chang-Min Yu's chapter, "Live Streaming and *Present.Perfect.*: Digital Able-Bodiedness, Liveness, and Disabilities," examines the complex body politics of Chinese live streaming culture, highlighting its gendered construction of able-bodiedness through feminized beauty filters and demonstrations of masculine agility in video game live streams. Yu illuminates how these platforms perpetuate specific ideals of physical standards, intricately intertwining gender norms with able-bodied expectations in the digital sphere. Taking Shengze Zhu's found-footage documentary *Present.Perfect* (*Wanmei xianzaishi*, 2019) as his object of study, Yu demonstrates

45. David Harvey, *A Brief History of Neoliberalism* (Oxford: Oxford University Press, 2005), 122–50.

how Zhu's curation of an archive of live streaming footage can destabilize digital "ableism." This approach not only features subjects with disabilities at the level of representation but also explores how negating idealized images in accordance with capitalist logic might transform cinema, or the moving image more broadly, into an ontologically disabled medium. As Zhu's film illustrates how representations of environmental and bodily disabilities undergo transformation and remediation through the process of voluntary broadcasting, it contemplates how the infrastructure of information storage can either facilitate or impede live interactions and transactions on screen. On this note, the film initiates a meaningful dialogue between digital media studies and critical disability studies in an era where self-images are readily searchable and accessible, enabling the highly profitable performance of the private-made-public. Yu's analysis underscores the transformative potential of documentary filmmaking in challenging prevailing norms and fostering a nuanced understanding of digital able-bodiedness within the contemporary media milieu.

Complementing Yu's critique of prevalent practices of self-objectification, self-exhibition, and self-appropriation in the live streaming industry, Lilian Kong's chapter, "'The Most Calming Thing You Have Done on the Internet': Healing Vlogs and the Aesthetics of Li Ziqi," studies the serene aesthetics of Chinese vlogger Li Ziqi's portrayals of everyday life in rural China. Kong situates Li's globally popular vlogs within the conventions of vlogging and East Asian healing culture, to explore what Li's international acclaim reveals about the role of online healing content. Kong's analysis emphasizes how Li's videos circulate transregionally alongside other global "healing" vlogs, shedding light on the commodification of (mental) well-being in capitalist societies. The chapter critically examines the formal elements of Li's style, encompassing natural imagery, processual representation, and slow aesthetics. It illustrates how the combination of these affective components creates an atmospheric field with a therapeutic effect, accommodating manifold—even contradictory—tensions, anxieties, and desires for viewers to experience, rather than advocating any singular mood or means of escape. This atmospheric quality in Li's videos suggests that online healing content can offer comfort to individuals navigating the anxieties of capitalist societies by aesthetically mediating and transforming the complexities of their lived experiences and subjectivity formations.

Beyond the concepts discussed in *Socializing Medicine*, contemporary East Asia confronts pressing medical and health concerns, notably an aging population and plummeting fertility rates. The region now has some of the world's lowest birth rates, raising widespread anxiety in Japan, South Korea, Taiwan, and mainland China about future development and family structures. This phenomenon results from delayed and fewer marriages, increased exposure to endocrine disruptors in food and environmental pollution, and economic uncertainty and insufficient welfare support.[46] In China, the current "socialist market" health care system reflects the collision and convergence of market values, neoliberal strategies, and state-led socialism. The profit-driven market approach since the 1980s has resulted in exorbitant medical expenses, patient-provider conflicts, and limited access to affordable care. In response, the 2000s saw gradual reforms emphasizing the state's responsibility in health care provision, signaling a belated recommitment to primary and preventive healthcare.[47] Japan's health care system, renowned for its efficiency and accessibility, grapples with financial strains due to its aging population and the associated expenses of chronic illness and long-term care. Policy reforms in the 1990s, including increased patient co-payments, limitations on free access to medical institutions, and stricter controls on medical supplies, failed to effectively reduce deficits in the health insurance budgets. Consequently, additional reforms in the early 2000s focused on the health care services sector.[48]

Taiwan's health insurance system, established in 1995, has been known for its affordability, extensive population coverage, and high patient satisfaction rates. However, it has long grappled with financial instability due to escalating medical costs, an aging population, and governmental reluctance to significantly adjust fees to meet financial demands for fear of political repercussions. Recently, medical professionals in Taiwan, particularly nurses, have struggled with burnout and low wages, leading to a high turnover rate (more than 11 percent in 2022).[49] Since the early 2000s, South Korea has improved its redistributive health policies, though high out-of-pocket spending remains a challenge. The policymaking process witnessed a solidarity coalition between grassroots activists (including labor unions, NGOs, and citizen organizations), medical experts, and bureaucrats, many of whom were student activists in the 1970s and 1980s democratization movements.[50] The enduring impact of this history persists. As we finalized the manuscript of this volume in early 2024, thousands of doctors from over a hundred teaching hospitals in South

46. Naohiro Ogawa, Iqbal H. Shah, and Gayl D. Ness, "Introduction," in *Low Fertility and Reproductive Health in East Asia*, ed. Ogawa and Shah (Dordrecht: Springer, 2015), 2–7; Francesca Bray, "Introduction," in *Gender, Health, and History in Modern East Asia*, ed. Angela Ki Che Leung and Izumi Nakayama (Hong Kong: Hong Kong University Press, 2017), 1–34.
47. Jiong Tu, *Health Care Transformation in Contemporary China: Moral Experience in a Socialist Neoliberal Polity* (Dordrecht: Springer, 2019).
48. Naohiro Yashiro, Reiko Suzuki, and Wataru Suzuki, "Evaluating Japan's Health Care Reform of the 1990s and Its Efforts to Cope with Population Aging," in *Health Care Issues in the United States and Japan*, ed. David A. Wise and Naohiro Yashiro (Chicago: The University of Chicago Press, 2006), 17–42.
49. "Night-shift Nurse Bonus Unhelpful: Survey," *Taipei Times*, October 21, 2023, https://www.taipeitimes.com/News/taiwan/archives/2023/10/21/2003808010.
50. Illan Nam, *Democratizing Health Care: Welfare State in Korea and Thailand* (New York: Palgrave Macmillan, 2015), 51–72.

Korea went on strike, protesting against the government's proposed changes to the number of trainee doctors and calling for improved pay and working conditions.[51]

We hope this volume serves as a foundation to inspire future scholarly dialogue on the intersection of health and mass media across diverse East Asian regions and temporal frameworks beyond our current purview. This includes an exploration of various contexts such as early Republican China, socialist North Korea, the colonial eras of Hong Kong and Taiwan, and contemporary settings in Japan and South Korea, among many other possibilities. Also meriting further exploration is the extensive corpus of East Asian fiction films, documentaries, television dramas, and other audiovisual media that engage with medicinal culture and health issues.[52] Adopting a more expansive methodological stance and scope will not only enrich our understanding of the historical nuances in East Asian media and health humanities but also encourage cross-disciplinary theoretical discourse to unravel the complex layers embedded within these domains.

51. Justin McCurry, "South Korea Doctors' Strike: Government Moves to Suspend Thousands of Medical Licences," *The Guardian*, March 12, 2024, https://www.theguardian.com/world/2024/mar/12/south-korea-doctor-strike-government-suspends-medical-licenses.

52. Just to name a few: the Japanese film *Dear Doctor* (Miwa Nishikawa, 2009), which highlights the shortage of medical professionals in rural areas; the South Korean film *Poetry* (dir. Lee Chang-dong, 2010) on such themes as aging and dementia; and the Chinese film *Dying to Survive* (dir. Wen Muye, 2018), about a man selling affordable Indian generic drugs to aid underprivileged patients battling Chronic Granulocytic Leukemia. Recently there has been a surge of Taiwanese films focusing on physical and mental health within domestic settings, including *The Falls* (dir. Chung Mong-hong, 2021), *American Girl* (dir. Roan Feng-I, 2021), and *Trouble Girl* (dir. Chin Chia-hua, 2023).

Section I

Medical and Media Imperialism

1

Contagious Disease and Visual Media in Colonial Korea

Jeehey Kim

Scholars have been investigating the intricate relationship between disease control and epidemics, revealing them as pivotal components of imperial endeavors. Within the context of the British Empire, leprosy emerged as a notable example of a disease that became entwined with notions of race and colonialism, largely due to the way its medical management was influenced by cultural constructs.[1] This chapter discusses how Japanese imperial power employed visual media—photographs, lantern slides, and moving images—to establish a culture of fear and ostracism as a mode of controlling contagious diseases, particularly cholera and Hansen's disease (often called leprosy, a term that conveys a derogatory connotation), the most threatening and widespread diseases at the time. A newspaper article from the 1930s suggests that disseminating portrait photographs of lepers prevents them from approaching villages where "normal" people reside, as the disease leaves visible markers on the infected.[2] In public lectures to colonial Koreans about the dangers of contagious diseases, photography and film were viewed as effective means of education by the Japanese colonial government and police units charged with enforcing public hygiene. Furthermore, characterizing these illnesses as "colonial diseases" was a tool to racialize and to "Other" colonial citizens.

Through exploring the use of visual media as apparatus of the state intended to mobilize colonial citizens, this chapter addresses complex ways in which photography and film served a system of authoritarian discipline by which imperial Japan

1. Rod Edmond, *Leprosy and Empire: A Medical and Cultural History* (Cambridge: Cambridge University Press, 2006); Jane Buckingham, *Leprosy in Colonial South India: Medicine and Confinement* (New York: Palgrave Macmillan, 2002).
2. I use the terms *leprosy* and *lepers* to retain the tone of the colonial media and bureaucracy and to show their linguistic mode of colonial violence.

ruled its colonies ideologically, politically, and culturally. The chapter starts with an analysis of the colonial government's official records of cholera control in 1919 and 1920, focusing on a shift of tone in the selection and order of photographs. Then, it explores propaganda films of hygiene education both from colonial Korea and the main island of Japan to shed light on the colonial ruler's use of the media for highlighting its achievements and concealing the dark aspects of its treatment of disease carriers. Through analyzing the colonial tactics of disease control, the chapter also aims to reveal the ways in which the colonial legacy of racializing and genderizing disease continues in the postcolonial Korean society.

Politics of Fear and Racialization of the Sick

Causing some 20,000 deaths on the Korean peninsula, outbreaks of cholera in 1919 and 1920 pitched the Japanese colonial government into a panic. As the disease originated from outside Korea—Manchuria and Russia from the north, Japan from the south—the colonial government began to quarantine visitors and cordon off afflicted areas. Isolation hospitals and the vaccination of civilians were considered crucial efforts to contain the epidemic. The colonial government published two meticulous records of its preventive measures against cholera in 1920 and 1921.[3] The opening pages of these books each include around twenty photographs illustrating the ways in which the colonial and local governments systematically enforced preventive measures throughout the peninsula. The photographs are carefully organized to elucidate orderly procedures to contain the disease, from inspecting travelers, establishing quarantine facilities, and surveilling civilians to tracing unreported infectors and vaccinating all colonial citizens. As the colonial government published these records as official documents of colonial governance, one can infer that the photographs were meant to offer evidence of successful containment of the disease. The books depict Koreans willingly conforming to the protocols despite inconvenience and oppression. While the isolation facilities in the records appear newly built, in reality, there was a severe shortage of such facilities, so most patients remained at home or were denied entry to isolation facilities due to poor management.[4] Thus, photography not only recorded administrative practices, but it also concealed a reality that would otherwise have disrupted the illusion of successful colonial rule. The colonial government's publications aimed to produce a manual

3. Chōsensōtokufu, ed., *Taishō hachinen korerabyō bōekishi* (Seoul: Chōsensōtokufu, 1920); Chōsensōtokufu, ed., *Taishō kyūnen korerabyō bōekishi* (Seoul: Chōsensōtokufu, 1921).
4. Seon Lye Baek, "1919–20nyeon singminji Joseonui kollera yuhaenggwa bangyeokwaldong" (MA thesis, Seoul, Hanyang University, 2011), 22–23.

of disease control as well as to glorify the achievements of the Japanese rule in its colonies.

Police departments were the major organs enlisted to control epidemics during the colonial period. Beginning in the 1880s, policing citizens' bodies and households was considered the most effective preventive measures against epidemics. These methods were systematized by the Japanese when the Protectorate was established in 1905.[5] The advent of "hygiene police forces" (*wisaeng gyeongchal* 衛生警察) signaled the emergence of a police state wherein police forces were the main organs of disciplining the public and surveilling individual hygiene under the guise of protection of the public from infectious diseases. This supported the notion that the health of the state depends on the health of individuals within the state. While precolonial measures—including the Gabo Reforms of 1894—embraced the use of police as disciplinary bodies of sanitation and hygiene, the Korean public resented the recent coercive strictures by police as painful reminders of Japan's forced annexation of Korea.[6]

Photographs published in the 1919 record of preventive measures against cholera show how Japanese hygiene police officers visited homes, carrying out medical examinations of individuals.[7] In one photograph, a man is lowering his trousers while a hygiene police officer collects a feces sample to determine whether he is infected (Figure 1.1). Another hygiene police officer in a white gown is taking a note, possibly of the identity of the barefoot Korean man lowering his head. The photograph offers the reader visual evidence of how thoroughly preventive measures were enforced. The Japanese police officers look into the lens of camera, willingly presenting themselves as doing their duty. In contrast, the two Korean men appear humiliated: the Korean man with his buttocks exposed turns his head away; the other Korean man's eyes are cast down. What appears to be an objective record of successful control of disease reflects subjugation, humiliation, and power hierarchy. The invisible photographer was given an authority to enforce the surrender of control over one's body and its representation. Photography here does not merely document a colonial reality but actively constitutes the social structure of governing the colonial bodies, because its use doubly reminds the subject of his colonial identity not only as a potential threat to the public hygiene of the empire but also as a being to be naked and vulnerable whenever authority deems it necessary.

In colonial Korea, photography often traumatized its colonial subjects by forcing them to stand before a camera. For instance, in the 1910s, Ryūzō Torii's

5. Keunsik Jung, "Singminji wisaenggyeongcharui hyeongseonggwa byeonhwa, geurigo yusan: Singminji tongchiseongui sigageseo," *Sahoewa yeoksa* 90 (2011): 223–26.
6. Kyung Moon Hwang, *Rationalizing Korea: The Rise of the Modern State, 1894–1945* (Oakland, CA: University of California Press, 2015), 220–46.
7. Chōsensōtokufu, *Taishō hachinen korerabyō bōekishi.*

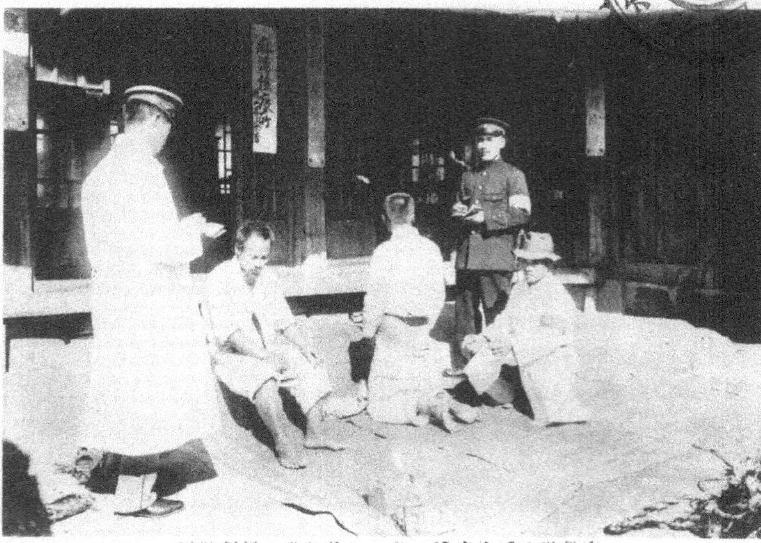

京畿道京城府麻浦ニ於ケル旅行者ノ採便状況

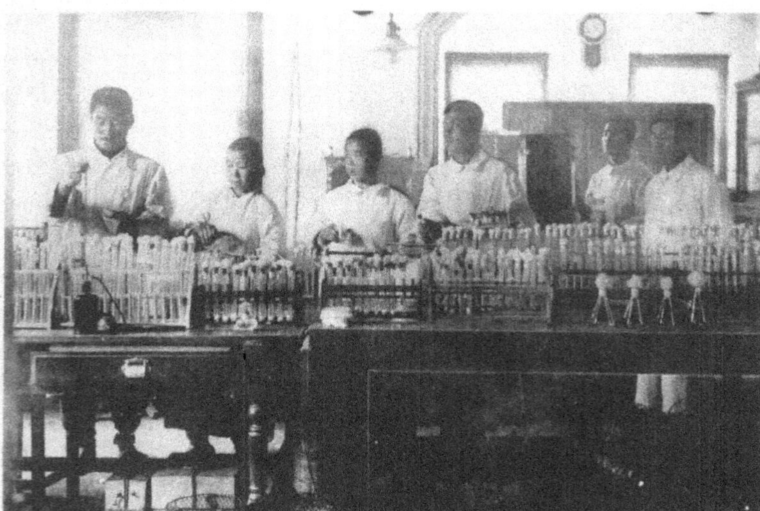

京畿道仁川府ニ於ケル細菌検査状況

Figure 1.1: Chōsensōtokufu, ed., *Taishō Hachinen Korerabyō Bōekishi* (Seoul: Chōsensōtokufu, 1920), unpaginated.

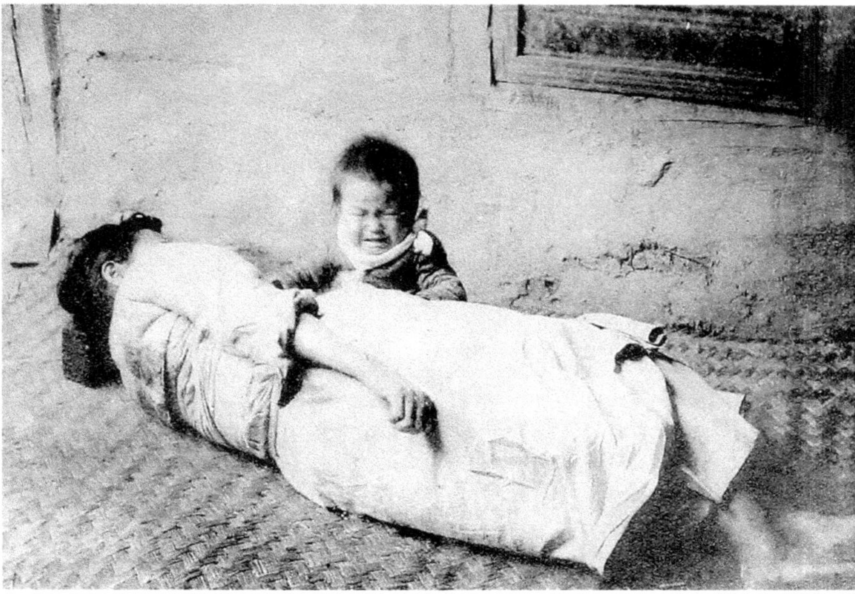

Figure 1.2: Chōsensōtokufu, ed., *Taishō Kyūnen Korerabyō Bōekishi* (Seoul: Chōsensōtokufu, 1921), unpaginated.

anthropometric photographs had made it permissible for the colonizer to undress the colonized before a camera.[8] Colonial administrators learned that photography created a community of colonial citizens as ethnographic subjects. As photography historian Abigail Solomon-Godeau notes, "dominant social relations are inevitably both reproduced and reinforced in the act of imaging those who do not have access to the means of representation themselves."[9]

The photographs in the 1920 record are more sensational than those of the previous year. Some images show corpses. One photograph shows a two-year-old baby crying next to his dead mother's body (Figure 1.2), although the image might have

8. For Ryūzō Torii's anthropological photographs of Koreans during the 1910s, see Hyung Il Pai, "Capturing Visions of Japan's Prehistoric Past: Torii Ryūzō's Field Photographs of 'Primitive' Races and Lost Civilizations (1896–1915)," in *Looking Modern: East Asian Visual Culture from Treaty Ports to World War II*, ed. Jennifer Purtle and Hans Bjarne Thomsen (Chicago: Center for the Art of East Asia, University of Chicago; Art Media Resources, 2009), 265–93. For more on the complex nature of racialization through photography during the colonial period, see Gyewon Kim, "Faces That Change: Physiognomy, Portraiture, and Photography in Colonial Korea," in *The Affect of Difference: Representations of Race in East Asian Empire*, ed. Christopher P. Hanscom and Dennis C. Washburn (Honolulu, HI: University of Hawai'i Press, 2016), 133–58.
9. Abigail Solomon-Godeau, *Photography at the Dock* (Minneapolis, MN: University of Minnesota Press, 1991), 180.

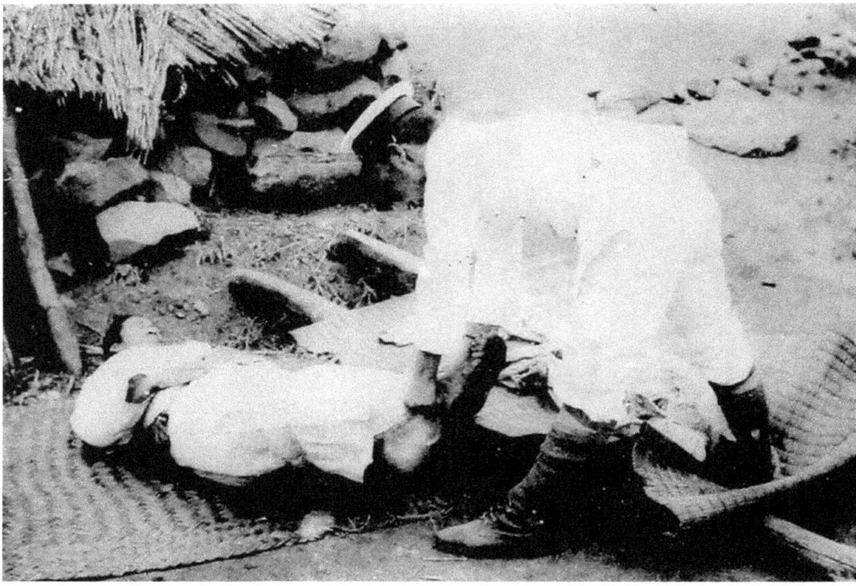

Figure 1.3: Chōsensōtokufu, ed., *Taishō Kyūnen Korerabyō Bōekishi* (Seoul: Chōsensōtokufu, 1921), unpaginated.

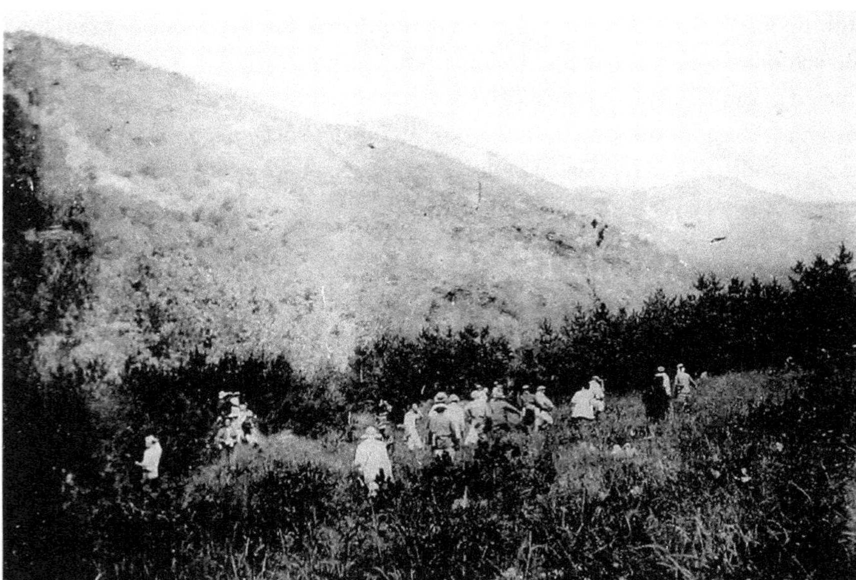

Figure 1.4: Chōsensōtokufu, ed., *Taishō Kyūnen Korerabyō Bōekishi* (Seoul: Chōsensōtokufu, 1921), unpaginated.

been staged in a similar way that colonial officials forced Koreans to take specific poses in most of ethnographic and social survey photographs. In another image, a hygiene police officer moves a corpse to a stretcher (Figure 1.3). The caption explains that the officer carries the body for cremation without having time for proper steps of disinfection. Another photograph shows a local military party searching for corpses that the bereaved have secretly buried in order to avoid cremation (Figure 1.4). These photographs reveal the challenges that colonial authorities confronted because Koreans refused cremation, which is against their tradition of burial for the dead. Moreover, photographing the dead family member must have caused humiliation and brought disgrace to Koreans, as traditional culture allows only close family members to view the deceased. That a police force took control of the dead reveals the ways in which colonial public health policy established what Achille Mbembe calls "necropolitics": sovereignty and politics defined by the control over death.[10] Once the infected died, their bodies fell under the control of the hygiene police. The colonial government was alarmed by bereaved families hosting funerals at home, where relatives and other guests were invited to enter contaminated space. The house was to be disinfected and the dead transferred to public crematoria. Thus, control of the (infected) dead was a form of governing the living in colonial Korea.

While photographs of the 1919 outbreak illustrate the orderly process of containing the disease, the 1920 images foreground the tragic results of an out-of-control epidemic. The 1919 images show the quarantining of arrivals at ports and train stations, followed by disinfection and isolation of the infected. The final images show Koreans receiving vaccinations. In contrast, the 1920 record starts with photographs of vaccination, followed by images of isolation, disinfection, and public education. The last photographs illustrate a desperate situation, where the dead bodies of the infected overwhelm the authorities. The order of the photographs in both records shows that the colonial government emphasized the efficacy of vaccination, as it required Koreans to carry vaccine certificates.[11] More importantly, the different order of photographs reveals that the colonial government tried to conceal the inefficiency of vaccination to contain the disease. The concluding photographs of devastated Koreans in the record of the 1920 outbreak place the responsibility for failed measures on "uncivilized" Koreans' unhygienic practices.

Most Koreans disliked the colonial officers' treatment of patients as criminals, while also distrusting Western and Japanese medicine as different from the Oriental practice. The photographs in the 1920 record do not reveal the frustration felt by

10. Achille Mbembe, "Necropolitics," trans. Libby Meintjes, *Public Culture* 15, no. 1 (2003): 11–40.
11. Yunjae Park, "Sanitizing Korea: Anti-Cholera Activities of the Police in Early Colonial Korea," *Seoul Journal of Korean Studies* 23, no. 2 (2010): 161.

Koreans who suffered from the colonial government's draconian measures. There were protests against transfer to isolation facilities, the most publicized one of which occurred in the summer of 1920, when thousands of Koreans attacked police officers transferring a Korean patient to an isolation hospital in Seoul.[12]

The colonial authorities' dominant view of Koreans as ignorant and negligent is also reflected in these photographs, while no image shows a Japanese-occupied residence under inspection or disinfection. These photographs were deployed to reinforce the boundary between the Japanese and Korean ethnicities. At the time of the epidemics, around 347,000 Japanese lived on the Korean peninsula, about 65,000 of them in Seoul.[13] According to the records, 175 Japanese residents died of the disease in 1919; 110 died in 1920. Though the number of the Japanese dead is a lot lower than that of the Korean (more than 10,000), the mortality rate is similar, which evidences colonial authorities' failure to contain the epidemic, not Koreans' ignorance or unwillingness to follow public health protocols. But with the exception of a photograph showing a few Japanese seated at an outdoor public education event, neither record provides photographs of Japanese suffering from the disease.

The 1919 and 1920 outbreaks were not the first to strike the Korean peninsula, as the disease had been widespread for some time. Under the Japanese protectorate (1905–1910), cholera broke out in 1907 and 1909. Nor was Korea the only region within the Japanese Empire to be affected, as Taiwan and the Japanese main island were heavily stricken in 1919 and 1920.[14] What motivated the colonial government to confine these extensive records to these two years and only to Korea? The photographs reveal a new mode of governing Koreans in the wake of the March First Movement of 1919. Cholera broke out around five months after the protest. The suspicious death of King Gojong in January and the continuing devastation by the 1918 Spanish flu led to growing unrest and complaints about Japanese rule.[15] The protest unsettled imperial administrators, who replaced militarized control with *naisen yuwa* (harmony between Japan and Korea). Through educational and

12. Baek, "1919–20nyeon singminji Joseonui kollera yuhaenggwa bangyeokwaldong," 37–41.
13. Jun Uchida, *Brokers of Empire: Japanese Settler Colonialism in Korea, 1876–1945* (Cambridge, MA: Harvard University Asia Center, 2011), 65.
14. Yuehtsen Juliette Chung, "Sovereignty and Imperial Hygiene: Japan and the 1919 Cholera Epidemic in East Asia," in *The Decade of the Great War: Japan and the Wider World in the 1910s*, ed. Tosh Minohara, Tze-ki Hon, and Evan Dawley (Leiden: Brill, 2014), 439–60.
15. It should be noted that the colonial government's handling of the Spanish flu was quite different from its management of cholera, despite the former's higher mortality rate. The policy derives from the government's categorization of infectious diseases, which excluded influenza from its nine diseases, but included cholera and smallpox. Thus, Spanish flu was not subject to legal procedures to prevent its spread. The government's coercive measures to identify the infected aggravated the Koreans' antipathy toward Japanese rule. Taek-joong Kim, "1918nyeon dokgamgwa Joseonchongdokbu bangyeokjeongchaek," *Inmun nonchong* 74, no. 1 (2017): 197.

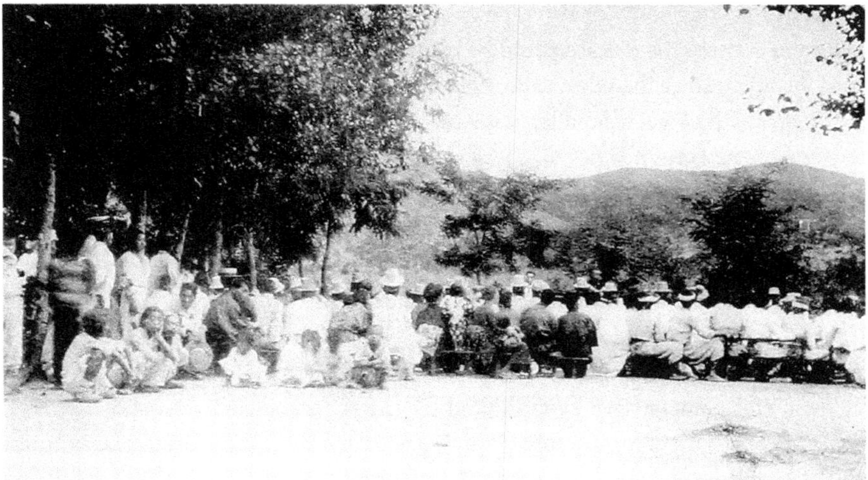

Figure 1.5: Chōsensōtokufu, ed., *Taishō Kyūnen Korerabyō Bōekishi* (Seoul: Chōsensōtokufu, 1921), unpaginated.

economic commitments, the colonial government promoted the idea of coexisting ethnicities within the peninsula via systemic integration.[16]

Compared to the 1909 cholera outbreak, when disease control was founded on coercing Koreans to sanitize themselves by imposing fines and hygiene taxes,[17] the colonial government devoted itself to enlightening the public to the dangers through lantern slide shows and public lectures. The authorities attempted to reduce public resentment that equated hygiene and sanitization measures with policing by implementing various modes of motivating colonial citizens to pay more attention to personal hygiene.

In 1920, the colonial government determined that the disease derived from Japan, in contrast to the 1919 incursion from China and Russia. In this context, Koreans were considered responsible for spreading the disease due to their poor hygiene rather than the colonial administration's failure to block the influx from Japan. A photograph shows a public lecture about the importance of hygiene and other personal measures to contain the disease (Figure 1.5). The colonial government was devoted to organizing such programs in 1920, including the distribution of booklets, as well as lantern slide shows and films on hygiene and cholera.[18] This contrast between subjects encapsulates the government's shift from control of the

16. Uchida, *Brokers of Empire*, 143–46.
17. Yun-Jae Park, "Hanmal, ilje cho hanseongwisaenghoeui hwaldonggwa singmin jibae," *Seoulhagyeongu* 22 (2004): 67–89.
18. Chōsensōtokufu, *Taishō kyūnen korerabyō bōekishi*, 87–88.

masses to making individuals responsible for their own health conditions. Thus, failure to contain the disease could be blamed on Koreans' ignorance of and disregard for rules rather than the authorities' failure to devise effective measures.

Koreans had been familiar with magic lantern shows since the 1890s, and hygiene magic lantern slides (*wisaeng hwandeung*) first came to be used for public education around 1906.[19] American missionaries presented slides of scenic views and industrial development in foreign countries along with biblical scenes. The magic lantern show was also a new form of entertainment and spectacle, often accompanied by music and dance performances.[20] As Todd Henry notes, hygiene lectures and lantern slide shows mobilized Koreans to hygienic modernity beginning in the protectorate period (1905–1910).[21] Though Henry points out that the didactic effect might have been diluted by entertainment between slide lectures, the performativity of magic lantern shows facilitated the combination of education and entertainment, which wielded a more propagandistic impact on mobilizing colonial citizens to attend events organized by the authorities. It appears that both books' photographs were deployed in hygiene lantern slide shows. The photographs reproduced for colonial record came to be mobilized to educate colonial citizens, demarcating trans-medial use of photographic images as efficient colonial tactics.

In 1920, the Department of Hygiene established its own magic lantern unit, dispatching it to warn the public of the coming threat.[22] Images of unsanitary living conditions were proposed as the major cause of contagious disease, creating fear and terror through images of infected victims, and slides of bacteria were shown to heighten public awareness of the importance of preventive measures. Compared to the display of bacterial images at the Industrial Exhibition of 1915, which served to provide Koreans with more advanced scientific and medical knowledge, these slides made the gravity of the disease seem more real, as they were sequenced with slides of the ill and deceased.[23] As the victims were always presented as Korean, the images of cholera bacteria came to be associated with Koreans. Keijō (present-day Seoul) was

19. Dong Hoon Kim, *Eclipsed Cinema: The Film Culture of Colonial Korea* (Edinburgh: Edinburgh University Press, 2017), 35.
20. Sunyoung Yoo, "Sigakgisulloseo hwandeunggwa singminjiui sigakseong," *Eollongwa sahoe* 24, no. 2 (2016): 191–229; Hye-ju Shin, "1900Nyeondae gisaeng hwandeunghoe yeongu," *Hangugeumaksahakbo* 58 (2017): 99–136. Yoo explores how magic lantern slide shows structured nationalism among Koreans in the early 1920s. According to Shin, *gisaeng* (female entertainer) performance accompanied magic lantern slide shows of their likenesses in popular theaters of Seoul in the 1900s and 1910s.
21. Todd A. Henry, *Assimilating Seoul: Japanese Rule and the Politics of Public Space in Colonial Korea, 1910–1945* (Oakland, CA: University of California Press, 2016), 144–45.
22. Yeong Hee Cho, "Geundae hanguk sigakgyoyuk midieoroseoui hwandeunghoe yeongu" (PhD diss., Seoul National University, 2018), 121–24.
23. For the display of bacteria and virus specimens at the 1915 Industrial Exhibition, see Dong Won Shin, *Hoyeolja, Joseoneul seupgyeokhada* (Seoul: Yuksabipyungsa, 2004), 59–64.

even called "the Empire's diseased city," which derives from racialized assumptions that it was Koreans' ignorance and unwillingness to civilize themselves that caused the outbreak rather than the colonial authorities' discrimination against Koreans by failing to provide social welfare programs and build sanitary infrastructure.[24]

What distinguishes the colonial government's hygiene project after the March First Movement is that it produced visual materials, including silent films, within the colony, rather than merely delivering knowledge provided by experts from the imperial metropole or the West. Due to the recognition by the colonial government that the primary catalyst for the uprising lay in its oppressive military governance, it embarked on a concerted effort to exert cultural influence over its colony through media channels. The colonial authorities began to recruit Koreans into its cultural production as an attempt to embrace the locality of its colony, while allowing Koreans to establish their own venues of cultural activities, such as newspapers and film production.[25] The colonial government also established the Moving Picture Unit in 1920 as a mode of cultural rule in reaction to the Koreans' protests against coercive Japanization. To promote peaceful coexistence, the unit produced films for Japanese and Koreans to understand each other's culture and history.[26] Unlike earlier performances that collected admission fees, these events were offered free of charge, not only to disseminate information as widely as possible, but also to monitor visitors and vaccinate them after the screening.[27] The 1920 establishment of lantern slide and moving picture units reveals how colonial officials incorporated visual media into public health education.

The so-called cultural rule, however, did not result in less emphasis on police power. A new mode of institutionalizing police power was injected into the daily lives of the colonized, who were expected to willingly discipline their bodies and personal conduct.[28] Beginning in late 1919, the number of police officers increased,[29] and from the early 1920s, police organized film screenings about cholera and smallpox. The emergence of "hygiene films" facilitated the spread of fear over contagious diseases under the name of educating the public on the dangers of poor personal

24. Henry, *Assimilating Seoul*, 146–67. Nationalist writers criticized ethnocentric approaches to regulating Koreans, promoting hygienic modernity as a form of self-governance and autonomy. Henry notes that the goal of improving sanitary and public health conditions, which both the Japanese colonialists and Korean nationalists shared, was "same bed, different dreams." He also points out that nationalists and colonialists were both aware of class issues as one of the major causes of poor sanitary conditions.
25. In 1920, the two Korean newspapers *Tonga ilbo* and *Chosun ilbo* were established.
26. Kim, *Eclipsed Cinema*, 41–50.
27. Henry, *Assimilating Seoul*, 161; Cho, "Geundae Hanguk sigakgyoyuk midieoroseoui hwandeunghoe yeongu," 137.
28. Henry, *Assimilating Seoul*, 158.
29. Park, "Sanitizing Korea," 165.

hygiene. The Japanese colonial government appropriated hygiene cinema for social guidance and enlightenment from Germany, where film was integral to disseminating knowledge of hygiene, medicine, and sanitation. Unlike in Germany, however, the Japanese implemented the use of police departments as the major organ for distributing and sponsoring hygiene films.[30] Beginning in 1921, police and local sanitation officers organized expositions where nightly screenings of hygiene films were offered free of charge.[31]

Hygiene films were the first films produced in Korea, as local audiences were accustomed to viewing motion pictures imported from Europe, the United States, and the metropole of Japan; and a film showing the devastating situation of the 1919 cholera outbreak was released in 1920.[32] Thus, the epidemic played an instrumental role in the establishment of local film culture. These early hygiene films have been lost, but details about them are recorded in contemporary newspaper and magazine articles. The Government-General sponsored films on cholera and smallpox, which were produced by Korean directors and starred Korean actors and actresses. As these were the first films in which Koreans could see their own faces, they were quite popular.[33]

The narratives of hygiene films were relatively simple: a beautiful woman contracts smallpox due to poor personal hygiene, which leads to disfigurement and subsequent abandonment by her lover; in despair, the woman takes her own life.[34] The enormous popularity of these hygiene films derives from their incorporation of trendy issues, such as free love and suicide from failed love, in addition to the excitement of watching Koreans on-screen for the first time.[35] The films present the diseases as gendered by positioning female protagonists as ignorant, uncivilized, and vulnerable to social stigma over appearance, attributing responsibility for infection to individual conduct rather than to medical and social systems. The genre reveals the ways in which diseases were not only racialized but also gendered, with stereotypes based on rural/urban divide in terms of education and sanitation.

---

30. Keum Dong Kim, "Dogil wisaengyeonghwareul tonghae bon Joseon kollerawisaengyeonghwa(1920)wa cheonyeonduwisaengyeonghwa(1922)ui teukjinggwa hangye," *Yeonghwa Yeongu*, no. 55 (2013): 39–40.
31. Jae-Seong Choe, "Ilje gyeongchalgiguui wisaeng seonjeon," *Hanilminjongmunjeyeongu* 40 (2021): 13–17.
32. Hyun Hee Park, "Tears in the Imperial Screen: Wartime Colonial Korean Cinema, 1936–1945" (PhD diss., University of Chicago, 2017), 28–29.
33. Kim, "Dogil wisaengyeonghwareul tonghae bon Joseon kollerawisaengyeonghwa(1920)wa cheonyeonduwisaengyeonghwa(1922)ui teukjinggwa hangye," 67–69.
34. "Wisaenggangyeonhwaldongsajin," *Maeil sinbo*, June 18, 1922. Other details of the film, including the title and the name of director, are not known.
35. Kim, "Dogil wisaengyeonghwareul tonghae bon Joseon kollerawisaengyeonghwa(1920)wa cheonyeonduwisaengyeonghwa(1922)ui teukjinggwa hangye," 70–73.

Hyesook Bok (1904–1982), one of the earliest Korean film actresses, notes that her debut was *Bangyeok* (*Prevention of Epidemics*), a hygiene film sponsored by the Government-General in 1923.[36] In the film, a girl is infected with cholera after drinking lemonade sold by a street vendor. Her family, ignorant of modern hygiene and medicine, brings a shaman to treat the disease. The girl dies after being transferred to a hospital too late. Another hygiene film, *Nama no hokori* (*The Pride of Life*), was released in 1922.[37] The original film is believed to have been lost, but its full script was published in *Keimu iho*, a monthly bulletin of the Government-General's Police Bureau, as its hygiene department sponsored the production. All the characters were Korean, and the police bureau organized a public screening at its lecture hall. Around 6,000 people attended the event, where, in an attempt to allay fear among the public, a speech was given about the role of police officers as protectors of the people. Newsreels were shown on cholera prevention, current affairs of Tokyo and Korea, firefighting training, and memorial services of policemen.[38] Rather than physicians or public health officials, police officers were the speakers, which shows that public health was a crucial project of policing colonial bodies.

The Pride of Life tells the story of a beautiful woman taking her own life in despair over her disfigured face after recovering from smallpox. She lives in the countryside and visits her uncle in Seoul. Her fiancé is a student living in her uncle's house while attending medical school. The film mobilizes the fictional narrative for the purpose of hygiene education. Incorporating an educational motif, the scenes of medical facilities are instrumental in showing the advancement of the public health system established by Japanese colonial rule. There is a scene of the female protagonist amazed at what she sees on a visit to a hospital operated by the Government-General. During her stay, smallpox breaks out and inoculation is encouraged. The film introduces the development of the vaccine by showing two medical students visiting a vaccine manufacturing facility in Busan.

---

36. Hyesook Bok, "Naui gyoyurok wolloyeoryu-ga yeongneun hoego <83> yeonghwa debwi (13)," *Donga ilbo*, May 6, 1981. According to Bok, the film was directed by Baeknam Yun (1888–1954), who is known to have made *Wolhaui maengseo* (*The Vow Made Below the Moon*) the same year, another film sponsored by the Government-General to encourage savings among the public. *Vow under the Moon* is known to be the first Korean feature film, but Bok's memoir suggests that hygiene films of the early 1920s predate it.
37. Scholars confused *Nama no hokori* with other hygiene films, which is based on research of newspaper articles of the time and memoirs written by filmmakers, actors, and actresses. According to the script published in *Keimu iho*, the 1922 film is different from other hygiene films produced in previous years. For the discussion of *Nama no hokori* as the first hygiene film in Korea, see Sang Eon Han, "1920nyeondae choban Joseonui yeonghwasaneopgwa Joseonyeonghwaui tansaeng," *Yeonghwa yeongu*, no. 55 (2013): 659–62; Sangeon Han, "1892–1925: Yeonghwa yuipgwa yeonghwasaneobui hyeongseong," in *Hangukgeundaeyeonghwasa: 1892nyeoneseo 1945nyeonkkaji*, by Hyoin Yi, Chonghwa Chung, and Sangeon Han (Paju: Dolbaegae, 2019), 68–69.
38. "Honkai shusai katsudoshashinkai," *Keimu iho*, October 1922.

The female protagonist and her cousin's wife go to get vaccinated, but she refuses because she had not imagined having to expose her skin in public. The film contrasts her naive rural perspective with her cousin's educated urban views as someone who accepts modern medicine. Upon returning to her home, the protagonist finds that her maid has contracted smallpox. Her father brings in a doctor of traditional Asian medicine who is ignorant of how to treat the disease. Due to exposure to the infected maid, the protagonist also contracts smallpox and is hospitalized. She recovers, unlike her mother who died of the disease many years ago, but her face is scarred with pockmarks. Her fiancé, who had felt pride that his future wife is prettier than his friend's wife, is disappointed. In the end, the female protagonist drowns herself in the Han River after witnessing the anguish of her fiancé. The film ends with her fiancé setting out on a journey of propaganda (*senden*), finding pride in saving the lives of others after realizing the importance of inoculation. Thus, "the pride of life" is to be found in educating others to the importance of public health, with the woman as sacrifice.[39]

The film's patriarchal narrative represents a Korean woman from a rural area where the colonialist program of "civilization" has yet to be practiced, while positing a Korean man as ready to join the colonial project. The Japanese colonial authorities expected that localizing the hygiene film with Korean characters would have a more powerful impact on colonial citizens. Local people were indeed enthused by the experience of watching Koreans on screen, and the film was a great success owing to its combination of educational content with a melodrama. The Korean audience might have been attracted to the tragic aspect of the film rather than its didactic message, but the government's new tactic of propaganda enthusiastically embraced the medium's ability to clothe the educational program as a type of entertainment. The Japanese police force, which published the full script in its bulletin, had an important role in realizing popular entertainment as a means of social education. Policing how films were produced, circulated, and consumed confirms that mass culture was under full state control.

The number of hygiene films submitted for censor's approval dramatically increased to around seventy-six between August 1926 and July 1927.[40] Keum Dong Kim points out that hygiene films were enlisted not only for public education but also for demarcating the boundary between the colonizers and the colonized, as Japanese were shown to prevent disease with expert knowledge, while Koreans were subject to contract diseases due to their ignorance, poor sanitation, and poor

39. Keimukyoku eiseika, "Kyakuhon *Nama no hokori* (jō)," *Keimu iho*, June 1922; Keimukyoku eiseika, "Kyakuhon *Nama oo hokori* (ge)," *Keimu iho*, July 1922.

40. Keum Dong Kim, "Dogil wisaengyeonghwaeui suyongwa suneunghaneun shikminji juche hyeongseong," *Yeonghwa yeongu*, no. 51 (2012): 23–25.

personal hygiene.[41] Thus, the films served as racial markers in a way similar to photographs published in government records of disease. Visual media were actively used to conceal the reality that the Japanese colonial government neglected to establish medical facilities or develop a system of public health, while justifying surveillance and law enforcement under the guise of improving personal hygiene and public sanitation.

Politics of Fear and Segregation of the Sick

The colonial government utilized visual media not only for educating colonial citizens about public health, but also for securing social stability that might be endangered by the failure of disease control. In addition to cholera and tuberculosis, the Japanese authorities endeavored to control Hansen's disease. The terms *leprosy* (*nabyeong*) and *lepers* (*nahwanja* or *mundungi*) were commonly used during the colonial period. Isolation of the afflicted was promoted as the best way to contain the disease. In articles about lepers committing murder based on a superstition that eating a child's raw liver would cure the disease, newspapers and popular magazines described the disease as a social threat.[42] Public fear of leprosy was thus not only about its communicability but also fear of one's child being kidnapped and killed. Lepers were dangerous criminals, which justified the state's discipline and surveillance of leprosy patients' bodies.

Medical doctors also expressed concerns over leonine-faced lepers loitering in groups on the streets, suggesting that since leprosy is chronic, segregation is the best solution.[43] The disease is signaled not as an issue of public hygiene, but as a social and national threat, because it is contagious and hereditary, which necessitated exclusion of the infected from the "normal" population. Biomedical experts sustained discriminatory treatment of the infected, justifying forced lifelong segregation. In a 1930 magazine article, a dermatologist asserts that leprosy is not found in civilized countries that have effective isolation policies, such as in the United States, where the infected were moved to Hawai'i.[44] Estimated at one million, those infected with leprosy were described as social parasites in colonial Korea because, being crippled, they had lost the capacity for labor. The colonial government's protocol of leprosy prevention and control followed the global initiative of isolation of lepers, which the Norwegian physician Gerhard Hansen had proposed in Berlin during the first

41. Kim, "Dogil wisaengyeonghwaeui suyongwa suneunghaneun shikminji juche hyeongseong," 26.
42. "Mundungbyeongeyakdoendago eorinaeganeulppaeeo," *Chosun ilbo*, July 5, 1927; "Saengganmeogeunnabyeongnyeo sahyeongeulguhyeong," *Donga ilbo*, September 7, 1928.
43. Sangyong Kim, "Nabyeongui yeongu geup chiryobeop," *Gaebyeok*, June 1923.
44. "Hakjayeongusilsullye(1), baengman mundung gujecha segyunyeongu jungui ouihakbaksa," *Samcheolli*, July 1930.

International Conference on Leprosy in 1897.[45] The Japanese endeavor to control the disease was one of its projects to align the imperial power with European countries that categorized leprosy as Asian and African problems. In 1916, Sorok Island was designated to isolate Korean leprosy patients with the establishment of a hospital (*jahyeuiwon*). In 1939, expansion was completed with a sanatorium (*gaengsaengwon*) to accommodate around 6,000 patients.[46]

As Gijae Seo points out, the colonial authority visualized Sorok Island as a paradise while reinforcing leprophobia through mass media to justify the isolation policy.[47] Outside of Sorok, lepers were viewed as subjects to be hunted and apprehended, but on the island they were purported to be beneficiaries of a joyous life courtesy of a benign government.[48] Because newspaper articles often sensationalized false rumors of cannibalism by lepers, patients' presence among "normal" populations was viewed as a threat to law and order. There was no analysis of what caused lepers to become vagrant or what gave rise to outlandish superstitions or public misconceptions about unfounded cures. Social discrimination against lepers led to ostracism from employment, community, and even their own families, forcing them into cities where they could subsist through begging. In addition, the lack of medical facilities for leprosy was not acknowledged, much less the potential curability of the disease.[49]

Sorok Island is around 1.7 square miles in area. Thousands of patients and staff were unable to support themselves and had to depend on government support. Following the mobilization for war in 1938, the government decreased food rations and medicine, even forcing the patients to contribute to the imperial war effort through financial donations or labor.[50] Belying the horrors of forced labor, sterilization through nonconsensual vasectomy, and rising fatalities, Sorok was visualized in mass media as a paradise and utopia (*nakwon* and *byeolcheonji*). It seems unimaginable to include images of disease in travel magazines promoting trips to Korea, but

45. Eunjung Kim, *Curative Violence: Rehabilitating Disability, Gender, and Sexuality in Modern Korea* (Durham, NC: Duke University Press, 2017), 170–72. Kim also points out that American medical missionaries' arrival in Korea before Japanese colonization was enabled by Western imperialism.
46. Kim, *Curative Violence*, 172–74.
47. Gijae Seo, "Hansenbyeongeul dulleossan jeguguihagui geundaesa: Ilboneo midieoreul tonghae bon daejunggwanri jeollyak," *Uisahak* 26, no. 3 (2017): 417–54.
48. Eiji Takio, ed., *Shinbun kiji ni miru Hansenbyō 1*, vol. 4, 8 vols., Shokuminchika Chōsen ni okeru Hansenbyō shiryō shūsei (Tokyo: Fuji Shuppan, 2002); Eiji Takio, ed., *Shinbun kiji ni miru Hansenbyō 2*, vol. 5, 8 vols., Shokuminchika Chōsen ni okeru Hansenbyō shiryō shūsei (Tokyo: Fuji Shuppan, 2002); Seo, "Hansenbyeongeul dulleossan jeguguihagui geundaesa," 432. Seo bases his research of the colonial media on Eiji Takio's compilation of newspaper articles on leprosy in Japan and Korea during the colonial period.
49. Jae-Hyung Kim, "Singminjigi Hansenbyeong hwanjareul dulleossan jugeumgwa saengjon," *Uisahak* 28, no. 2 (2019): 480–90.
50. Kim, 498–99.

Sorok was promoted as a destination for Japanese tourists as a part of the southern islands trips.[51] *Kankō Chōsen* (Tour Joseon), published by a Korean branch of the Japan Tourist Bureau from 1939 to 1944, ran several articles about the island, devoting its 1942 May issue to the "leprosy paradise." Changing its name to *Bunka Chōsen* (Culture Joseon) in December 1940, the bimonthly magazine was distributed at department stores and train stations in Korea and Japan.[52] The coverage of Sorok as paradise in mass media went along with the colonial ruler's endeavor to advertise its disease control as successful. Sorok as a tourist spot was visualized as a beautiful island with beaches, where visitors could enjoy sea bathing without any contact with leprosy patients, whose living quarters are located on the other side of the island.

Media coverage of Sorok as a utopia began in the early 1930s, when Masasue Suwa (1885–1942), a Japanese physician, was appointed fourth director of Sorok Island Leprosy Hospital in 1933. Suwa immediately embarked on an expansion project to make the sanitarium the world's largest leprosy treatment facility, drafting the patients to perform forced labor in a brickyard. He became the inaugural director of the new Sorok Island Sanatorium. When the sanatorium was completed in 1939, a series of picture postcards were made to show a serene landscape absent human presence. A set of ten postcards were enclosed in an envelope, the inside of which was printed with information on transportation and the sanatorium. The postcards may have been produced to commemorate the completion of the sanatorium, providing photographic images of newly built residences for patients and a Shinto shrine. Marketed to outsiders, the postcards served as propaganda for the government's purportedly successful control of the disease. Yasutoshi Mizuguchi (1915–1949) was appointed as a doctor at the sanatorium in 1941, immediately after obtaining a medical degree from Keijō Imperial University.[53] Two years later, he was transferred to a camp for Allied prisoners of war in Incheon. After the war, he was sentenced to death by hanging for his mistreatment of prisoners in his charge.[54] Mizuguchi reminisced about his time on Sorok during his term at Sugamo prison, particularly after receiving the picture postcards of the sanatorium from a nurse

51. "Bandoui mulsangwa munhwa, sipsamdo gakdoreul jeonmanghamyeo," *Samcheolli*, May 1940; "Sorokutō tanbōki: Chōsen'no *Kojima No Haru*," *Modan Nippon Chōsenhan*, 1940; Modan Nihonsha, *Ilbonjapji modeonilbongwa Joseon 1940*, trans. Seunyoung Hong et al. (Seoul: Eomunhaksa, 2009), 189–95.
52. Gijae Seo, *Joseon yeohaenge tteodoneun jeguk* (Seoul: Somyeong chulpan, 2011), 295–334.
53. "Sotsugyōsei: Keijōteikokudaigaku," *Chōsensōtokufu kanpō*, April 5, 1941; Chōsensōtokufu, ed., *Chōsensōtokufu oyobi shozokukansho shokuinroku* (Keijō: Chōsensōtokufu, 1941), 155.
54. Sarah Kovner, "Allied POWs in Korea: Life and Death during the Pacific War," in *The Dismantling of Japan's Empire in East Asia: Deimperialization, Postwar Legitimation and Imperial Afterlife*, ed. Barak Kushner and Sherzod Muminov (London: Routledge, 2018), 116–20; Eiji Takio, *Chōsen Hansenbyōshi: Nihon shokuminchika no Sorokuto* (Tokyo: Miraisha, 2001), 278–84.

he had worked with.[55] For Mizuguchi, the memory of the island was full of good moments, such as fishing and playing baseball games, but he did not write about Korean leprosy sufferers and staff in the memoir. As in the picture postcards, the doctor's memories of the colony focus only on joyful moments. The production and circulation of Sorok's picture postcards reveal the ways in which the Japanese colonial power contextualized the leprosy island as its imperial achievement, while colonial officials romanticized their experience with the sanatorium.

When *Kankō Chōsen* ran several photographs of Sorok, it described the island as a realization of *Kojima no haru* (*Spring on the Small Island*), a 1938 bestselling memoir by Masako Ogawa, a Japanese physician.[56] The small island refers to Nagashima, where Aisei-en Sanatorium is located, and Sorok came to be depicted as a Korean version of paradise for lepers. In 1938, twenty-three leprosy sufferers were "repatriated" to Korea from Osaka, allegedly because they had spread the disease by wandering around and stealing from passersby.[57] The Koreans were described as criminals threatening the public health and security of Mainland Japan, where sick colonials were denied status as imperial citizens. While Ogawa reminisced about her endeavor to persuade leprosy sufferers to move to a sanatorium, Korean sufferers were transferred off the mainland to Sorok.

In February 1940, when the 14th Congress of the Japanese Leprosy Association announced that it would hold its meeting on Sorok in September, renowned Korean film director Kichae Park proposed a plan to produce a film on the island.[58] The hygiene department of the Government-General was moved to hear Park's plan, deciding to sponsor its production the next year.[59] However, the film was never realized. Instead, a Japanese film adaptation of Ogawa's memoir became a megahit when it was released in the summer, its propagandistic message corroborating the public's embrace of sanatoria as the ideal solution to leprosy.[60] Kathryn M. Tanaka's argument in this volume (Chapter 2) regarding the provocative nuances conveyed through the inclusion of tanka (short Japanese poem) in the film did not resonate with the Korean audience, who were not familiar with the genre, much less the

55. Yasutoshi Mizuguchi, *Sugamo senpan kōshukei: Aru senpan no gokuchū shuki*, ed. Fuyuko Kamisaka (Kyoto: Mineruva Shobō, 1981), 86.
56. "Sorokutō no haru," *Kankō chōsen*, March 1940.
57. "Nabyeonghwanjareul daepanseo songhwan," *Maeil sinbo*, June 28, 1938.
58. "Yakjin Joseonyeonghwagye munhwayeonghwajejak chaksu," *Chosun ilbo*, February 20, 1940. Around the same time, Japan passed the National Eugenics Law that required compulsory sterilization of those infected with hereditary diseases such as leprosy and mental illness. The law was not enforced in Korea, but leprosy patients were subject to vasectomy on Sorok Island.
59. "Sorokdo yeonghwahwae chongdokbu wonjo," *Maeil sinbo*, January 10, 1941.
60. Susan L. Burns, *Kingdom of the Sick: A History of Leprosy and Japan* (Honolulu, HI: University of Hawai'i Press, 2019), 224–25.

literary works of the Japanese leprosy patients. The colonial government mobilized the film to link its effort of the Korean leprosy control to the one of Mainland Japan.

Yong-Kyu Yoon, who played a crucial role in the post-liberation film scenes of North and South Koreas, served as assistant director.[61] The film was also released in Korea in September 1940,[62] with its didactic message providing knowledge on leprosy through the female protagonist's presentation and microscopic images of leprosy bacillus. The female physician travels around to persuade leprosy sufferers to move to the sanatorium in Nagashima, where she treats patients. Unlike other hygiene films that dramatized death of the infected so that the public would attend to their personal hygiene, this film promoted the government's successful control of the disease by isolating the patients.

Photography also plays an important role in the film. The colonial power recognized how efficient photography and film could be in mythologizing its self-acclaimed achievements through foregrounding the media's truth value. The female physician takes pictures of a girl whose father lives in a sanatorium and worries about his daughter's well-being, but notably, she does not bring pictures of the father to his daughter. In another scene, the personal photography album of a young woman infected with leprosy stops at the page where she enjoys school life before infection. In the original memoir, photographs show the landscape instead of leprosy patients in the sanatorium on Nagashima.[63] In both the film and the memoir, the audience will find no images of lepers' deformities: the film's director replaces the faces of lepers with landscape images when the physician engages in conversation with them, while one patient is identified only by his wearing sunglasses rather than by revealing his deformed body parts.[64] When patients of Nagashima sanatorium had a chance to watch the film, they expressed their disappointment that the film failed to represent them.[65]

The colonial government also reinforced its mode of representing the disease in the yearbooks of Sorok sanatorium, which contain no images of afflicted individuals.

61. Taewoo Lee, "Joseonyeonghwaui baljeon," *Kyunghyang sinmun*, January 6, 1949. Lee notes that Yoon was an apprentice to the director Shirō Toyoda. In the film, Haruyama Jun (Yoon's Japanese pseudonym) appears in the credits as an assistant director.

62. Ryeo-Sil Kim, *Tusahaneun jeguk tuyeonghaneun singminji: 1901–1945nyeonui hanguk yeonghwasarul doejibda* (Seoul: Samin, 2006), 317. Toyoda directed *Portrait of Youth* (*Wakaki Sugata*) in 1943, which was produced by Joseon Film Production Company to promote the conscription of Korean men to the war.

63. Tae-Woong Kang, "Jeonjeon ilbonui Hansenbyeong hwanja gyeongnijeongchaekgwa gukchaegyeonghwa jageun seomui bom," *Ilbonyeoksayeongu* 54 (2021): 191–92.

64. Kang, "Jeonjeon ilbonui Hansenbyeong hwanja gyeongnijeongchaekgwa gukchaegyeonghwa jageun seomui bom," 192–95. Kathryn M. Tanaka points out the gender and class divide in the film's visualization of leprosy sufferers in her contribution to this volume (Chapter 2).

65. Kang, "Jeonjeon ilbonui Hansenbyeong hwanja gyeongnijeongchaekgwa gukchaegyeonghwa jageun seomui bom," 205–7.

Most photographs are panoramic views of the island and images of the sanatorium. The patients are always shown in groups from a distance, their individual names never noted. The yearbook does not provide information about who took pictures. Thus, photography does not reproduce the reality of the sanatorium; it produces what the state wanted to be visualized and foregrounded. Photographs conceal rather than reveal what the government does to leprosy sufferers. What one sees in these images are the ways in which the state intervenes in the lives of the sick. The photographs of the Shinto shrine and the leprosy patients lining up to hear the director's speech suggest that the sick persons are enjoying a normal life as imperial citizens and residents of the sanatorium.

Popular media incorporated the state's mode of representing persons afflicted with leprosy. The cover image of the 1942 special issue of *Bunka Chōsen* is a photograph of a nurse, rather than one of the patients, who looks up to the sky and receives sunshine as if her duty is divinely given (Figure 1.6). Her pose reminds one of the Japanese physician in the film *Spring on the Small Island*, where the protagonist often appears with her face angled up to the sky in full sunlight. The audience was familiar with the pose, as it was often appropriated in films and popular magazines to spotlight the protagonist or the main model. Leprosy sanatoria, both in Japan and its colony, were represented by female medical staff as symbols of beneficence.

Enshrining and bowing to imperial portrait photographs was an important part of structuring imperial citizenship. The Japanese Empress Dowager (1884–1951) was a major benefactor of leprosy relief. A monument was erected, inscribed with a poem composed by the empress, to celebrate the completion of the Sorok sanatorium expansion in 1939,[66] and the Sorok yearbook often reproduced photographs of the empress's gifts. An imperial portrait shrine housing a photograph of the empress dowager was built on the island in 1941, as she distributed her photograph to all public leprosy sanatoria.[67] Thus, leprosy patients on Sorok were obliged to follow the state protocol of showing respect to the imperial family, while they were denied the right to live freely in that empire.

By the time *Bunka Chōsen* devoted its May 1942 issue to the Sorok Island sanatorium, the complaints of the patients had reached their peak. Suwa's bronze statue was falsely promoted as a plea by patients and paid for by their forced donations, the same patients whose labor had been exploited to build the sanatorium since 1933.[68] The death rate began to increase from the late 1930s, reaching 432 deaths in 1941, while 41 patients fled the island. In contrast to state images of the island, life in the

66. Takio, *Chōsen Hansenbyōshi*, 213–25.

67. "Kōtaigōhēka gokinei gokashi kaku kokuryū rairyōyōjohe," *Chōsen shinbun*, July 17, 1941.

68. Keun-Sik Jung, "Ilje malgiui Sorokdogaengsaengwongwa Ichunsang sageon," *Yeoksabipyeong*, no. 72 (2005): 336–37.

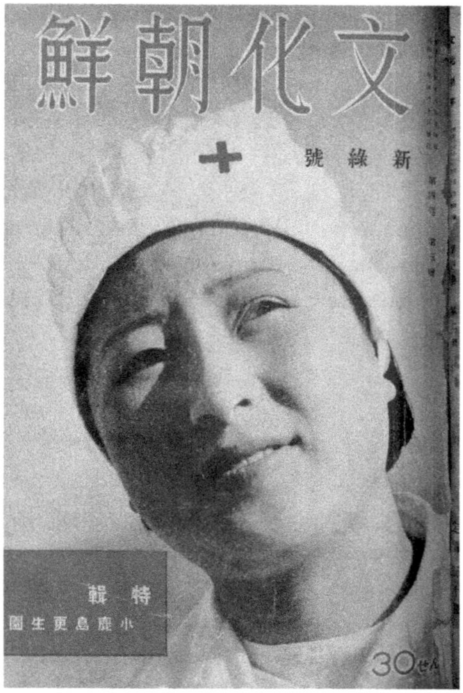

Figure 1.6: Cover of *Bunka Chōsen*, May 1942.

sanatorium was dystopic, with forced labor and decreasing financial support from the government due to the war effort.[69] There were two murders in 1941 and 1942: one involving a leprosy patient killing a patient representative who forcibly collected "donations" for Suwa's statue.[70] The other murder was perpetrated by a patient who stabbed Suwa in front of his statue.[71] *Bunka Chōsen*'s special issue, published around a month before Suwa's death, included an article praising his achievements.[72]

Death is never visualized in representations of Sorok, though newspaper articles often covered suicides and homicides of leprosy sufferers and their relatives in the 1920s and 1930s.[73] Death on the island was noted only as numbers in the sanatorium's yearbooks. Nor for that matter can one find a tomb on Sorok, a notable exception to the familiar reminder of the presence of the dead found in every Korean

69. Jung, "Ilje malgiui Sorokdogaengsaengwongwa Ichunsang sageon," 337–40.
70. Jung, "Ilje malgiui Sorokdogaengsaengwongwa Ichunsang sageon," 340–42.
71. Takio, *Chōsen Hansenbyōshi*, 266–77; Jung, "Ilje malgiui Sorokdogaengsaengwongwa Ichunsang sageon."
72. Kaji Hajime, "Suō Masasue enchō wo kataru," *Bunka chōsen*, May 1942.
73. Kim, "Singminjigi Hansenbyeong hwanjareul dulleossan jugeumgwa saengjon," 472–79.

community. Burial was not allowed for leprosy patients: their bodies were autopsied and cremated, and their bones were interred in a charnel house built in 1937.[74] Practicing sterilization and cremation, the sanatorium was a place of eternal death, where leprosy sufferers did not have descendants to commemorate them yet were not allowed to leave the island even after death, much less to be remembered. While the bodies of living cholera patients were under state ownership, leprosy patients' lives and afterlives were entirely governed by the colonial government. One could still commemorate those who died of cholera within his or her family, but those who died as leprosy patients were not to be memorialized either on or outside of the island.

Conclusion

Hansen's disease sufferers are said to die three times: first, social death through isolation when they contract the disease; then, when their body is dissected after death; and finally, when their body is cremated. These leprosy sufferers wished to die on a Sunday, the only day when there would be no autopsy.[75] The colonial institutionalization of these "multiple deaths" continued during postcolonial Korea until the 1990s, while the Institute for Leprosy Research was established in 1976 with the donation of Ryōichi Sasakawa, a war criminal who later established the Nippon Foundation.[76] The Korean military dictator Park Chung-hee, seeking amicable relations with Japan and Sasakawa's support of Korean leprosy research, promoted the policy as a component of anti-communism.[77] Thus, Cold War politics institutionalized the disease, inheriting the colonial mode of controlling the sick. However, there were films protesting the government's unjust treatment of leprosy patients in the 1970s, unlike those hygiene films produced during the Japanese colonial period. *Ingandanji* (*Strong Will of Cut Fingers*), directed by Won-se Lee, offers a poignant portrayal of leprosy patients' struggle for autonomy and representation in the face of marginali-

74. Sorokutōkōseien, ed., *Sorokutōkōseien nenpō* (Sorokutō: Sorokutōkōseien, 1937), 39. The report on building the charnel house notes that the bones of 249 among 559 dead patients since 1916 were placed in the newly built charnel house. These 249 dead were those whose bones were not collected, but the report does not specify whether the others' remains were taken off the island or kept by bereaved fellow leprosy sufferers. A joint memorial service was held during the opening of the charnel house, but there may have been no funerals for individual deaths.
75. "Apeun 100nyeonui yeoksa donghaenghaneun Sorokdo," National Sorokdo Hosptial Museum of Hansen's Disease, accessed October 21, 2021, http://www.sorokdo.go.kr/museum/html/content.do?menu_cd=05_04&depth=mi.
76. "Hangungnabyeongyeonguwon jungongsik," *Donga ilbo*, September 25, 1976; Franziska Seraphim, "Spaces of Punishment," in *The Tokyo Tribunal: Perspectives on Law, History and Memory*, ed. Viviane E. Dittrich et al. (Brussels: Torkel Opsahl Academic EPublisher, 2020), 369–70.
77. "Jeong-jaegyeui sillyeokja . . . 'Burussiseojulsu itgireul'," *Chosun ilbo*, September 25, 1976.

zation and manipulation. While the film succeeds in highlighting the indomitable spirit of its characters, it ultimately fails to significantly impact the discourse surrounding leprosy institutions with poor audience figures. Throughout the 1970s, newspaper articles predominantly portrayed leprosy patients and Sorok Island in the context of Young-soo Yuk's compassionate role as the First Lady, casting her as a wise and motherly figure intent on reshaping the perception of her husband's stern governance.

Beginning in the early 2000s, leprosy patients and their families began to seek compensation from the Korean and Japanese governments.[78] The postcolonial Korean government was never willing to discontinue the colonial legacy of stigmatizing Hansen's disease sufferers but found it effective to inherit the colonial mode of disease control through inciting fear and hatred toward the marginalized. The endeavor to decolonize the social structure of postcolonial Korea was often criticized as the Communist engagement throughout the 1960s and 1970s, as those who worked for the Japanese colonial power continued to serve as public officials of the newly established Korean government after the liberation. More importantly, the colonial habits of mind that racialized and genderized disease under the Japanese rule tenaciously sustained the postcolonial Korean society's vision of healthy and powerful nation-state during the Cold War era. The COVID-19 breakout summoned the specter of colonial rule when the media presented the disease as originating from China, and the LGBTQ community was targeted as the spreader of the disease in its early stages.

78. Jeff Kingston, "Compensating Colonial Lepers, Slave Laborers and Hibakusha: Troubling Legacies and Evolving Standards of Postcolonial Justice in Japan," *The Asia-Pacific Journal: Japan Focus* 3, no. 11 (2005), https://apjjf.org/-Jeff-Kingston/1579/article.html.

2

Ink on the Silver Screen

Medical Culture and Poetic Voices in *Spring on the Small Island*

Kathryn M. Tanaka

In October 1940, a film from the Tokyo Hassei Company directed by Toyoda Shirō (1906–1977), *Spring on the Small Island* (*Kojima no haru*) screened at Nagashima Aisei-en, the first national sanatorium for the treatment of Hansen's disease.[1] The film, distributed by Tōhō Cinema, was based on a 1938 best-selling travel diary or memoir of the same name by Aisei-en doctor Ogawa Masako (1902–1943).[2] The book, which described her travels around the Inland Sea to diagnose sufferers of Hansen's disease and raise awareness about the illness, became a bestseller.[3] It went from an initial print of 500 to a run of 30,000 copies.[4] In the wake of this phenomenon, Ogawa's life and work were taken up, and often celebrated, in media across the archipelago.[5] This media attention was due in part to both contemporaneous public health campaigns across the Japanese Empire targeting Hansen's disease and legislation aimed at controlling people diagnosed with Hansen's disease. Indeed, by the late 1930s, when the book was written, Hansen's disease was a global concern, with

1. The research for this chapter was conducted with the support of Grant-in-Aid for Early-Career Scientists 20K12936. Matsuoka Hiroyuki, *Hansen-byō ryōyōjo to jichi no rekishi* (Tokyo: Misuzu shobō, 2020), 352. Hansen's disease is the preferred nomenclature for the illness more pejoratively known as leprosy. In this chapter, I use the term Hansen's disease in my own writing, and use terms derivative of *leprosy* when translating materials that also used the more discriminatory Japanese term *rai* (癩).
2. Ogawa Masako, *Kojima no haru—Hansen-byō chiryō ni, shōgai wo sasageta aru joi no shuki* (Tokyo: Nagasaki shuppan, 2009).
3. This paper differentiates people with Hansen's disease undergoing treatment by using the term *patients*. For those living at home and treating their condition themselves, I use the term *sufferer*.
4. Matsuoka, *Hansen-byō ryōyōjo to jichi no rekishi*, 333.
5. For more on Ogawa Masako's book and its celebration in media, see Kathryn M. Tanaka, "For the Purity of the Nation: Ogawa Masako and the Gendered Ethics of *Spring on the Small Island* (*Kojima no haru*)," *U.S.-Japan Women's Journal, no* 50 (2016): 93–114.

the disease often serving as a locus to negotiate colonial power and racial or ethnic tensions.[6] The treatment of the disease and popular response to it was imbricated in imperial health systems, and *Spring on the Small Island* and its popularity was a reflection of these global tensions.[7]

Yet, even within global contexts the film was unique not only in its treatment of Hansen's disease, but also in what many have described as its "humanistic" elements in the face of cinema and media projects becoming increasingly propagandistic and militaristic as the Japanese empire continued its aggressive expansion.[8] When the film was first released in July 1940, the media attention on Ogawa and her work reached fever pitch, with many in popular media celebrating Ogawa as a heroine devoted to her work of saving people suffering from Hansen's disease by encouraging institutionalization at Nagashima Aisei-en.

Prior to the release of the film, Hansen's disease had become an increasingly frequent topic in the media as a threat to public health that needed government intervention. Its sufferers faced discrimination because of the illness' debilitating physical effects and its incurability prior to the 1941 discovery that the drug Promin could cure the condition. Thus, in the first half of the twentieth century, Hansen's disease in Japan was targeted by a series of laws designed to provide palliative care for those diagnosed with the illness. In 1907, the "Law Concerning the Prevention of Leprosy" was passed. This legislation established five regional public hospitals designed to receive itinerant patients, such as those who begged for alms at temples or shrines.[9] The hospitals established under this law began accepting patients in 1909.

---

6. There is a growing body of work about the intersections of Hansen's disease and colonial projects, beginning with Rod Edmund, *Leprosy and Empire: A Medical and Culural History* (Cambridge: Cambridge University Press, 2006). See also, for example, Michele T. Moran, *Colonizing Leprosy Imperialism and the Politics of Public Health in the United States* (Chapel Hill, NC: The University of North Carolina Press, 2012) and Stephen Snelders, *Leprosy and Colonialims: Suriname under Dutch rule 1750–1950* (Manchester: Manchester University Press, 2017).
7. Jeehey Kim studies the film's reception in colonial Korea in Chapter 1 of this volume: "Contagious Disease and Visual Media in Colonial Korea."
8. The idea of *Kojima no haru* as a humanist film is prominent in both Japanese and English-language scholarship; Joseph L. Anderson and Donald Richie wrote the film was "a cry for humanism in an age marching toward militarism" in their *The Japanese Film: Art and Industry* (Princeton, NJ: Princeton University Press, 1982), 141.
9. Both Hirokawa Waka and Susan Burns have explored the ways in which Hansen's disease policies were created and contested. See Hirokawa Waka, *Kindai Nihon no Hansen-byō mondai to chiiki shakai* (Osaka: Osaka daigaku shuppankai, 2011) and "A Colony or a Sanatorium? A Comparative History of Segregation Politics of Hansen's Disease in Modern Japan," in *Science, Technology, and Medicine in the Modern Japanese Empire*, ed. David G. Wittner and Philip C. Brown (London: Routledge, 2016), 117–29 and Susan Burns, *Kingdom of the Sick: A History of Leprosy and Japan* (Honolulu, HI: University of Hawai'i Press, 2019).

By 1930, Mitsuda Kensuke (1876–1964), Japan's most prominent leprologist and an influential doctor often credited with pioneering the government's treatment policies, had successfully lobbied the government to open a national sanatorium on an island in the Inland Sea. When Aisei-en opened on the island of Nagashima, Mitsuda was appointed the first director. He was the official who hired Ogawa in 1934 to work at the institution. It was he who sent Ogawa on her travels into Japan's rural areas to both raise awareness about Hansen's disease, and to encourage sufferers there to seek treatment at Aisei-en. Her diary recording these travels became the book *Spring on the Small Island,* which was then adapted into the 1940 film.

Hagiographic descriptions of Ogawa and her work exploded across popular media in the wake of the book and the movie, accelerated by the fact that in 1937 Ogawa had contracted tuberculosis and subsequently resigned her position at Aisei-en. Popular media consistently depicted her as a heroine who sacrificed herself to serve national health interests. This celebration of her life and work became grounds for criticism by later scholars; historians such as Fujino Yutaka, Arai Eiko, Narita Ryūichi and others treat her work as propaganda in service of Hansen's disease relief work that contributed to increasing stigma and accelerating "total quarantine" and the "Leprosy-Free Prefecture movement," a public campaign wherein Japan's prefectures competed to see which could achieve zero patients outside the sanatorium.[10] In short, contemporary scholarship has often treated the book and the film as complicit in continued violations of human rights of survivors of Hansen's disease. Much contemporary scholarship treats the history of Hansen's disease as one of patient struggle to regain their human rights in the face of an oppressive government that continued to deny them, even after the discovery of a cure. And while more recent scholarship, such as Hirokawa Waka, Matsuoka Hiroyuki, and Susan Burns have complicated this binary view, Ogawa's work and the film it inspired is still often treated as a tool of oppressive government policies.[11]

This chapter builds on Matsuoka Hiroyuki's more recent reexamination of Ogawa's book, film, and her own responses to her depiction in media and her deployment in Hansen's disease relief work propaganda. In contrast to earlier scholars, Matsuoka demonstrates that while Ogawa remained committed to quarantine as the most appropriate measure to eliminate Hansen's disease from Japan, her

10. Fujino Yutaka, *"Inochi" no gendai shi* (Tokyo: Kamogawa shuppan, 2001); Arai Eiko, *Hansen-byō to kirisuto-kyō* (Tokyo: Iwanami shoten, 1996); Narita Ryūichi, "*Kojima no haru* no manazashi," in *Nihon kindai shisō taikei 22: sabetsu no shosō furoku, Geppō* 15, vol. 22, ed. Katō Shūichi (Tokyo: Iwanami shoten, 1990), 4–7; *"Rekishi" wa ika ni katarareruka: 1930 nendai "kokumin no monogatari" hihan* (Tokyo: Nihon hōsō shuppan kyokai, 2001). See also Arai Yuki, *Kakuri no bungaku: Hansen-byō ryōyōsho no jiko hyōgen-shi* (Tokyo: Shoshi arusu, 2011).

11. Hirokawa, *Kindai Nihon no Hansen-byō mondai to chiiki shakai*; Matsuoka, *Hansen-byō ryōyōjo to jichi no rekishi*; and Burns, *Kingdom of the Sick*.

letters reveal her ambivalence—and indeed, displeasure—with the sensationalized version of her life and propagandistic uses of her work that appeared in newspapers and magazines.[12] Building on this, I argue that rather than being a simple film that promoted policies of Hansen's disease relief work, Toyoda's film in fact includes subtle ambiguities in the treatment of patients based on both social class and gender through its visual depictions of sufferers.

Second, this chapter demonstrates the importance of the tanka that appear onscreen in the film as both cinematic innovation and vehicles of patient experience.[13] While previous scholarship has attributed the poems in the film to Ogawa or the famous poet Akashi Kaijin (1901–1939), the poems included as text superimposed over montage come from at least three authors, two of whom were sufferers of Hansen's disease residing at Nagashima Aisei-en. Furthermore, the tanka and the stories of the sufferers featured in the film come not just from the travelogue *Spring on the Small Island,* but from at least five different literary sources and two patient authors. I argue the inclusion of patient voices and the centering of locality through poetry further serve to complicate understandings of this film as simple propaganda. Seen as a literary adaptation that includes multiple voices and evokes mixed responses from critics and sufferers, *Spring on the Small Island* becomes a much richer cinematic text.

In the consideration of multiple voices in cinema, it is useful to consider the work of Russian philosopher Mikhail Bakhtin, in particular his concept of heteroglossia. While Bakhtin developed this idea out of literary discourse in his *Discourse in the Novel,* the concept of heteroglossia is also useful in a consideration of the film *Spring on the Small Island.* For Bakhtin, heteroglossia referred to "a diversity of social speech types . . . and a diversity of individual voices" intersecting in a multiplicity of languages, speech genres, and ideological discourses, as well as the dialogic nature of their use.[14] Each of these different "languages" represents "specific world views, each characterized with its own objects, meanings, and values" that may "be juxtaposed to one another, mutually supplement one another, contradict one another and be interrelated dialogically."[15] Thus, heteroglossia inherently reflects resistance against a hegemonic urge to impose a single interpretation on any intersection of "languages" or voices.

A consideration of heteroglossia is particularly useful in the case of this film, both in understanding how a dominant interpretation has shaped our understanding

12. Matsuoka, *Hansen-byō ryōyōjo to jichi no rekishi,* 333–66.
13. Tanka is a style of Japanese poetry that follows a syllabic pattern of 5-7-5-7-7 mora per line, for a total of 31 mora. The short length of the poem allows it to be easily written in a small space.
14. M. M. Bakhtin, *The Dialogic Imagination,* ed. *Michael Holquist.* trans. Caryl Emerson and Michael Holquist (Austin, TX: University of Texas, 1981), 262–63.
15. Bakhtin, *The Dialogic Imagination,* 292.

of it, and how other voices are included within it. For film critic Robert Stam, attention to heteroglossia in film and television allows viewers to "bring out the text's muffled voices" rather than accepting a mass interpretation, which is precisely what this chapter accomplishes.[16] Heteroglossia, for Stam, introduces a "social semiotic of the cinema" and allows attention to "the coincidences and competitions of languages and discourses."[17] This chapter highlights the fact that the treatment of sufferers and the inclusion of the poems by patients are part of the heteroglossia of the film. Attention to them identifies the ways in which Toyoda draws on extant poetic film techniques to create a piece meant to provoke thought in his viewers, rather than inspire blind agreement with government policies.

Spring on the Small Island: Hansen's Disease Relief Work and the Establishment of Dominant Narratives

Spring on the Small Island as a film is a realistic adaptation of several episodes from Ogawa Masako's memoirs, with considerable embellishment and textual additions from other sources. Despite this, the film has been treated primarily as a faithful cinematic adaptation of Ogawa's text, and dominant understandings of the film based on this assumption have emerged. At the same time, there were a variety of responses to the film when it was first released. This section explores the reception of the film and identifies two dominant interpretations: those who hail the film as a humanistic melodrama, and those who treat it as a tool in the fight for Hansen's disease relief work. These two interpretations continue to frame most criticism of the film today. Complicating this binary were multiple and varied interpretations of the film that postwar criticism frequently overlooks. In particular, despite being renowned for his literary adaptations of authors such as Mori Ōgai (1882–1916), Kawabata Yasunari (1899–1972), and Tanizaki Jun'ichirō (1886–1965), Toyoda Shirō's work in *Spring on the Small Island* has rarely been listed among his literary adaptations, but the use of literary source materials in this film cannot be overlooked.[18]

The film *Spring on the Small Island* highlights the episodic structure of the original text. It follows the travels of Dr. Koyama Masako (played by Natsukawa Shizue, 1909–1999), from the first national sanatorium for Hansen's disease, Nagashima Aisei-en, and includes four main families she visits: the Yokogawa family, the Miyata family, a woman in a peach orchard, and the Horiguchi family. In doing so, the film

16. Robert Stam, *Subversive Pleasures: Bakhtin, Cultural Criticism, and Film* (Baltimore, MD: The Johns Hopkins University Press, 1989), 221.
17. Stam, *Subversive Pleasures*, 50.
18. Kyoko Hirano, "A Case Study of Japanese Film Exhibition in North America: The Japan Society, New York," in *Routledge Handbook of Japanese Cinema*, ed. Joanne Bernardi and Shota T. Ogawa (London: Routledge, 2019), 318.

underscores the way in which treatment of Hansen's disease was impacted by gender and class through the way in which the body of the sufferer is depicted in the film. In particular, the reticence of the camera to show the faces of women suffering from Hansen's disease, while showcasing the faces and bodies of male sufferers struggling with poverty, reflects gendered or class-based experiences of Hansen's disease.

Recent scholarship has sought to complicate narratives about *Spring on the Small Island* through attention to the era in which it was produced, such as film critic Fujii Jinshi's attention to the way the film depicts roles of women and children as Japan mobilized during World War II. Yet recent criticism still relies heavily on the idea that the film was essentially on some level a propagandistic piece, be it for Hansen's disease relief work or the contributions of women to the Japanese empire.

Indeed, modern critiques of the film draw on its initial reception in the media. Medical professionals reviewed the film at the time it came out, and in general their responses outlined what became dominant understandings of the film: they viewed it in general as both propaganda for Hansen's disease relief work on one hand, and an artistic, humanist narrative on the other. For example, an anonymous review published in *Chiryō Kusurihō* stated that the "adaptation was made to appeal to the public during wartime," a "humanistic" narrative.[19]

Despite the film's humanist impulses, for many doctors it was still useful as publicity for Hansen's disease relief work. Shikiba Ryūzaburō (1898–1965), a psychologist who specialized in art and frequently published comments on patient writing, perhaps summed up the feelings of many medical professionals when he argued that *Spring on the Small Island* fell short as a "medical film" (*igaku eiga*) or a "prevention film" (*yobō eiga*) because of its sentimentalism. But despite this, many argued that it was still useful for prevention work: "Rather than films that are blatant prevention films or advertisements for leprosy relief work, this type of thing is much more effective. Although lacking in direct action and weak in its depiction of leprosy medicine, the public will realize what is behind that theme. Thus, indirectly, it must be useful as a preventive medical film."[20]

Perhaps more strongly than other medical professionals, Mitsuda Kensuke also argued for the value of the film as a promotional tool, pointing specifically to the efficacy in the realism of the scenes where Dr. Koyama examines sufferers, as well as the scene where the doctor hosts an informational lecture for village heads. Mitsuda writes that these things mean that: "This is more effective as a film promoting leprosy relief work than hundreds or thousands of lectures would be."[21] Mitsuda's cooperation was essential in giving the crew access to film on location at Nagashima

19. "Eiga *Kojima no haru*," *Chiryō Kusurihō* 485 (1940): 19.
20. Shikiba Ryūzaburō, "Igakuteki ni mita *Kojima no haru*," *Nihon eiga* 5, no. 9 (1940): 38.
21. Mitsuda Kensuke, "*Kojima no haru* no kansō," *Nihon iji shinpō* 935 (1940): 59.

Aisei-en. In his writing and his cooperation with the production, it is clear that Mitsuda intended the film to be part of Hansen's disease relief work (Figure 2.1).[22]

That *Spring on the Small Island* was effective in publicity for Hansen's disease relief work and was in fact actively used by the institution to promote its activities is clear from the archives. Records in Nagashima's archives show that the institution received a copy of the film, which they then lent out to be shown as part of Hansen's disease relief work. One letter that accompanied the return of the films from Tottori prefecture notes that both *Spring on the Small Island* and *The Story of Bacteria* (*Saikin Monogatari*, 1950) were borrowed from the entertainment offices at Aisei to show for "Leprosy Relief Day," referring to both as "educational publicity films" (*keimō senden eiga*).[23]

Mitsuda was likely aware of the potential of *Spring on the Small Island* to be a film that promoted Hansen's disease relief work even before the production. After

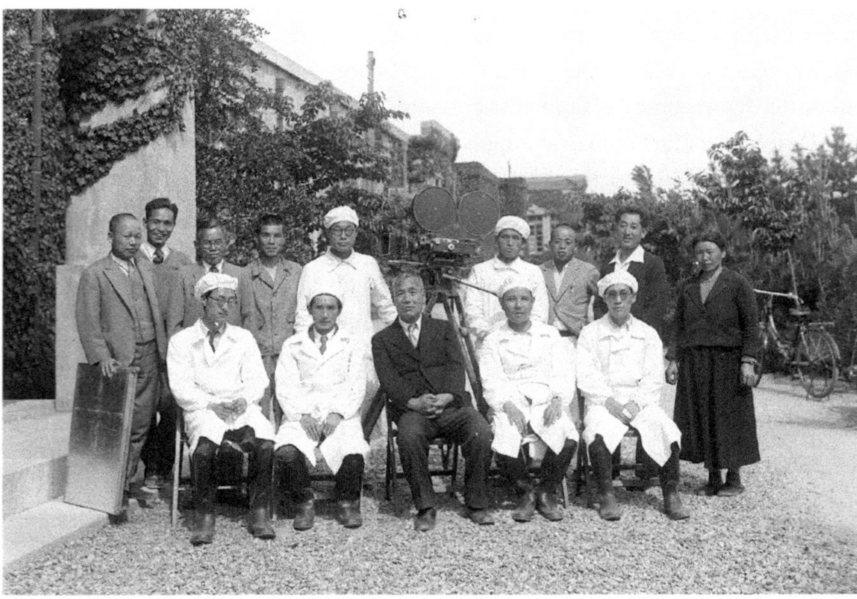

Figure 2.1: Film crew and Aisei-en staff on location at Nagashima Aisei-en. Courtesy of Nagashima Aisei-en Archives.

22. I thank Hiroshi Kinoshita and Tomohisa Tamura, curators and archivists at Nagashima Aisei-en for their assistance in locating this photograph and the other the materials from Nagashima archives mentioned here.
23. "Tottori ken kōshū eisei kacho," Letter to Nagashima Aisei-en Entertainment Committee Chief returning two borrowed films, July 25, 1951. Nagashima Aisei-en Archives. *Iji kankei ippan*, Showa 26–27.

the book was released, readers of the text were motivated to send in donations to the institution. After the film came out, seeing the depiction of the sufferers on-screen promoted more letters and donations from viewers, ranging from one or two yen to as many as 5,000 yen, a considerable amount of money at the time.[24] Many letter writers shared that they had been moved by both the pitiable circumstances of the sufferers and Ogawa's compassion.

In addition to the donations and letters of support, after reading the book or seeing the film, a small number of sufferers actually wrote to the institution, seeking admission. One such sufferer wrote that they had believed the institution to be akin to a prison, but reading the book had changed their mind, and they asked for more information about "patients' lives" in the institution, and the procedure to be admitted.[25] A second letter mentioned that the deep benevolence shown by Ogawa and the country confirmed for the writer that for the sake of their children's future they should seek institutionalization.[26] In addition, at least one person sent a letter to Aisei-en stating that after reading the book they suspected they had Hansen's disease but were unsure and requested advice.[27]

The letters of support, requests for institutionalization and the donations made in the name of Ogawa Masako and *Spring on the Small Island* demonstrate the affective appeal of the book and film that Mitsuda Kensuke likely understood. It is clear that Mitsuda had a purpose in supporting this film and using it in Hansen's disease relief work as he did. It also seems likely that because of Mitsuda's prominence in medicine in Japan, his assessment of the film had weight; it has likely colored the reception and subsequent analysis of the film, creating the dominant narratives around it.

Among the viewers of the film when it was released, however, were two who viewed the film as a tanka film, or poetic film. A doctor who also worked at Aisei-en, the ophthalmologist and poet Uchida Mamoru (pen name Uchida Morito, 1900–1982) offered a different take on the film, describing it as a *tanka eiga*, or tanka film. He writes, "It seems this film is the first tanka film since the film about the poet Takuboku. There are fourteen poems that appear; Ogawa's poems, Akashi Kaijin's poems, and Hayashi Yukiko's poems."[28] Uchida is the only contemporaneous critic

---

24. One yen in 1940 would be roughly equivalent to a little over 1,000 yen in 2019. The letter enclosing a donation of 5,000 yen was acknowledged on May 16, 1943. [Name Redacted]. Letter to Dr. Mitsuda. Nagashima Aisei-en Archives. May 6, 1943.
25. "Nyūengan ni kan suru ken." Letter. Nagashima Aisei Archives. Undated. Likely sent in fall of 1940.
26. "Nyūengan ni kan suru ken." Letter. Nagashima Aisei Archives. September 4, 1940.
27. "Rai yōgisha mishindan ni kan suru ken." Letter. Nagashima Aisei Archives. August 16, 1940.
28. Uchida Morito, "Eiga *Kojima no haru* no zakkan," *Nihon dangi* 3, no. 10 (1940): 50. The film he refers to is Kumagai Hisatora's 1936 film *Takuboku, Poet of Passions* (*Jōnetsu Shijin Takuboku*), now believed to be lost. See Peter B. High, *The Imperial Screen: Japanese Film Culture in the Fifteen Years' War, 1931–1945* (Madison, WI: The University of Wisconsin Press, 2003), 227.

to note the poems were a means of incorporating different voices into the film, a point that is elaborated in the next section. While Uchida is not a film critic, his use of the term *tanka eiga* is interesting in that it reminds us that what is lost in calling *Spring on the Small Island* a sentimental melodrama or a propaganda film is the fact that it was also a literary adaptation, and the inclusion of tanka reminds viewers of that fact.

In addition to Uchida, critic Aoki Bunzō (dates unknown) also argued that the film itself reminded him of a tanka poem in its use of affective imagery.[29] He wrote: "The tendency to critique this film and view it as an interesting example of a leprosy relief culture film (*kyūrai no bunka eiga*) is frightening," because the film was a great deal more literary and artistic than that phrase implied.[30] A *bunka eiga*, or culture film, was defined by the Film Law of 1939 as "films that are specifically useful to the education of the people," or a film that contributed "to the nurturing of the people's knowledge or the cultivation of (their) national spirit."[31] For Aoki, the film was primarily aesthetic, and to treat it as a culture film or documentary offering solutions to Hansen's disease relief work in Japan was misguided.

Finally, after the screening of the film at Aisei-en, a special section of the institutional magazine *Aisei* recorded how residents responded to the work. Of course, this publication was subject to censorship by hospital officials, and the responses selected for inclusion would have been carefully screened. But many of the reflections praise the way in which Natsukawa Shizue excelled in the role of Dr. Koyama Masako and captured Ogawa's empathetic manner perfectly.[32] While most patients who responded in *Aisei* also stated their belief that the film would be a powerful tool to help sufferers, several also expressed a concern that the tragic depiction of sufferers in the film would make life harder for uninstitutionalized sufferers and their relatives, and that it was a difficult film to watch because the memories it recalled were too painful.[33] For patients watching the film in Aisei-en, the story was more personal, and the pain they expressed for themselves and concerns about their families in their responses reflected this.

The responses from film critics, medical professionals, and patients highlight the fact that the discourses and criticisms surrounding the film all sought to impose different interpretations onto it, and from its appearance *Spring on the Small Island* invited debate and defied easy categorization. The complexity of the film is reflected

---

29. Aoki Bunzō, "*Kojima no haru* to tanka no sekai," *Eiga hyōron* 22, no. 9 (1940): 61.
30. Aoki, "*Kojima no haru* to tanka no sekai," 63.
31. Daisuke Miyao, "What's the Use of Culture? Cinematographers and the Culture Film in Japan in the Early 1940s," *Arts* 8, no. 42 (2019): 4–5.
32. For a collection of the reactions of thirteen patients to the film, see "Eiga hihyō—*Kojima no haru* kansō tokushū," *Aisei* 11, no. 3 (1941): 7–17.
33. "Eiga hihyō—*Kojima no haru* kansō tokushū," 7–17.

in the responses to it, and this is erased in contemporary criticisms of the film that continue to reduce it to either propaganda or a humanistic film about women working for medicine during the war. In particular, the importance of poetry in the film, pointed out by Uchida and Aoki, has been largely overlooked.

Poetry, Locality, and Patient Voices on the Screen

This section draws on the points Uchida in particular makes about poetry to demonstrate the way in which poetry allows the film to adapt some patient narratives not included in Ogawa's original text for melodramatic effect. In doing so, Toyoda moves the film away from easy interpretation as a cinematic adaptation of Ogawa's memoir. He adds a layer of fictionality, while at the same time representing the struggle involved as sufferers comply with the health ideologies. Furthermore, I argue that the tanka seeks to complicate the medical gaze that guides the film through the introduction of patient voices and perspectives.

In particular, the tanka is one prominent way the film introduces heteroglossia. This is because in addition to allowing for the inclusion of multiple voices, the poems also introduce a different form of discourse—written in some cases, written and chanted in others—into the film. Second, the use of the poems allows the depiction of at least three voices whose experiences are not always congruous. Ogawa's own tanka and tanka by famed patient poet Akashi Kaijin (1901–1939) are the two most prominent voices in the film. While critics have noted that the film is based on a memoir by Ogawa and includes some poems by Kaijin, apart from the single mention in the article by Uchida, the inclusion of poems by a second patient writer, Hayashi Yukiko (married name, Kitada Yukiko, 1909–1993), went unnoticed and has been completely overlooked in contemporary discussions of the film. This may be because, unlike Kaijin, whose book of tanka poetry *Hakubyō* (Ink *Sketches*, 1939) had been published to acclaim, Hayashi Yukiko's poems and essays only appeared in larger collections of patient writing that did not receive much popular attention.[34]

The way the multiple texts were incorporated into the film likely depended on the collaboration of several men. Toyoda and scenario author Yagi Yasutarō (1903–1987) make several important interventions into the story that further fictionalize Ogawa's original travelogue text. It should not be lost on viewers that Toyoda is known for his literary adaptations, as was the screenwriter Yagi Yasutarō.[35] And it is likely that the two men collaborated on the way to bring poetry to the screen in

34. Akashi Kaijin, *Hakubyō* (Tokyo: Kaizōsha, 1939). Hayashi's work appears in a collection of women's writing. See Hayashi Yukiko, "Tanka," in *Hagi no shimazato*, ed. Uchida Morito (Tokyo: Fujokai, 1939), 61–78; and "Zakuro no nageki," in *Seto no Akebono*, ed. Uchida Morito (Tokyo: Fujokai-sha, 1939), 139–73.

35. Izawa Jun, "Yagi Yasutarō ron," *Shinario* 14, no. 3 (1958): 26–27.

Spring on the Small Island; the cinematographer Ogura Kin'ya made clear the director was involved in how the sequences featuring poetry were shot and superimposed.[36] But there are other important techniques in the way *Spring on the Small Island* is told that gives voice to the costs of the treatment and the unevenness with which it is applied.

There have been several important studies into the use of tanka in *Spring on the Small Island*. Fujii has argued that they are included as a device to distract viewers from the grim reality of Hansen's disease, describing the superimposition of tanka as "an effective step, both dramatically and to avoid instinctive repulsion."[37] To Fujii, the poems are a code that deploy images of cherry or peach blossoms to distract the viewer from the reality of the sufferers. Similarly, in his consideration of the representation of sufferers in the film, Ishii Hironari argues that the poems are "used as a device to evoke sympathy from viewers."[38] Neither develop further arguments about the use of poems in the film.

More recently, Matsuoka Hideaki has examined the use of tanka in the film, arguing that the inclusion of tanka was a device to sanitize the realities of Hansen's disease. For him, tanka allowed filmmakers to make the tragic subject matter more palatable to audiences by creating sympathy between sufferers who were segregated and those who enforced segregation. Viewers are able to sympathize with sufferers of Hansen's disease through "their fascination with the purity of Koyama's actions."[39] Rather than emphasize physical suffering, Matsuoka argues that the film emphasizes how sufferers can be helped through institutionalization. In his analysis, this emphasis is reinforced through tanka that allows for sympathy while ultimately reinforcing the boundary between the sick and relief workers even as they shared a common goal.

Matsuoka further argues tanka was likely used in the film because of the concomitant popularity of a literary genre of writing by patients at the time referred to as *rai bungaku* (leprosy literature).[40] He also points to the heteroglossia of tanka in the text: "The tanka poems that appear in the film were composed by Ogawa (these

36. Tamura Yoshihiko, Tanaka Toshio, Ogura Kin'ya, Ikeda Kazo, Nishimura Masami, and Tomiogi Masao, "*Kojima no haru* no zadankai," *Eiga to gijutsu* 15, no. 8 (1940): 21–22.

37. Fujii Junji, "Kashi to fukashi no poritikusu—eiga *Kojima no haru* to sōryoku taisei-ka ni okeru kattai no hyōshō (4) Metsubo no yūtopia," *UP* 364 (2003): 26. See also Fujii Jinshi, "'Joshi domo' no hanran—*Kojima no Haru* ni okeru sōryokusenka no shintai to sei," in *Eiga to shintai/sei*, ed. Ayako Saitō (Tokyo: Shinwa-sha, 2006), 171–95.

38. Ishii Hitonari, "Hansen-byō byōzō to shite no eiga *Kojima no haru*—1940 nen ni okeru kakuri no egakarekata to sono mirareru kata," in *Kindai Nihon no "tasha" to mukiau*, ed. Kurokawa Midori (Tokyo: Kaihō shuppan sha, 2010), 157.

39. Matsuoka Hideaki, "Hansen-byō to tanka: Eiga *Kojima no haru* wo megutte," *Communication Design* 12 (2015): 49.

40. For more on this genre, see the groundbreaking work Arai, *Kakuri no bungaku*.

appear in several places throughout the film), by the leper Yukiko[41] (appearing in the scene where Dr. Koyama meets Yukiko), and by Akashi Kaijin (appearing and being recited in the scenes that show Nagashima Aisei-en."[42] However, he seems to assume that Yukiko is an entirely fictional character and largely treats the poems by Ogawa, Yukiko and Akashi as having a similar function. Thus, critics have missed an important point: they have attributed all of the poems in the film to Ogawa, Akashi, or a fictional patient. These understandings erase the fact that a young woman named Hayashi Yukiko contributed her poems to the film as well.

Hayashi Yukiko is important to an analysis of *Spring on the Small Island* because, more than her poetry, the film in fact adapted her story, perhaps for the melodramatic effect of a young woman afflicted in the prime of her youth with an incurable illness. At the same time, the inclusion of Hayashi's story as she told it, not as it was told in Ogawa's best-selling diary *Spring on the Small Island,* adds an unmistakable layer of heteroglossia, of intertextuality between several texts: Akashi's *Ink Sketches* (*Hakubyō*), Hayashi's poetry and autobiographical essay, and Ogawa's poetry from *Spring on the Small Island* and the institutionally published magazine at Nagashima Aisei-en that included poetry and sections of patient writing, the journal *Aisei.*[43]

The slip between texts was intentional, as Uchida Mamoru noted in a short essay he published in response to the film. After stating he accompanied Yagi, Toyoda, and Ogura on their trips to the Inland Sea, he added: "I was consulted about a number of aspects related to the film's presentation, and it seemed that a great deal of effort had been put into the medical representation of leprosy, but another major problem was how to present patients in the film without attracting public outcry. Personally, I was thankful to Mr. Yagi for accenting the film with *tanka.*"[44] For Uchida—the only source to confirm that the film uses the voices of three poets—tanka seems to be a way to represent patients in the film: Ogawa, Akashi, and Hayashi. Out of the fourteen poems featured in the film, Ogawa wrote six, as did Akashi, and Hayashi contributed one. I have been unable to identify or confirm the source for two poems, one of which was likely written specifically for the film. The second poem seems from its position in the film and its contents to be inspired or written by Hayashi. In the screenplay, however, a larger selection of poems by Hayashi (seven) and Akashi (sixteen) was included, that did not make the final film. Finally, while scholars

41. He uses 雪子, which are the characters for Horiguchi Yukiko (堀口雪子) in the film. The name of the author of the poems, Hayashi Yukiko (林由貴子), was written 由貴子, although both are read Yukiko.

42. Matsuoka, "Hansen-byō to tanka: Eiga *Kojima no haru* wo megutte," 48.

43. For a transcription and translation of each poem that appears in the film, as well as the author and sources that are identified, see the Appendix.

44. Uchida Morito, "Eiga *Kojima no haru* no zakkan," 50.

assume the poems attributed to Ogawa are taken directly from her travel diary, in fact one poem that opens the film was published by Aisei-en's in-house publication, *Aisei*, and a second may have been written specifically for the movie.

There are also subtle differences between the way the poems by each author are presented. The voices shift as the film progresses; the film opens with two poems by Ogawa, the text superimposed as the camera pans over a sea dotted with islands, as women sing in harmony over orchestral music. Each poem appears for around ten seconds, and the scenery shifts as the text remains unmoving. The next six poems are all written by Ogawa, and each is used as a scene cut. The third poem appears after the screen fades to black after a scene in which Dr. Koyama examines schoolchildren to check their health; it is displayed in silence on a dark background painted with flowers. This is the only poem written by Ogawa that is presented in silence; the others are accompanied by music and shown superimposed either over long, panning, scenic shots or over a dark, flowered background.

In general, the poems written by Ogawa are used to cut scenes and shift the location of the film. They also serve to underscore the dramatic episodes in the film, in that two are about people: the children of a sufferer, and the woman in the peach orchard. Ogawa's poems highlight her movement through references to "the small island," or Nagashima, and the locales in which she travels, but they also foreground her gaze over the scenery as well as over the patients she treats. Ogawa's gaze is clinical, and her words serve as final, cutting scenes as the film fades to black and reopens on a new scene.

Ogawa's voice ends when the patient poetry begins, complicating the narrative as one voice picks up where another one has left off. Ogawa's last poem appears thirty-eight minutes into the film, and Akashi Kaijin's first poem appears at fifty-nine minutes. His poems serve as a frame for Hayashi's narrative, and the poetry written by patients themselves are highlighted in the film in different ways. The poems of both Hayashi and Kaijin are superimposed over montage scenes of people working and moving around Nagashima Aisei-en, rather than the shots of idyllic Seto Inland Sea scenery that was used under Ogawa's poems. This is an immediate and jarring contrast: while Ogawa's poems are associated with scenry and poetic landscapes, then, patient voices are associated with laboratories, and the shots of patients going about their daily lives in the sanatorium.

Akashi Kaijin was a best-selling poet who was institutionalized at Aisei-en and died there in 1939. He is mentioned by name in the film as Dr. Koyama visits Horiguchi Yukiko, a sufferer in a well-to-do family, hidden in a dark room in her family's house. Dr. Koyama sees a poem by Akashi hung on the wall, and Dr. Koyama begins to speak of him. In that sense, Kaijin and his poetry mark a shift in the narrative and away from Ogawa's best-selling text. In the film, Dr. Koyama then begins to question Yukiko about her illness, and Yukiko's life story is introduced. Horiguchi

Yukiko, as she is introduced in the film, has no parallel episode in Ogawa's original text. Instead, she is based on the experiences of another patient at Aisei-en, Hayashi Yukiko.

There are undeniable parallels between Horiguchi and Hayashi. Both were young, educated women from a comfortable background when they were diagnosed, and both shared an affinity for poetry. In real life, Hayashi Yukiko shared a friendship with the famous Nagashima poet Akashi Kaijin, whereas in the film Horiguchi Yukiko is inspired by Kaijin's poems. The mise-en-scène of the room where Horiguchi Yukiko lives moreover mirrors poetic descriptions Hayashi Yukiko gives of her life in quarantine at home before she entered a private hospital (Figure 2.2).[45] In her autobiographical writings, Hayashi describes a small, damp room with a single high window and mice.[46] In the cinematic adaptation, as Koyama awaits admission into Horiguchi's room, a mouse darts down the stairs, and the room is shadowy, with water dripping in places. Hayashi's poems refer to the mice in her room as a relief from loneliness:

> Hiding in the darkness of the backroom
> I gained the friendship of the mice
> 奥の間の闇きが中に隠れつついつしか鼠の友を得にけり[47]

> On days when even the mice are quiet
> Lonesome, I, Yukiko, look out the small window
> 鼠等の静かなる日は由貴子われ何かさびしく小窓見て居り[48]

By using imagery from Hayashi's own poems and by recreating the scenes she described within them, the film introduces the story of a patient from their own point of view, rather than through Ogawa's mediated, medical gaze. In the film, we only see Horiguchi Yukiko in the present from behind, hidden in shadows. In Figure 2.2, Yukiko does not face the camera or Koyama, but instead has her back to the camera, and her face is only visible to her mother. In the case of both Horiguchi and the woman in the peach orchard, the camera shows shadows and glimpses of their bodies, but never reveals their faces.

---

45. I thank Tomohisa Tamura, curator and archivist at Nagashima Aisei-en, for his assistance in locating this photograph.
46. In addition to Hayashi's poetry that was published in a collection of women's writing, *Hagi no shimazato*, Horiguchi Yukiko's story draws on Hayashi's autobiographical essay published the same year. See Hayashi, "Zakuro no nageki," 139–73.
47. Hayashi, "Tanka," 62. A version of this translation was also published in Kathryn M. Tanaka, "Contested Histories and Happiness: Leprosy Literature in Japan," *Health, Culture, and Society* 5, no. 1 (2013): 99–118.
48. Hayashi, "Tanka," 62.

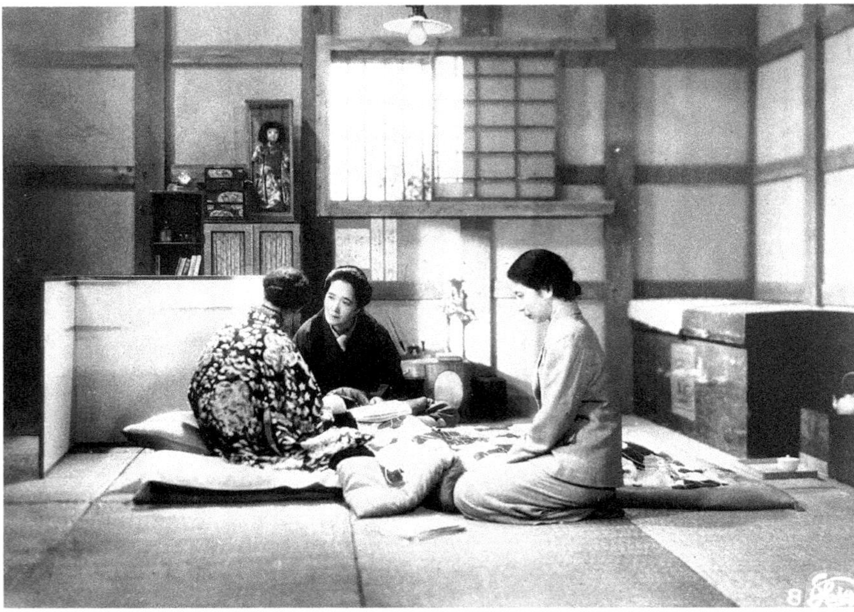

Figure 2.2: A still from an album of images from the film showing the mise-en-scène of the room of Horiguchi Yukiko. Courtesy of Nagashima Aisei-en Archives.

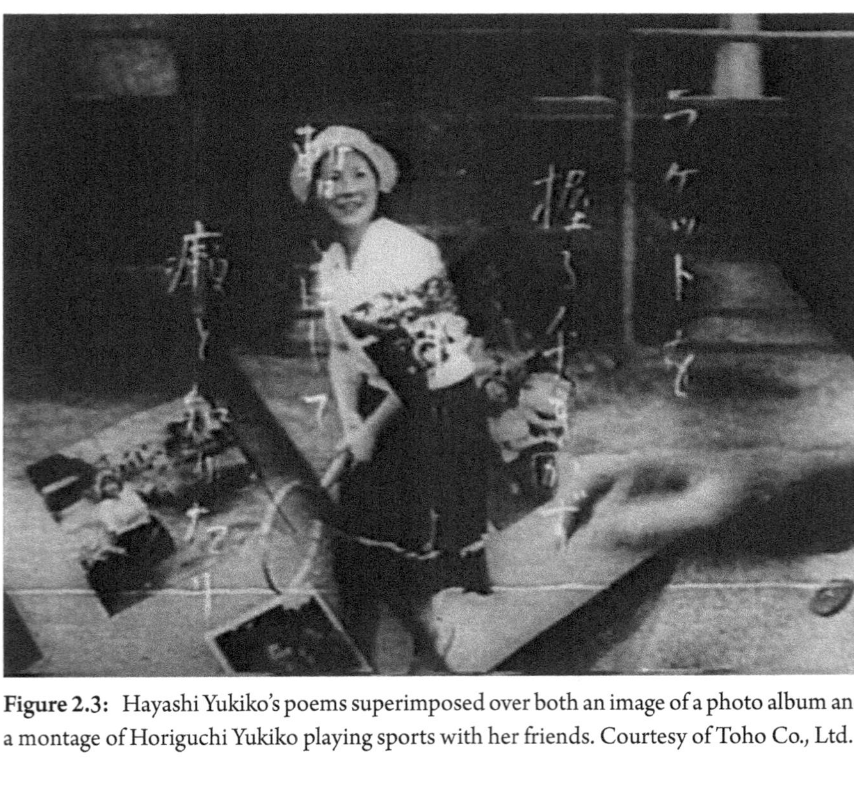

Figure 2.3: Hayashi Yukiko's poems superimposed over both an image of a photo album and a montage of Horiguchi Yukiko playing sports with her friends. Courtesy of Toho Co., Ltd.

We do, however, see Horiguchi's face and body on full display in flashback, as she recalls her life before her diagnosis. As she talks to Dr. Koyama, Hayashi's poems are shown over two superimpositions. In the case of poems by Hayashi Yukiko, the poems are twice superimposed: a scene shows Dr. Koyama flipping through a photo album, containing images of Yukiko when she is healthy. A montage of flashbacks of a young, beautiful girl playing tennis and then basketball is superimposed over the photo album. Then, over both the photo album and the montage, the poem is superimposed (Figure 2.3). The poem superimposed here reads:

Soon after becoming unable to grip my racket
I found out it was leprosy
ラケットを握る手利かずなりてより暫くにして癩と知りたり[49]

This is similar to a poem included in the 1939 women's poetry collection, *Hagi no Satojima*. There, Hayashi begins by writing about finding out about her diagnosis and quitting her job at the post office:

Soon after becoming unable to flick the beads of the abacus
I found out it was leprosy
算盤をはじく手利かずなりてより暫くにして癩と知りたり[50]

The difference between the two poems is two words in Japanese—the verb *hajiku*, or flick, is changed to *nigiru*, to grip, and the noun *abacus* is changed to *racket*. This switch—from the abacus Hayashi used in her job at the post office—to a tennis racket again underscores the class tensions underpinning the different treatment of patients. Tennis was a leisure sport for those who could afford it, and the montage reveals the wealth of the Horiguchi family. Indeed, the fact that in the film Dr. Koyama arranges a discrete, private transport to Aisei-en for Yukiko is in stark contrast to the travel arrangements for Yokogawa, for example, whose poverty and body are on display as he is paraded in front of the crowd of villagers to the boat bound for Aisei-en. The contrast between these two treatments is an example of gendered and class difference in the treatment of Hansen's disease in the film.

The second poem included in the film during Yukiko's story is one that I have been unable to trace in any of Hayashi's published work:

I decide to die, and quietly stand up and go out
My mother is outside the shoji sliding doors
死ぬましとひそやかにして立ち出ずる障子の外に母はいましぬ[51]

49. Yagi Yasutarō, "Kyakyuhon *Kojima no haru*," *Kinema Junpō bessatsu Nihon eiga daihyō shinario zenshū* 2 (1958): 91.

50. Hayashi, *Hagi no satojima*, 61.

51. Yagi, "Kyakyuhon *Kojima no haru*," 91.

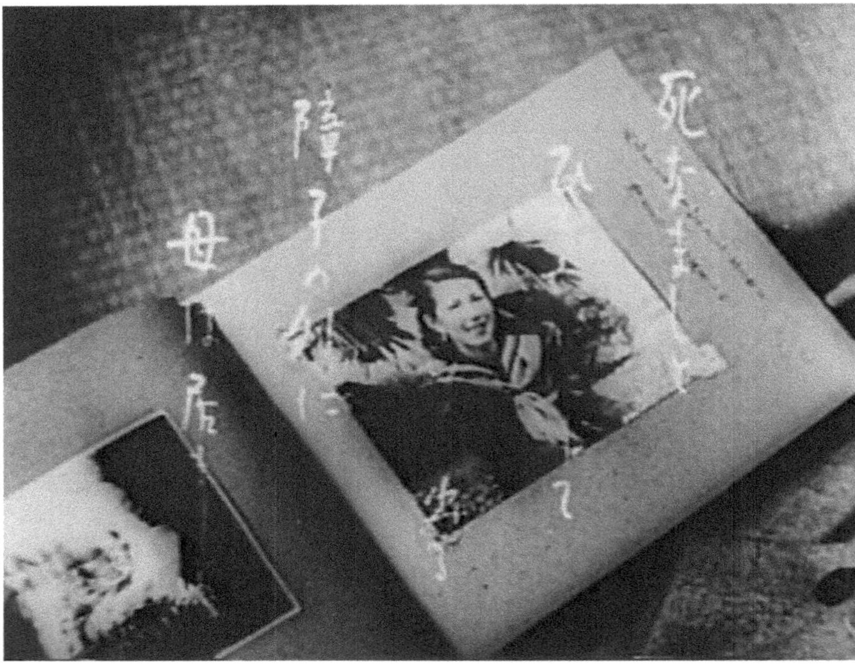

Figure 2.4: A poem possibly written by Hayashi Yukiko superimposed over Horiguchi Yukiko's photo album. Courtesy of Toho Co., Ltd.

In the script, the poem appears in the scenario in the middle of a block of eight poems, all written by Hayashi and taken from the same poetry collection. And in that collection, there is a poem by Hayashi that is similar to the one that appears in the film:

> The life that is left to me is given over to my mother
> Ill, collapsed on the bed
> かにかくに生きねばならぬ生命が母にまかせて床に臥し居り[52]

Given the position of the poem in the film and the script, it seems reasonable to attribute authorship of the second poem to Hayashi; or at least it was meant to be understood to be in her voice. Parts of Hayashi's story, as told through her tanka and autobiographical essay, were woven into the cinematic version of *Spring on the Small Island*, perhaps to elicit sympathy or to showcase how truly anyone could suffer from this illness, even beautiful young, wealthy women.

52. Hayashi, "Tanka," 62.

The inclusion of Hayashi's poetry in a film that was purportedly adapted from a text by Ogawa gives patients a place in popular media to represent their own experiences, using heteroglossia to complicate the dominant medical voices. The montage, assembling Yukiko on-screen as a vibrant, beautiful, healthy young woman created affective interplay when contrasting these fragments with the mise-en-scène of Yukiko in a dark, lonely room, speaking to Dr. Koyama. The gap between the healthy young woman and the sufferer, marked by poetry, allows audience members to identify with Yukiko as healthy and create sympathy for her when she is sick. The poems from Hayashi and the cinematic techniques of the montage foreground the moment of transformation, when she goes from healthy to a sufferer of a stigmatized illness, and they give voice to the shock of this moment. Finally, the poems by Hayashi mark a shift away from Ogawa's voice. The remainder of the poems in the film are by Akashi.

Hayashi's poems allow the viewer to sympathize with a sufferer who is in a liminal space: sick, but giving voice to the moment of transition where she learns her body is no longer healthy. Liminal, in that she is sick, but quarantined at home in a dark, dirty, and secret room rather than receiving treatment in a facility. If Hayashi Yukiko's poems and her montage emphasize this moment of liminality between sickness and health, then Akashi Kaijin's poems represent the voice of the sufferer who is sick and isolated from society.

Being in a liminal space also allows the film to show the body of a female patient. Once the disease had progressed, the bodies of women suffering from Hansen's disease are hidden from the viewer. Diane Wei Lewis has argued that in interwar cinema, "women's bodies in extremis are used to repel and attract," which she argues makes "cinema the site of a radical act of identification with suffering women."[53] Women sufferers in *Spring on the Small Island* arguably also serve to repel and attract. The nature of their illness makes them abject figures, but hearing their stories without seeing their bodies marred by illness allows viewers to identify with the women—and indeed, the way the camera follows the female sufferers who always remain partially obscure has elements of voyeurism. Thus, while the two women sufferers (the woman from the peach orchard and Horiguchi Yukiko) do appear on-screen, their figures and their faces are never shown in full. They are presented on-screen as shadowy figures, whose faces are always obscured by quilts, by half-open doors, by shadows. As in Figure 2.2 above, Yukiko is shown from behind, her face and body obscured by shadows.

Akashi Kaijin's poems, like Yukiko's, are also shown over a montage, a perspective of the process of institutionalization and life in Aisei-en. The dialogue between

53. Diane Wei Lewis, *Powers of the Real: Cinema, Gender, and Emotion in Interwar Japan* (Cambridge, MA: Harvard University Asia Center, 2019), 202–3.

Dr. Koyama and Yukiko fades out with Dr. Koyama saying, "Akashi Kaijin lived in poetry. He truly put his life into his poems. He started writing poetry after he came to Nagashima. So, his home, as a poet, is Nagashima."[54] As she concludes, the scene fades in with a long shot panning over the buildings and the beaches of Aisei-en.

In the case of poems by Akashi Kaijin, the poems are superimposed over scenes filmed on location at Aisei-en and read aloud. The cinematographer, Ogura Kin'ya, stated that all of the poems were set to be read aloud by a patient: "At Aisei-en, there was a patient who was good at reciting. We intended to have them record [the poems], but there was opposition, so we gave it up."[55] Furthermore, Uchida wrote that he urged the director to include recitation for all the tanka, but Toyoda apparently thought that was not a good decision for the film.[56] This makes it more curious that in the final version of the film, Akashi Kaijin's poems are in fact read aloud by a child. In contrast to Ogawa and Yukiko's poems, which are superimposed across the entire scene, the poems superimposed over Aisei-en are only on half the screen, giving the viewer an unimpeded view of the images on the other side of the screen. The child's voice is jarring, as they recite poems about blindness, medical treatments, and death.

The montage over which Akashi's poems are superimposed traces the process of institutionalization, showing the institution from afar, then doctors on a pier. Medical professionals, clothed from head to foot in white protective clothing, are shown mingling in front of the administrative building, on the staff-side of the institution that was off-limits to patients, and walking into a laboratory ward. A shot in the laboratory shows prominent Erlenmeyer flasks labelled as "Chaulmoogra oil" (*Taifūshi*, a widely used palliative medicine), with two women in masks and white garb working on them. The superimposed poem reads:

> To treat my unhealed illness, today again
> The yellow oil is injected into my body[57]
> 癒えがてぬ病を守りて今日もかも黄なる油をししむらに射つ[58]

The montage continues, shifting outside again and into the patient area of the institution: a blind man is shown walking with a cane, a nurse rides a bicycle through a residential area, nodding to residents in their yards. The camera pulls out over the residences to follow the cyclist through the institution before cutting to a shot of

54. Yagi, "Kyakyuhon *Kojima no haru*," 91.
55. Tamura et al., "*Kojima no haru* no zadankai," 21.
56. Tamura et al., "*Kojima no haru* no zadankai," 21.
57. The yellow oil refers to chaulmoogra oil, a thick, odorous oil from the chaulmoogra tree that was one of the few palliative treatments for Hansen's disease at the time Kaijin wrote. Patients typically got injections three times a week.
58. Akashi, *Hakubyō*, 33.

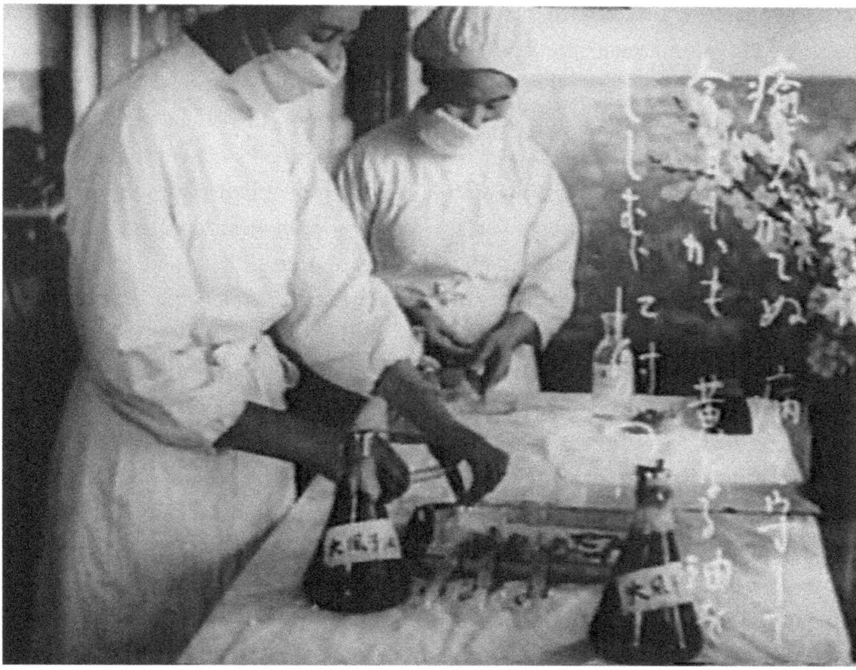

Figure 2.5: A poem by Akashi Kaijin on one side of the screen over a montage including shots of doctors filling syringes with chaulmoogra oil in a laboratory. Courtesy of Toho Co., Ltd.

crowds of children playing, patients tending to pigs and cows, and others working in vegetable fields. The final shot in the montage is of the bell at Nagashima, used for marking time and ceremonial purposes, being rung. The entire montage sequence, with five poems, lasts only about three minutes.

The residents that are shown is a man walking with a cane, and men working in fields. As is the case in the stories of Yokogawa and Miyata, the male bodies of patients are on display for the public, allowing the viewer to see the effects of the illness. In the Nagashima montage, the man is blind and walks with a cane; Yokogawa wears tattered clothing that mark his poverty and dark glasses that show his weakening eyes. Miyata is introduced to the viewers as the camera pans down dramatically, slowly revealing bandaged hands holding crutches and bandaged feet. In the treatment shown during the montage on Nagashima, and the stories of Miyata and Yokogawa during the film, the camera gaze is gendered, and the men's bodies reveal the reality of the disease to the public while women diagnosed with the disease remain hidden in shadows.

Kaijin's poems, included in the Appendix here and read aloud as the montage flickers beneath them, both echo and belie the images on the screen. As doctors are shown coming up from the pier, Akashi's poem mourns losing his identity and the name his parents gave him through institutionalization. The shot of the women working with chaulmoogra oil in the lab has Akashi's poem about the oil, the word "unhealed" subtly contradicting the medical efficacy on display in the laboratory. As patients' daily lives are shown on-screen, Akashi's poems lament his worsening illness and his separation from his family. The final poem that closes the sequence over the bell—and the final poem in the movie—looks toward Akashi's eventual death and the return of his bones to his wife and children.

While Yukiko's story is layered through superimposition—the photo album, the montage, and her poems—Akashi's are layered in a different way. They take half the screen, with the action on-screen moving around the superimposed poetry. The poems exist alongside, but separate, from the action happening on the other side of the screen. This, together with the fact that Akashi's poems speak to the shots on-screen as they tell a different story, serves to highlight the heteroglossia in the film.

In the end, Akashi's poems are the only ones recited in the film, and they are the only ones to feature the footage shot on location at Aisei-en. The voiceover of the poems shot on location ultimately serves to both highlight the montage and emphasize the content of the poems, thus highlighting the dialectic between the medical gaze, and the lived experience of patients. The shooting on location at Aisei-en showcased the cutting-edge medical treatments available there and the neat facilities that allowed patients to live happily there, but at the same time the poems of patient experience hint at the futility of this treatment and the layers of different patient experiences.

Although the final sequence from Nagashima is quite short, and there was some hesitancy to be on location there, the footage shot was fairly intensive. Cinematographer Ogura recalled: "It was very difficult. We had to wear long boots and masks to enter certain areas. I didn't wear a mask, and I also couldn't cover my reflex, tripod, and other equipment, so I had a hard time taking care of them."[59] Uchida Mamoru, the ophthalmologist who wrote about the film, also assisted on location for four days and noted the six-member film crew was afraid of shooting in the patient area, although ultimately they managed to do so. He writes: "At Nagashima, they shot thirteen cuts. At the same time this film was shot, they were shooting a different *bunka eiga* film of Nagashima, so they shot about two reels, and over three days they shot about sixteen thousand feet of film."[60] The shooting ratio between footage shot and that which appears in the final cut again hints at the fact that the footage selected and used in the end was likely chosen to highlight the content of the poems.

59. Tamura et al., "*Kojima no haru* no zadankai," 21.
60. Uchida, "Eiga *Kojima no Haru* no zakkan," 50.

If Yukiko's story traces the bodily transformation from health to sickness in poetry and montage, Kaijin's poems and the accompanying montage trace the journey of the patient, from institutionalization to worsening condition and futile medical treatment to death. Their voices serve to decenter Ogawa's voice and her story. While they speak, Dr. Koyama is displaced by a montage that foregrounds the poems and patient voices in very different ways. These poems subtly acknowledge that medical treatment alone is insufficient to heal what ails the writers—a loss of health and family.

The patients recognized their own stories in those shared on the screen. A special screening of the film was held at Nagashima, and after seeing the film, Hayashi Yukiko acknowledged her story had been told when she wrote: "Everything was just as it had been in the days of my past, and seeing it recalled to mind painful memories."[61] She even captured her feelings in a poem about watching the film:

> かたゐ我れ映画の中に病む人の面は見難く眼をそらす
> As I suffer from leprosy, it is difficult to watch the scenes with invalids in the film
> I avert my eyes[62]

Yukiko does not acknowledge more explicitly that it was in part her story, or that the film used her poems. But she writes that she was choking on tears as she watched the film and remembered the sorrow she had in leaving her mother. For Hayashi, the film was a tanka film (*tanka eiga*), and its use of heteroglossia was a way to help the public understand that the plight of sufferers was more than just illness, and to view sufferers and patients with sympathy rather than with prejudice.

Conclusion

This chapter has argued that *Spring on the Small Island* is in fact a more nuanced film than a humanist story or a propagandistic piece. I have argued that attention to the heteroglossia of the tanka, the gendered gaze of the camera, and differences in class make the film a complex work that cannot be reduced to propaganda. The work instead takes at times a more provocative approach to the government's policies of institutionalization than appears on a superficial viewing of the film. Toyoda uses the inclusion of tanka, references to class, use of location, and the film's gendered gaze as elements to provoke thought about the narrative and resist easy identification or approval of the policies the film was taken to promote. Perhaps in part due to Mitsuda Kensuke's intentions in backing the production, and his subsequent use of the film in Hansen's disease relief work, critics at the time, and since, have viewed

61. "Eiga hihyō—*Kojima no haru* kansō tokugō," *Aisei* 11 no. 3 (March 1941): 12.
62. "Eiga hihyō—*Kojima no haru* kansō tokugō," 12.

the film primarily through the social contexts in which the Leprosy-Free Prefecture and other relief work was promoted. This reductionist viewing of the film ignores techniques used by Toyoda in his direction. In addition, Yagi's screenplay is a far more complex and nuanced text, in dialogue not only with the rhetoric of the relief works, but also drawing on writing by the patients themselves to create a compelling film and complicated narrative of the treatment of Hansen's disease in Japan. The richness of this intertextual layer, as well as the debates around the reception of the film at the time it was released, have been erased by attention to the dominant messages in this film. This chapter has been a first step to rethink the reception of the film and the importance of the heteroglossia and the nuances of camera gaze within it.

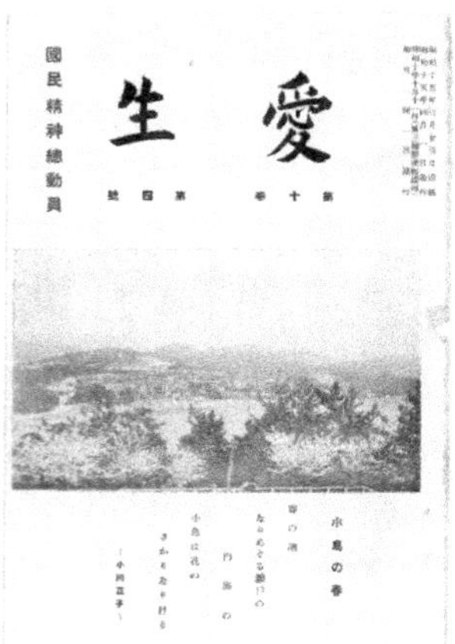

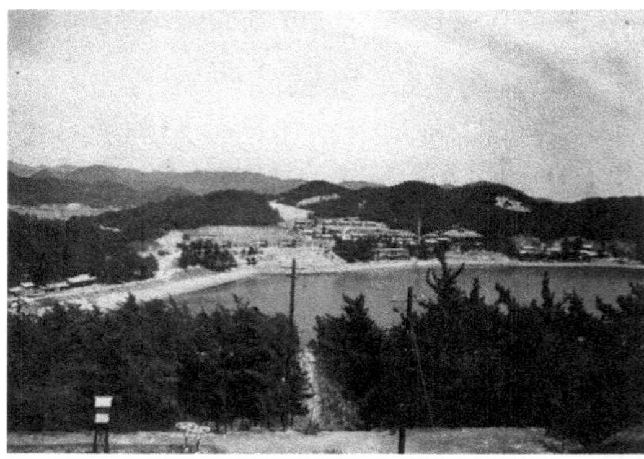

Figures 2.6 (left): Cover of *Aisei* 10(4); **Figure 2.7 (right):** The source of the first poem in the film, together with an image of the institution similar to the one on the cover. Courtesy of Nagashima Aisei-en Archives.

Appendix: The Fourteen Poems Included in the Film *Spring on the Small Island*

2:39
春の潮なりめぐる瀬戸の内海の小島は桃の花さかりなり[63]
The spring tide comes in, and the peaches on
The small island in the Inland Sea are in full bloom

2:58
桃の花さける小島の丘の上に幸せ住むと我はおもひも[64]
I believe happiness resides on the hill on the small island
Where the peach blossoms bloom

11:03
癩患者の児と云う子らの我が前に目をそらせて立つにいとしさ湧くも[65]
Said to be children of a leper, standing before me,
Averting their eyes, the darlings

30:31
桜散る窓辺に火桶かこみをり孤島の春の雨のさむきに[66]
The cherry blossoms fall near the window while we crowd around the braizer
The cold of the spring rain on the lonely island

38:45
おもへ人はなれ小島の山陰に癩女がひとりする雛祭りを[67]
On an isolated island in the shade of the mountains
A leper woman celebrates the Doll Festival alone

39:11
阿波池田吉野の川の橋に立ち仰ぐ箸蔵寺順礼の鈴[68]
Standing on the bridge over the Yoshino River in Awa-Ikeda
The ringing of the prayer bell at Hashiozoji Temple

59:15
雨一日訪う人もなく夕暮れて塒すずめは鳴きひそまるぬ[69]
A day of rain, no one comes to visit
At dusk, the sparrows call from their roosts

63. Ogawa Masako, "Tanka," *Aisei Special Issue Kokumin Seishin Sōdōin* 10, no. 4 (1940), cover. This was edited from Ogawa's original to change "flowers" to "peach blossom."
64. Unconfirmed poem, but given its focus on peach blossoms and the happiness of life on Nagashima, it may have been written specifically for the film.
65. Ogawa Masako, *Kojima no Haru—Hansen-byō chiryō ni, shōgai wo sasageta aru joi no shuki* (Tokyo: Nagasaki shuppan, 2009), 196.
66. Ogawa, *Kojima no haru*, 213.
67. Ogawa, *Kojima no haru*, 225
68. Ogawa, *Kojima no haru*, 13.
69. Akashi Kaijin, *Hakubyō* (Tokyo: Kaizōsha, 1939), 141.

1:01:06
ラケットを握る手利かずなりてより暫くにして癩と知りたり[70]
Soon after becoming unable to grip my racket
I found out it was leprosy

1:01:20
死ぬましとひそやかにして立ち出づる障子の外に母は居ましぬ[71]
I decide to die, and quietly stand up and go out
My mother is outside the shoji sliding doors

1:02:37
父母のえらび給ひし名をすててこの島の院に棲むべくは来ぬ[72]
I have given up the name that my parents chose for me,
And I have come to dwell in this island's hospital

1:03:07
癒えがてぬ病を守りて今日もかも黄なる油をししむらに射つ[73]
To treat my unhealed illness, today again
The yellow oil is injected into my body

1:03:33
盲ひてはおのれが手になつくらね庭のトマトの伸びをたのしむ[74]
I enjoy the growth of the tomatoes in the garden
Though blind, I take them in my hand

1:04:10
すこやかに育てばまして嘆かるる幼き命わが血をぞ曳く[75]
Growing up healthy, the young life is still lamentable
As my blood runs through their veins

1:04:42
わが骨の帰えるべき日を嘆くらむ妻子等をおもう輪夕凪ひととき[76]
A moment of calm in the evening
As I think of my wife and children, greiving the day when my bones will return to them

70. Hayashi Yukiko, "Tanka," in *Hagi no shimazato*, 61.
71. Unconfirmed poem, likely by Hayashi Yukiko.
72. Akashi, *Hakubyō*, 32.
73. Akashi, *Hakubyō*, 33.
74. Akashi, *Hakubyō*, 133.
75. Akashi, *Hakubyō*, 125.
76. Akashi, *Hakubyō*, 202.

3

Deformed Bodies in Nuclear Family Rhetoric

The Hiroshima Maidens Project in the Early Cold War

Yuki Obayashi

> It is not so much what we have done for them [Hiroshima Maidens], but what they have done for us. They come to this country to be mended of the outward scars which the world put upon them and in coming they healed in many of us the inward scars and wounds of our own selves.
>
> —Host family in Shrewsbury-Red Bank, NJ[1]

In May 1955, twenty-five female victims of the US atomic bombing—*hibakusha* (explosion-affected people)—of Hiroshima, aged seventeen to thirty-one years old, were flown to the United States and received extensive plastic surgery to correct severe deformity from keloids.[2] Initiated by the American journalist Norman Cousins and the Japanese Methodist minister Tanimoto Kiyoshi, this one-and-a-half-year project was supported on multiple civilian fronts in the United States: free medical treatment at Mount Sinai Hospital in New York City; housing secured by Quakers in suburban areas in New York, New Jersey, and Connecticut;[3] and successful fundraising through the popular TV program *This Is Your Life*.[4]

---

1. New York Friends Center, "A Report on Our Guests from Hiroshima." April 11, 1956, RG2/NY/N456, series 1, New York Friends Center Records, Friends Historical Library, Swarthmore College.
2. This chapter is a revision of a section in my dissertation, "Unsettled Empires: Japanese and U.S. Cultural Imaginaries of the 'South Pacific,'" accepted to the University of California, Santa Cruz, in 2023. I appreciate my professors, Christine Hong, Noriko Aso, and Karen Tei Yamashita, for their thorough feedback and support.
3. Paul Tobenkin, "Hiroshima Girls Here for Surgery," *New York Herald Tribune*, May 10, 1955. Archived in Hiroshima Maidens: Correspondence, Memos folder, Office of the Director (Martin Steinberg) Records, 1939–1969, The Arthur H. Aufses, Jr. MD Archives, Icahn School of Medicine at Mount Sinai.
4. Dr. William Hitzig, Norman Cousins's physician and friend, and Dr. Arthur Barsky at Mount Sinai Hospital, joined the project to conduct surgeries for the Hiroshima Maidens. The chairman of its board of trustees, New York lawyer Alfred Rose, personally donated all the costs for hospitalization.

From the moment the Hiroshima Maidens set foot in the United States, the media walked in lockstep in offering up a narrative of the project that enabled Americans to avoid grappling with the devastating consequences of US wartime antagonism toward Japan. A widely circulated image of two Hiroshima Maidens smiling inside a bus at the Mitchell Field military airport in New York underscored the futural orientation of the Hiroshima Maidens project.[5] Yet, Americans indeed witnessed the first visual images of *hibakusha* of Hiroshima and Nagasaki, published in an article titled "Uncensored Photos Show Atomic Bombing Through Victims' Eyes" on the September 19, 1952 issue of *Life*, seven years after the original photos were taken. Having survived the US government's censorship during its occupation of Japan, the images of the destroyed cities, gruesome corpses, and shell-shocked *hibakusha* were revived from the repressed past. However, unlike the blurred images developed from damaged negative film, Hiroshima Maidens appeared in front of American eyes as the actual human being who was living in the present, where the past continued to be carried over through their deformed bodies. The images of Hiroshima Maidens that were taken upon their arrival in New York reinforced the sunny outlook of these visitors to the United States.[6] Although one woman had keloid burns on the left side of her face, and the other completely covered her right eye, unable to close due to burns, with a patch, they hid not only their fatigue following a long trip with stopovers in Hawai'i and San Francisco, but also a decade of suffering with smiles in front of the camera. The implication was that these "maidens," now safely in the United States, would benefit from superior American medical technology and thereby secure the possibility of a "normal" future *as women*.

When the brutal Pacific War was referenced at all, US media took pains to highlight Hiroshima Maiden Sako Michiko's comments on Japan's Pearl Harbor attack.[7] *The World Telegram* quoted an extended version of her comments: "It got us to thinking of the beginning of war that the Japanese Navy took the first step in the war. We in Hiroshima got a terrible destruction visited upon us, but we show our repentance

He requested that his name be anonymous and that the hospital take credit for the donation. Rodney Baker, *The Hiroshima Maidens: A Story* Rodney Barker, *The Hiroshima Maidens: A Story of Courage, Compassion, and Survival* (New York: Penguin Books, 1986), 70. The reality documentary series, *This Is Your Life*, was initially broadcasted on NBC Radio between 1948 and 1952 and was televised on NBC between 1952 and 1961.

5. See Tobenkin, "Hiroshima Girls Here for Surgery," for the photo image.
6. Theo Wilson, "25 Hiroshima Maids Here for Surgery," *Daily News*, May 10, 1955. Archived in RG2/NY/N456, series 3, New York Friends Center Records. Friends Historical Library, Swarthmore College.
7. It seems that Sako was inspired by her and other Hiroshima Maidens' visit to Pearl Harbor on their way to the US mainland. Because the US Air Force agreed to transport the Hiroshima Maidens, they ironically had a layover at Pearl Harbor.

rather than hatred and we begin to hate war in general."[8] Sako's emphasis on Pearl Harbor as precipitating the atomic holocaust the United States perpetrated against Hiroshima arguably mitigated any hesitation and guilt Americans might have felt about the Hiroshima Maidens. Rather, Americans could see themselves—through the eyes of a *hibakusha*—as victims and justify their nation's war crime as a reaction to Japanese aggression. Whether or not Sako's juxtaposition of Pearl Harbor and Hiroshima was meant to argue historical equivalence, her comments, widely broadcast over US media, served to soothe the American conscience toward the Hiroshima Maidens.

The Hiroshima Maidens project, in the early Cold War, demonstrated how Americans succeeded in collectively transforming their anti-Japanese sentiments into a form of humanitarian rescue that was aimed at their former enemy.[9] In an example of what Michael J. Yavenditti calls "American benevolence," the Hiroshima Maidens project allowed Americans to heal from their wartime guilt over the atomic bombings in Japan by successfully painting them as a savior of innocent women.[10] Furthermore, despite the desperate need for money and resources to operate the project, Cousins sidestepped help from Jewish organizations that would emphasize his Jewish background.[11] Avoiding the easier route for donations, Cousins intentionally presented this initiative in studiously national terms as an American humanitarian project. By emphasizing American "generosity" during a sensitive Cold War juncture, with the war in Korea fresh in the global imagination, US media and contributors to the project objectified Hiroshima Maidens to fit into the American Cold War logic that highlighted their moral superiority as a nation.

---

8. Carol Taylor, "25 A-Burned Girls Here for Surgery," *The World Telegram*, May 9, 1955. Archived in RG2/NY/N456, series 3, New York Friends Center, Friends Historical Library, Swarthmore College.
9. The women themselves initially came up with the moniker "Atomic Maidens" [*genbaku otome*], which was then used by the Japanese media back in 1952 when they first underwent extensive surgeries in Tokyo. The Japanese word *otome* was translated into English as "maidens." Naoko Shibusawa, *America's Geisha Ally: Reimagining the Japanese Enemy* (Cambridge, MA: Harvard University Press, 2006), 227. Norman Cousins constantly used the phrase "Hiroshima Maidens" in his *Saturday Review* articles. The New York Friends Center that coordinated Quaker host families first referred to their work as the Hiroshima Project. Only midway through the project did they switch the name to the Hiroshima Maidens project in their newsletters and memoranda.
10. Michael J. Yavenditti, "The Hiroshima Maidens and American Benevolence in the 1950s," *Mid-America: An Historical Review* 64, no. 2 (1982): 21. Also see Amanda Jane Graham for a similar claim that Cousins contributed to Americans more than the Hiroshima Maidens by providing an opportunity to ease their minds over the atomic bombings, namely, "write a cheque, send it in, and feel better." Amanda Jane Graham, "Re-Covering the Hiroshima Maidens," in *Medicine, Healing and Performance*, ed. Effie Gemi-Iordanou et al. (Oxford, PA: Oxbow Books, 2014), 130.
11. Shibusawa, *America's Geisha Ally*, 242.

The sense of American geopolitical superiority over Japan in the early Cold War reflected the racialized and gendered rhetoric of Hiroshima Maidens. The *hibakusha* women were all portrayed as single, and their unwed, "innocent," and "vulnerable" status was central to the affective economy the project organizers hoped to foster.[12] Viewed to some degree as blank slates, the women, who had to have visible keloids on their faces to be accepted for the project, functioned as objects of active American sympathy *and* intervention.[13] The rhetorical emphasis on young, unwed Japanese women suppressed the previous images of militant, patriarchal Japan, a US rivalry in the Pacific Theatre during World War II. As Christina Klein argues, the feminized Hiroshima Maidens rhetorically reinforced "Japan's postwar status as ally and subordinate partner" with the United States.[14] As malleable figures, they could be productively made over. It is important to note that the project originated in Cousins's sympathy for *hibakusha* women who had formed a support group at Tanimoto's church in Hiroshima. Resistant at first to Tanimoto's proposal that these women be taken to the United States for cosmetic and other medical treatment, Cousins changed his mind after conversing with women at the church, who resigned themselves never to become the prospects of love or marriage.[15] It was, in other words, the foreclosure of their heteronormative futurity that impelled Cousins to act on their behalf. Identifying this group of *hibakusha* women with his daughters who were around the same age, Cousins refashioned himself as their father/savior figure, an ideological turn reflected in the ethos of the Hiroshima Maidens project in which doctors and host families would take part.

US cultural ideas of the Hiroshima Maidens should be scrutinized as an extension of its geopolitical interventions and dominance in Japan and East Asia. In framing the Hiroshima Maidens project as transnational, I consider that the US imaginations of female Asian bodies cannot be separated from examinations of East Asia media, since the images are products of self-portrayals and responses to perceptions by others. Thus, in this chapter, I analyze American responses to their nation's

12. The omission of male *hibakusha* speaks to the project's gender bias. However, project organizers did not seek out only single women, according to the archivist Barbara Niss of Mount Sinai Library. A married *hibakusha* woman had to turn the offer down, unable to commit to the initially one-year project and leave her family behind in Japan. Contradicting the media portrayals of the *hibakusha* women as all singles, one of them was, in fact, engaged; however, her planned marriage was not revealed in public.
13. Chujo Kazuo, *Genbaku otome* (Tokyo: Asahi Shinbunsha, 1984), 61–62.
14. Christina Klein, *Cold War Orientalism: Asia in the Middlebrow Imagination, 1945–1961* (Berkeley, CA: University of California Press, 2003), 150.
15. Selma Robinson, "A Maiden from Hiroshima," *Redbook* (December 1956): 80. Archived in Hiroshima Maidens: Correspondence, Memos folder, Office of the Director (Martin Steinberg) Records, 1939–1969, The Arthur H. Aufses, Jr. MD Archives, Icahn School of Medicine at Mount Sinai.

role as a perpetrator of nuclear atrocity in Japan to examine how they negotiated and contested this history during the Cold War, a period in which the United States sought to establish the legitimacy and supremacy of its global domination. In Cold War propaganda, Hiroshima Maidens were imagined as a valuable entity to promote American democracy. However, contrary to the racialized and gendered rhetoric of "maidens," Hiroshima Maidens' deformed bodies in the US media were downplayed as if Americans avoided discussing and looking at their physical and emotional pains. I examine these oppositional media perceptions of the Hiroshima Maidens by considering the early Cold War as a sociocultural juncture whereby the US government strategically embraced the American nuclear family to discredit the Soviet Union's critique of the inequality American women faced. Rather than improving the social problem in question, the US government emphasized that women in the Soviet Union had to endure physical labor in order to secure employment and work equally with men.[16] The US government promoted the nuclear family as the embodiment of democratic values, where women were economically protected by their husbands.

The Hiroshima Maidens represented an antithesis of the nuclear family where women were expected to be wives and mothers in the divided gender roles because of their deformity. The "unattractiveness" that assumably prevented them from getting married created unsettled narratives of the Hiroshima Maidens in US media. First, I argue that those who directly helped the Hiroshima Maidens, such as project organizers and host families, promoted the gendered and racialized rhetoric that the Americans rescued the innocent "maidens" from their misery. Nonetheless, more than simply being feminized, the women were collectively called "girls"—like daughters—in paternal America. Interpreting the word "girls" as social perceptions of relations to others, rather than defined by actual ages, I ask if the fixated image resulted from their deformed bodies that were not imagined as the women in the nuclear family rhetoric. Second, I examine a visual marginalization of Hiroshima Maidens in the TV program, *This Is Your Life*, aired on May 11, 1955, which further presents their unsettled positionality in early Cold War America. The episode, featuring Tanimoto Kiyoshi, the cofounder of the Hiroshima Maidens project, introduced two Hiroshima Maidens who stood behind the screen, hidden because of their disfigurements. In contrast to their invisibility, *This Is Your Life* excessively celebrated the well-being of the Tanimotos, an ideal nuclear family, who appeared as surprise guests. Revealingly, the positionality of the Hiroshima Maidens projected the American response to their deformed bodies that did not fit into the feminized images of women—wives and mothers—in the early Cold War, when nuclear families were celebrated as an embodiment of American democracy.

---

16. Laura A. Belmonte, *Selling the American Way: U.S. Propaganda and the Cold War* (Philadelphia, PA: University of Pennsylvania Press, 2008), 137.

Japanese "Daughters" in American Nuclear Family Imagined

A *New York Times*' article, published on November 7, 1956, "Hiroshima Victim Was Won by U.S.," describes a Hiroshima Maiden, Zomen Michiyo, and her emotional farewell to Americans on her way back to Japan.[17] Capturing Americans' hearts by appreciating the love that she received, which the article title suggests, she was presented in the article as a Japanese *hibakusha* who allowed Americans to obliterate the United States' role in her suffering. Conveniently, her emotional recollection alters historical accounts of the atom bombing by situating Americans as her saviors. As part of the geopolitical shifts in the Cold War, former Japanese foes—whom US media caricatured as "subhuman" creatures, such as "apes and vermin," during World War II—became America's new democratic allies and innocent girls or "maidens," who were free from the politics that divided the two nations.[18] The article begins, "A small young girl who had been crippled by an atom bomb dropped in World War II stood in tears before an American-Japanese audience today."[19] By simultaneously referring to the grown woman and her childhood self, the equivocal description, "a small young girl," was a canny American rhetorical intervention that pictured Zomen and the other "maidens" as though they were still children frozen in the late-war moment of 1945. The article, however, overlooked that Zomen was already twenty years old at the time of the atomic bombing.[20] This misconception revealed that Americans retroactively recast themselves as helping Japanese "children" out of misery in the rhetoric of the paused temporality. Infantilized not just in media coverage and in official project rhetoric, the Hiroshima Maidens were consistently imagined as daughters who needed to be nurtured by American parents. In this way, Americans scripted the twenty-five *hibakusha* as unfortunate girls who needed not only medical procedures but also love and rearing in the United States.

The Hiroshima Maidens, aged seventeen to thirty-one years old, were expected to become a part of their host families as daughters. Japanese American Helen Yokoyama, who worked as an interpreter and go-between on the American side,

---

17. The Hiroshima Maidens Project was initially planned as a one-year project. However, because some women still required extensive surgery after the year had passed, Norman Cousins decided to send the Hiroshima Maidens back to Japan separately. The *New York Times* article covers the latter group's return in November 1956, one-and-a-half years after they flew to the United States. Hailey Forster, "Hiroshima Victim Was Won by U.S.," *New York Times*, November 7, 1956, https://www.nytimes.com/1956/11/07/archives/hiroshima-victim-was-won-by-us-back-in-japan-girl-tells-tearfully.html.
18. John Dower, *War Without Mercy: Race and Power in the Pacific War* (New York: Pantheon Books, 1986), 9.
19. Hailey, "Hiroshima Victim Was Won by U.S."
20. Zomen and other Hiroshima Maidens recollected when the atomic bomb was dropped in interviews by Japanese journalist Chujo Kazuo. There, Zomen mentioned her age at that time. Chujo, *Genbaku otome*, 34.

encouraged the Hiroshima Maidens to behave like "daughters" by doing the dishes and giving massages to their "American parents."[21] These domestic chores reflected the American expectation toward the Hiroshima Maidens to fit into a stereotypical gender role in the patriarchal society. In this context, gratitude to the host families was reinforced by the Hiroshima Maidens' dependency on their "parents," who were their means of surviving in an unfamiliar country. Yet, Yokoyama's remark raises the question if it was possible for these *hibakusha* to show their appreciation as mature women outside this imposed parent-daughter rhetoric.

According to the rhetoric whereby the Hiroshima Maidens were "daughters" in the American host families, their affections to their host families' young children and grandchildren were explained as "natural" reactions to their siblings and nieces and nephews, as they reportedly displayed "genuine affection" toward them.[22] However, I interpret that as a sign of motherhood, which none of the scholars and contributors to the Hiroshima Maiden Project alike have pointed out. Lisa Yoneyama argues that Japanese women in postwar Japan fought against United States' nuclear testing in the Pacific to protect their families.[23] These gestures of motherhood contrasted with the Hiroshima Maidens' infantilized "pur[ity]" and "virgin[ity]" in "paternalized America."[24] In their daughter-like capacity, the Hiroshima Maidens were granted an opportunity to develop instincts for motherhood. Indeed, the limitation of the infantilizing daughter rhetoric was apparent in the Maidens' objection to studying with children at regular schools.[25] A series of the Hiroshima Maidens' acts and behaviors suggest that their maturity did not fit the image that the Americans constructed.

The multiracial family of American parents and Japanese daughters was imagined within a framework of an affluent suburban nuclear family that emphasized a divided gender role in the patriarchal society. The New York Friends Center placed the Japanese "daughters" in suburban nuclear families, whose affluence was signaled by the fact that mothers in these households did not need full-time jobs. Ida Day of the New York Friends Center specifically requested that potential host families have stay-at-home mothers.[26] Not only did all the host families have enough room in their

21. Shibusawa, *America's Geisha Ally*, 247.
22. New York Friends Center, "A Report on Our Guests from Hiroshima." April 11, 1956, RG2/NY/N456, series 1, New York Friends Center Records, Friends Historical Library, Swarthmore College.
23. Lisa Yoneyama, *Hiroshima Traces: Time, Space, and the Dialectics of Memory* (Berkeley, CA: University of California Press, 1999), 193.
24. Yoneyama, *Hiroshima Traces*, 202.
25. The host families sent the Hiroshima Maidens to various schools and provided private lessons in English and other subjects. New York Friends Center, "A Report on Our Guests from Hiroshima."
26. Letter from Ida Day to Friends, May 5, 1955, RG2/NY/N456, series 3, New York Friends Center, Friends Historical Library, Swarthmore College. Friends indicate the Quaker members.

homes to accommodate a guest, but also, the wives were at home during the day.[27] The aim of Day's request may have been to enable the Hiroshima Maidens to experience good American lives to supplement their intense care. However, Day was not the only person who pictured this kind of "perfect" American host family for the Hiroshima Maidens. Three months after they settled in, Director Arnold Vaught pointed out that some host families were concerned that the *hibakusha* women had not seen "typical American homes" that had "more young people" yet enough.[28] The New York Friends Center and the Quaker members thought it could be most beneficial for the Hiroshima Maidens to stay with host families who could not only satisfy their guest's material needs and ensure their comfort, but also introduce American social values of the nuclear family that celebrate gender divisions in the family.

Consequently, Ida Day and the Quaker members in host families therefore engaged with Cold War propaganda by matching the Hiroshima Maidens with typical American nuclear families. The early Cold War multicultural rhetoric that fashioned the Hiroshima Maidens as American daughters suggests that American social norms were embedded in the project. The Hiroshima Maidens were gendered and racialized to promote the paternalistic authority of the United States over its major Asian client state, Japan.

Deformed Bodies Hidden behind the Screen

Circulated a week before the Hiroshima Maidens arrived in the United States, a press release featured an anecdote about their weekly habit of viewing American films at a local theater in Japan, quoting one of them who explained, "We like to see the pretty girls and imagine that we are them."[29] This *hibakusha*'s praise underscored the special quality of American beauty for the US public, while neglecting Japanese standards of beauty that they could also observe through booming Japanese films in the post–World War II and post–US occupation years. This internalized normalization of American beauty excluded Japanese women from beauty standards in the racial hierarchy. Moreover, the screen in the theater physically and metaphorically divides the *hibakusha* women from "the pretty girls." While American actresses on the screen received all the spotlights from the filmgoers, not only the existence of the *hibakusha* women in the theater was erased in the darkened space, but also their invisible presence emphasized their actual social isolation. The *hibakusha* woman's

27. Ida Day, "Hiroshima Project—Hospitality Program." June 19, 1955, RG2/NY/N456, series 3, New York Friends Center, Friends Historical Library, Swarthmore College.
28. Minutes of New York Friends Center, July 12, 1955, RG2/NY/N456, series 1, New York Friends Center, Friends Historical Library, Swarthmore College.
29. Press Release by Sallie L. Parler, April 4, 1955, RG2/NY/N456, series 3, New York Friends Center Records, Friends Historical Library, Swarthmore College.

imagination that "we are them" like the actresses reveals their longing to become the subjects being filmed.

In this section, I examine the visual marginalization of the Hiroshima Maidens in the TV program *This Is Your Life*, aired on May 11, 1955.[30] Contrary to the already-circulated media coverage in newspapers and magazines, the Hiroshima Maidens who appeared in the show were hidden behind a screen. Aired on Wednesday nights on NBC between 1952 and 1962, the thirty-minute documentary reality series *This Is Your Life* created a vibrant atmosphere with the live audience, featuring celebrities and ordinary people and introducing their life stories; however, the program's proceedings were presumptuous in the sense that the featured guests were not informed of anything in advance, including guests as witnesses of parts of their lives. The host, Ralph Edwards, proceeded the program giving congratulating remarks to the featured guests for their life accomplishments, while the live audience in the studio cheered, laughed, and clapped their hands, responding to Edwards's celebratory proceeding. On the surface level, *This is Your Life* was meant to empower the guests, as it first featured the suffering veterans at hospitals in Los Angeles as a tribute to their courage.[31] However, as the title suggests, Edwards defined their life stories by controlling the narratives and selecting the highlights of stories and witnesses. The featured guests turned to become the objectification of their own life stories through Edwards's facilitation. In this reversal of subjectification/objectification, Edwards revealed sensitive personal stories of the guests, with what Joan McGettigan calls "ambush tactics," and forced them into the awkward position that their raw feelings were broadcasted nationally.[32] In this sense, *This Is Your Life* exploited the featured guests for viewer ratings, namely capitalistic gain.

The episode, which featured the Japanese minister Tanimoto Kiyoshi, who had recently arrived in the United States with the Hiroshima Maidens, highlighted American humanitarian absurdity that dehumanized the *hibakusha* women for the complacency of being a savior. While the TV program successfully raised $56,000, with the TV host urging viewers to show the "American way" by donating to the project, this generosity fostered an illusion of American humanitarian superiority towards its former enemy, which could be accomplished through financial help. Yet the fantasy propelling viewers to donate was much more subtly staged than the host Ralph Edward's overt calls for viewer contributions. In an episode which infamously staged a "reencounter" between one of the Enola Gay bombers, Robert A. Lewis, and Tanimoto, a visibly undisfigured *hibakusha*, for its television audience, the

30. *This Is Your Life*, season 3, episode 32, "Rev. Kiyoshi Tanimoto," aired May 11, 1955, on NBC, https://www.dailymotion.com/video/xl3jx5.

31. Stuart Lenig, *The Bizarre World of Reality Television* (Santa Barbara, CA: ABC-Clio, 2017), 214.

32. Joan McGettigan, "'The Whole World Shares Your Heartache': 'This Is Your Life' and 1950s Stardom," *Studies in Popular Culture* 35, no. 1 (2012): 110.

show's producers elected to keep two of the Hiroshima Maidens behind the partition separating the back stage from the front stage. By *not showing* the faces, much less the bodies, of these two Japanese women outright, *This Is Your Life* contributed to their racialization in a way that drew on the logic of the Hiroshima Maidens project itself; presenting these two *hibakusha* as silhouettes on an otherwise blank screen, the show invited its American audience to project gendered fantasies of rescue and rehabilitation onto them.

This Is Your Life created an exceptional *hibakusha* narrative by centralizing Tanimoto's life story, which was far from evoking the antagonistic relations between Japan and the United States during World War II. Tanimoto was one of the six historical figures featured in John Hersey's journalistic account, *Hiroshima* (1946), to serve as its central focus for telling the story of the US atomic bombing of Hiroshima.[33] Tanimoto's Buddhist family, as the show revealed, indeed cut ties with him because of his devotion to Christianity. Although he would subsequently fall under US national security scrutiny because of his peace activism, Tanimoto, who was US-educated and fluent in English, was portrayed in *This Is Your Life* as a figure to whom American viewers could easily relate. By contrast, the show left untold the stories of other *hibakusha*, including those of the Hiroshima Maidens, the very group whom Tanimoto had accompanied to the United States.

Of course, the success of the Hiroshima Maidens project turned on their exposure in the US media. In his *Saturday Review* article on their impending visit, "The Maidens Are Coming," Cousins gave his American readers a glimpse of the women in two photos that conveyed their suffering in objectifying ways. In the first photo, one of the unnamed *hibakusha* faces the viewer, revealing a keloid burn that stretches from her torso to her face. Her severely burned mouth and neck appear as a dark shadow in the black-and-white photo. She pulls her dress down to her breasts. Her privacy may be violated, but her gaze at the camera portrays her courage and strength. Undermining her gaze, however, the caption under the photo describes the women as "so badly disfigured that they felt self-conscious about appearing in public," a message that *This Is Your Life* would reinforce.[34] As with the TV show, this partial visual exposure is implicitly framed as necessary for supporting the project. Indeed, the caption to this photo insensitively interprets the woman's gaze as a plea for supporting the project. In the second photo, the woman, most likely the same person, presents her disfigured hands, her fingers swollen and twisted. Her disfigured body is displayed like a specimen whose purpose is to be looked—if not

33. *Hiroshima* was initially published in the August 31, 1946 issue of *the New Yorker*. It was republished by the publisher Alfred A. Knopt that same year.
34. Cousins, Norman. "The Maidens Are Coming." *The Saturday Review*, April 9, 1955, 24, www.unz.org/Pub/SaturdayRev-1955apr09-00024.

gawked—at. This *hibakusha* may have courageously agreed to appear half naked for the American public—something that no Hiroshima Maiden consented to do in the Japanese press—yet in so doing, she pleaded for the necessity of the project through her bodily vulnerability to the American readers.[35]

The images of the *hibakusha* women's disfigured bodies reinforced the American viewers' recognition of their own healthy bodies: a legitimate premise of the guaranteed subjectivity that allowed them to gaze at the *hibakusha* women's vulnerable bodies. In *This Is Your Life*, Dr. Marvin Green—a former classmate of Tanimoto back in Emory University, who was one of the earlier surprise guests—with Edwards's cue, explained Tanimoto's humanitarian mission for the twenty-five *hibakusha* women whose bodies were "badly disfigured and maimed." Along with Green's talk were three visual images of the *hibakusha* women introduced for the corroboration: two group photos and a close-up image, the one published in *Saturday Review*. Tellingly, as this visual exposure of the women emphasized their physical disfiguration, the US media excessively invited the fantasy of the transformative power of American intervention on Asian lives through gaze.

As the program proceeded, the Hiroshima Maidens whose disfigurements did not fit into standards of "normative" bodies were visibly marginalized. After Dr. Green's introduction, the scopophilic spectatorship got suddenly blocked by a white screen. Namely, *This Is Your Life* strategically concealed its two *hibakusha* women guests from the viewers by presenting solely their silhouettes.[36] In contrast to the visual images of the Hiroshima Maiden's bodily exposure during Dr. Green's introduction, host Ralph Edwards introduced Minowa Toyoko and Emori Tadako, as follows: "Tonight, we would like you to meet two of these girls. Both have lived through the terror of an atomic bombing. To avoid causing them any embarrassment, we will not show you their faces." Edwards's remark distorts the definition of a meeting by impeding the encounter between the viewers and the *hibakusha* women. Far from directly encountering the *hibakusha* who have come to the United States with the Hiroshima Maidens project, the viewers are confronted with a screen shielding them from view. By ascribing "embarrassment" to the women behind the screen, Edwards paternalistically "protects" them while piquing the viewers' curiosity in their disfiguration. However, the word "embarrassment" indeed reveals the unsettled image of the *hibakusha* women that Edwards projects in his controlling narratives during the program. Robert J. Edelmann observes from a psychological standpoint that embarrassment "results when a perceived discrepancy occurs between one's current self-presentation and one's standard for self-presentation,

35. It should be noted that Cousins voiced his carefulness about not exploiting the Hiroshima Maidens by "parading the girls around." Shibusawa, *America's Geisha Ally*, 237.
36. Graham, "Re-Covering the Hiroshima Maidens," 126.

as a result of an undesired and unintentional social accident or predicament."[37] In this segment that the *hibakusha* women are forced to be invisible, Edwards is the subject who discerns the "discrepancy" that divides between the *hibakusha* women and the American viewers. Edwards unconsciously claims the physical deformity of the *hibakusha* women as a deviant form, in this case, in contrast to the healthy American viewers.

By positioning the first-person plural as the subject who makes the decision, Edwards's statement "we will not show you their faces" reveals the power differential at play. In contrast to *The Saturday Review* image in which the *hibakusha* preserves her "womanly" modesty by holding her dress just above her nipples, *This Is Your Life* frames the wounds and scars of US atomic warfare as requiring cover. The decorous nondisclosure of US-inflicted nuclear violence thus emerged from the gendered purview of these "maidens" from Hiroshima. By decontextualizing victims' suffering, popular culture allows viewers to indulge in "fantasies of witnessing the pain of others" while imagining the fiction of happy endings.[38] Distancing the viewers from the reality of how the atomic bomb devastated the Hiroshima Maidens' lives, the rehabilitative fantasy in *This Is Your Life* turned on the function of the silhouette itself as a kind of blank screen that sanitized the gruesome reality for TV entertainment.

The two Hiroshima Maidens, Minowa and Emori, played their expected roles by adapting to a racializing plot that enabled Americans to skirt national guilt by intervening, through their donations, in the benevolent makeover of Japanese victims of the atomic bomb. Cloaked by the silhouette, they said in Japanese, "We are really happy to come to the United States. And we appreciate what everybody has done for us."[39] Their expression of appreciation not only accentuated a racial/geopolitical hierarchy positioning Americans as saviors but also left unmentioned the complexity of physical and emotional suffering they endured. Erasing their individuality, the silhouette hindered the audience from knowing which woman (Minowa or Emori) actually spoke. That they were adhering to a script was obvious: Edwards knew what they would say beforehand, asking Tanimoto to confirm if the speaker said that they were happy to be in the United States and appreciated Americans. While Minowa and Emori's presence granted authenticity to the story of the Hiroshima Maidens, they remained hidden behind the silhouette, on the margins of a conversation centered on Tanimoto.

---

37. Robert J. Edelmann, *The Psychology of Embarrassment* (New York: John Wiley & Sons, 1987), 6.
38. Rothe argues that media representations of trauma in popular culture minimize the sufferings of victims, à la Susan Sontag's critiques of war photography in *Regarding the Pain of Others*. Anne Rothe, *Popular Trauma Culture: Selling the Pain of Others in the Mass Media* (New Brunswick, NJ: Rutgers University Press, 2011), 6.
39. Translation mine.

The visual erasure of the *hibakusha* women's body in the silhouette does not operate without intervention. Robert Lewis—a former pilot of the Enola Gay—who awkwardly encountered Tanimoto in an earlier segment was scapegoated to complete the plot. Tanimoto was not notified about the special guest in advance; his smile disappeared and he slightly postured backward while they shake hands. Comparably, in a matter-of-fact way, Lewis described the decisive morning of August 6, 1945, being unable to look at the eyes of Tanimoto and Edwards. His uneasiness on the stage was apparent in his pose, holding his hands back the entire time. Urged to mention by Edwards what he wrote on a log that day, Lewis almost choked himself and said with trembling voice, "Oh, my god. What have we done?" Lewis was heavily drunk and skipped the rehearsal, understandably nervous about his guilty feeling being broadcast on the national TV program. The problem here is NBC's exploitation of Lewis's decade of suffering from his guilt. As Tanimoto later recollects in his memoir, Lewis was, on his way to the stage, guided to pass through a waiting room where the *hibakusha* women were staying.[40] While the viewers were shielded from the deformed bodies of the *hibakusha* women for "protection," Lewis was contrarily forced to witness them, then later, the camera could capture him emotionally agitated by his further guilt.

In this context, the viewers can shoulder all their guilt onto Lewis—a sole scapegoat of the atomic atrocity—without looking at the actual physical deformity of Minowa and Emori. Instead, they can be entertained by the happiness of the Tanimotos that Edwards set up through the surprise reunion. After the "appearance" of the two *hibakusha* women, Edwards wholly switches the program's direction from the war trauma to the nuclear family fantasy by introducing Tanimoto's four children who appear holding each other's hands. While Tanimoto picks up the youngest child to hold, the rest of the three children sit on the couch with Mrs. Tanimoto. By changing the program's focus to the joyful Tanimotos, *This Is Your Life* celebrates the prosperity and futurity of the nuclear family, cutting the *hibakusha* women out of the screen. Worse, Lewis is unbearably forced to stand behind the Tanimotos along with two other guests and participate in this celebration of the nuclear family as a passerby of Tanimoto's life. With the celebratory segment of the Tanimotos, *This Is Your Life* divulges its limitation of dealing with the American guilt embodied in the disfigurement of the *hibakusha* women.

Contrary to the Hiroshima Maidens' marginalized status, the final segment centralized the Tanimotos as the subject through whom Americans could heal the guilt, presenting lavish gifts. Edwards excitedly gives a 16-mm sound projector and movie camera to the Tanimotos and a 14-karat gold charm bracelet for Mrs. Tanimoto. Not

---

40. Tanimoto Kiyoshi, *Hiroshima genbaku to Amerikajin: Aru bokushi no heiwa angya* (Tokyo: Nippon hoso shuppan kyokai, 1976), 179.

only does the TV program showcase American capitalistic generosity, but it also marginalizes the Hiroshima Maidens. If the Hiroshima Maidens are "embarrassed" by being looked at, as Edwards says, the movie camera defines the Tanimotos worthy subjects of recording that excludes the deformed Hiroshima Maidens from this conversation. Moreover, Mrs. Tanimoto, who dresses up in a kimono and smiles endlessly throughout the TV show, is presented with the jewelry that was specially ordered for her. Again, the Hiroshima Maidens are not considered here to receive the same luxury, as if they need to take care of their deformed bodies first before wearing gold bracelets. Accordingly, the TV program evaluates female bodies by deciding who is worthy of feminine luxury; in this case, Mrs. Tanimoto, as she fits into the idealistic female image—wife and mother—of the nuclear family, unlike the unwed *hibakusha* women with deformed bodies.

Newly Deformed Bodies Created in the Pacific

Norman Cousins, although well-known as a critic of the US decision to drop the atomic bombs and the nuclear arms race more generally, made a distinctively Cold War political pitch to prospective donors to the Hiroshima Maidens project by framing it as an instrument to discredit the Soviet Union. In his letter, he warned that the Atomic Bomb Casualties Commission (ABCC), whose sole purpose was to collect *hibakusha*-based data without treating the victims themselves, was being used by the Soviet Union to smear the global reputation of the United States.[41] For Cousins, the Hiroshima Maidens project offered a salutary American counter to the purported heartlessness of the ABCC. By selectively treating a handful of *hibakusha*, the Hiroshima Maidens project represented a critical political opportunity to change the negative image of the United States as a depraved superpower that used the victims of its atomic attacks as nuclear experiments. By responding to the humanitarian dilemma posed by injured Japanese female bodies, Americans intervened with personal donations, an act that ultimately disavowed US culpability for the atomic bombs. Cousins's fundraising appeals, however, neglected the fact that, in the very same historical window, the United States was literally experimenting with Marshallese lives by conducting nuclear testing on their lands and waters.[42] The

41. Letter from Norman Cousins to Henry Kotkins, January 19, 1955, Hiroshima Maidens: Correspondence, Memos folder, Office of the Director (Martin Steinberg) Records, 1939–1969, The Arthur H. Aufses, Jr. MD Archives, Icahn School of Medicine at Mount Sinai.

42. The United Nations mandated the Marshall Islands as a trusteeship under the United States (Trust Territory of the Pacific Islands) in 1947. However, the United States conducted sixty-seven nuclear tests in the Marshall Islands between 1946 and 1958, instead of assisting them to recuperate from war-torn damages and gain independence for sovereignty. In the 1954 Castle Bravo test, a bomb 750 times more powerful than the atomic bomb in Hiroshima was detonated. See Jonathan M. Weisgall, "The Nuclear Nomads of Bikini," *Foreign Policy*, no. 39 (1980): 84.

Hiroshima Maidens project elevated the US national conscience while simultaneously revising the American narrative of the impact of its use of nuclear weapons. In her influential critique of militourism in the Pacific, Teresia Teaiwa importantly contrasts the bikini as a garment of the leisure classes to the US nuclear tests on Bikini Atoll, with the former obscuring the horror of the latter.[43] The Hiroshima Maidens project enabled Americans to turn a blind eye to the simultaneous nuclear atrocities the United States was committing in the Marshall Islands.

The Cold War politics that the Hiroshima Maidens project embodied thus revealed the markedly partial nature of American "generosity," with most Japanese and Marshallese *hibakusha* who were regarded as disposable lives. However, the Hiroshima Maidens project served ideologically to renovate the image of US nuclear power and was consequently successful in advocating Cold War propaganda, no matter what causes its contributors were driven by. After the project, Cousins received a letter from the White House stating that President Eisenhower was "especially gratified at the fine impression they [the Hiroshima Maidens] made on all the American families with whom they lived during their stay here."[44] It is a contradictory statement coming from the president who initially undermined the Hiroshima Maidens project by refusing to meet them in the White House during their visit to Washington, D.C.[45] The White House understandably circumvented political backlash of being accused of admitting the atomic bombing as a culpable deed by not inviting the *hibakusha* women. However, Eisenhower's official endorsement of Cousins at the end demonstrates that the American civilians elevated the Hiroshima Maidens project as a successful humanitarian project that the White House could no longer ignore.

43. Teresia K. Teaiwa, "Bikinis and Other S/pacific N/oceans," *The Contemporary Pacific* 6, no. 1 (1994): 92.

44. Letter from Dwight D. Eisenhower to Norman Cousins, November 16, 1956, RG4/066, box 69, Pendle Hill Records, Friends Historical Library, Swarthmore College.

45. "Hiroshima Maidens Coming to Capital," *Washington Post*, April 9, 1956. Archived in RG2/NY/M633 2.19, Montclair Monthly Meeting, Friends Historical Library, Swarthmore College.

Section II

Socialist Medicine in Revolution

4

A Battle for Life

Bacteriophage Therapy and Socialist Medicine in the Great Leap Forward

Lu Liu

Cinematic narratives of medicine in socialist China (1949–1976) adopt a critical stance toward Western medicine that is deeply inflected by the state's policies.[1] While Western medicine was promoted by intellectuals and reformers as an antidote to pseudoscientific and superstitious practices in traditional Chinese medicine in the first half of the twentieth century, the People's Republic of China (PRC) sought to transform both by "scientifying Chinese medicine and sinicizing Western medicine" in the 1950s to create a hybrid and unified form of socialist medicine.[2] As medical knowledge production and practices continued to be reconfigured throughout the 1950s, the "Western medicine learning from Chinese medicine" initiation in 1954 and Mao Zedong's call to integrate the two medicines in 1956 officially rehabilitated scientific legitimacy to Chinese medicine, putting it on par with Western medicine. In the Cultural Revolution (1966–1976), the professionalism of Western medicine was further challenged by the "barefoot doctor" program,

1. As the literal translation of *xiyi* 西醫, "Western medicine" refers to a complex assemblage of medical knowledge, practices, and institutions informed by the development of modern biosciences and imported into China in the nineteenth century. In this chapter, the use of "Western medicine" highlights what Volker Scheid calls the "etic Chinese perspectives" in the 1950s that perceived and theorized the distinctions between biomedicine and indigenous medical practices under the term "Chinese medicine." Volker Scheid, *Chinese Medicine in Contemporary China* (Durham: Duke University Press, 2002), 4.
2. For an analysis of the theme of medicine in socialist films and literature, see Xiaoping Fang, "Changing Narratives and Persisting Tensions: Conflicts between Chinese and Western Medicine and Professional Profiles in Chinese Films and Literature, 1949–2009," *Medical History* 63, no. 4 (2019): 454–74. For the self-fashioning of traditional Chinese medicine in the face of Western medicine, see Sean Hsiang-lin Lei, *Neither Donkey Nor Horse: Medicine in the Struggle Over China's Modernity* (Chicago: University of Chicago Press, 2014). For the CCP's transformation of traditional Chinese medicine, see Kim Taylor, *Chinese Medicine in Early Communist China, 1945–1963: A Medicine of Revolution* (London: Routledge, 2011).

which dispatched young students trained in basic Chinese and Western medical knowledge to the countryside with the aim of addressing the uneven rural–urban distribution of medical resources.[3] As an innovative form of collectivized health care and a "new born socialist thing," barefoot doctors' paraprofessional status called into question the monopolization of the medical sector by a small group of city-based Western medical professionals. The criticism of elitist Western medicine is echoed in Zheng Junli's *Spring Comes to a Withered Tree* (*Kumu fengchun* 枯木逢春, 1961), which dramatizes the anti-schistosomiasis campaign, and Sang Hu's *An Ode to the Silver Needle under a Shadowless Lamp* (*Wuyingdeng xia song yinzhen* 無影燈下頌銀針, 1974), which deals with acupuncture anesthesia. In both films, a theoretically oriented doctor adhering to biomedical methods is contrasted with a representative of socialist medicine, who is willing to integrate Chinese medicine and learn from indigenous medical practices. The tension escalates in Xie Jin's *Spring Sprouts* (*Chunmiao* 春苗, 1975), as the antagonist Qian, a medical expert and saboteur of socialist health care enterprise, denies the eponymous barefoot doctor access to Western medical knowledge. As a result, the protagonist Chunmiao has to study herbal medicine to care for villagers while struggling with the class enemy. Centering around the crucial question of the right to practice medicine, these films registered an ideal vision of socialist medicine, wherein practitioners possess political consciousness and synthetical expertise of both Chinese and Western medicine.[4]

However, socialist medicine as the integration of Chinese and Western medical traditions seems missing in an earlier film by Sang Hu, *Spring Reigns Everywhere* (*Chunman renjian* 春滿人間, 1959). With an exclusive focus on Western medicine, the film narrates the rescue of steel worker Ding Dagang based on the "saving Qiu Caikang 邱財康" event of 1958.[5] A team leader at Shanghai No. 3 Steel Factory, on May 26, 1958, Qiu was severely injured in an accident with molten metal, which resulted in 89.3 percent of his body receiving second- and third-degree burns. While it was rare to survive an injury of such magnitude and severity in the 1950s, through the collective efforts of Guangci Hospital, research and pharmaceutical institutes, and the masses, Qiu miraculously recovered after six months of intensive care and returned to work as a safety inspector—a position he held until his retirement. *People's Daily*, an official newspaper, praised the rescue as the "communist spirit's

3. As Xiaoping Fang's study reveals, barefoot doctors prescribed various kinds of Western medicine despite the government propaganda highlighting traditional Chinese medicine. Xiaoping Fang, *Barefoot Doctors and Western Medicine in China* (Rochester, NY: University of Rochester Press, 2012).
4. Miriam Gross, "Between Party, People, and Profession: The Many Faces of the 'Doctor' during the Cultural Revolution," *Medical History* 62, no. 3 (2018): 333–59. For an account of *Spring Comes to a Withered Tree* and *Spring Sprouts*, see Ban Wang's "The Mass Biopolitics of Medicine in Socialist Chinese Films" in this volume.
5. Qiu's name was sometimes printed 丘財康 in the 1950s.

victorious battle against the demon of death" and "an unprecedented miracle in the human history of medicine."[6] Created to celebrate the medical achievements of the new China for its tenth anniversary, *Spring Reigns Everywhere* shows four critical stages in the worker's treatment: a joint consultation of biomedical experts; the search for a scarce antibiotic, Polymyxin B; the homologous skin grafting surgery; and the use of phage therapy to contain *pyocyaneus* infection. Biomedical methods and drugs feature prominently, with no reference to Chinese or indigenous medicine.

Spring Reigns Everywhere invites a renewed understanding of socialist medicine in the 1950s outside of the Chinese–Western medical dyad. Despite the absence of Chinese medicine, an underlying tension between the elite and professionalized paradigm of Western medicine and the envisioned ethos of "socialist medicine" pervades the film and is manifest in the prolonged debates throughout the narrative about whether and how the worker can be saved. The ostensibly technical and medical procedures are profoundly inflected by contrasting interpretations of medicine's purpose, ethos, and content, as shaped by Marxist and capitalist ideologies. Instead of contesting who can practice medicine, the film and the "saving Qiu Caikang" event problematize and redefine the patient role by posing the question: Who is entitled to medical treatment?

In his anthropological study of patients and healers, Arthur Kleinman theorizes medicine as a "cultural system, a system of symbolic meanings" in Clifford Geertz's sense—i.e., the ways actors think about and deal with illness and treatment. The system includes health-related "beliefs" (knowledge production and ethics), "choices and decisions" (of both the doctor and the patient), "roles" and their "relationships" (e.g. doctor–patient relationship), "interaction settings" (e.g. hospital wards), and "institutions."[7] Kleinman's system of medicine would align well with the medical environment in socialist China, in which the Chinese Communist Party (CCP) regulated medical knowledge and practices, promoted new ethics, reconfigured doctor–patient and doctor–CCP relationships, and ultimately redefined illness and treatment. Following this framework, socialist medicine can be perceived as a complicated ecology of social relations—conspicuously underscored and amplified in the rescue of Qiu Caikang. Drawing on Kleinman's framework, this chapter investigates how socialist medicine as an ecology is narrativized vis-à-vis biomedical knowledge and expertise in the Qiu Caikang rescue and broadly explores interactions among 1950s media culture, medical knowledge production, and political campaigns. Furthermore, this chapter focuses on two forms of social relations that

6. "Gongchanzhuyi jingshen zhansheng sishen," *Renmin ribao*, June 29, 1958.
7. Arthur Kleinman, *Patients and Healers in the Context of Culture: An Exploration of the Borderland between Anthropology, Medicine, and Psychiatry* (Berkeley, CA: University of California Press, 1980), 24–70.

structure the rescue: the triangulated CCP–doctor–patient relationship shaped by the redistribution of medical expertise, and the interconnected relationship of the community informed by phage therapy.

Narrating the CCP–Doctor–Patient Relationship

The Great Leap Forward (1958–1962) is often perceived as having been detrimental to people's health. Irrational policies of industrialization and collectivization, exacerbated by unrestrained voluntarism, led to widespread famine from 1959 to 1962, with an estimated death toll of 30–45 million.[8] New medicine invented under the call for grassroots innovation also raises questions and invites ridicule if examined from a "scientific" perspective, such as "chicken blood therapy," where raw chicken blood is injected into humans to boost energy—a hybrid approach born from Soviet "tissue therapy" and Chinese folk practice.[9] An exception among inflated miracles of the time, Qiu Caikang's rescue is still remembered in the history of biomedicine for forging new treatment protocols in extensive burn care and for being one of the earliest successful trials of phage therapy on *pyocyaneus* infection. The case also received international recognition: in 1988, the American Burn Association conferred on Shi Jixiang, the leading surgeon in the rescue at Guangci Hospital, the Evans Award.[10]

The medical event became submerged in and inseparable from its narratives. Hailed as "medicine's leap forward," it inspired myriad cross-platform narrativization and kindled the "Qiu Caikang fever" well before Qiu's full recovery. A sanctioned idea of socialist medicine circulated through the texts via a standardized plotline as well as intertextual references that, together, constituted a transmedial ecology of socialist medical culture. An incomplete list of narratives includes Ba Jin's reportage literature "A Battle for Life" ("Yichang wanjiu shengming de zhandou" 一場挽救生命的戰鬥); children's literature *The Party Saved His Life* (*Dang jiuhuo le ta* 黨救活了他) and a single-episode TV drama under the same title; spoken dramas *Red Flags Flying* (*Hongqi piaopiao* 红旗飘飘) and *A Communist Song of Victory* (*Gongchanzhuyi de kaige* 共產主義的凱歌); and the educational film *A Song of Victory for Life* (*Shengming de kaige* 生命的凱歌), directed by Yu Qi and Du

8. Frank Dikötter, *Mao's Great Famine: The History of China's Most Devastating Catastrophe, 1958–1962* (London: Bloomsbury, 2010).

9. Liz P. Y. Chee, "'To Cure a Hundred Diseases': Animal Blood Therapies in Mao's China," *Science, Technology and Society* 23, no. 2 (2018): 195–213.

10. Hu Jun and Zhen Cheng, "Da yuejin qijian qiangjiu gangtie gongren Qiu Caikang: Zhang Disheng fangtan," *Zhongguo kejishi zazhi* 32, no. 2 (2011): 222–30; Zongcheng Yang, "Development of Burn Medicine in China," in *Chinese Burn Surgery*, ed. Zongcheng Yang (Dordrecht: Springer Netherlands, 2015), 1–7.

Shenghua.[11] *Spring Reigns Everywhere* is arguably the most successful adaptation, directed by veteran director Sang Hu and starring popular faces such as Bai Yang and Wang Danfeng, the latter widely acclaimed for her portrayal of a devoted, caring, yet also fashionable nurse in Tao Jin's 1957 *A Nurse's Diary* (*Hushi riji* 護士日記). The rescue also inspired folk songs, *pingtan* art, and local Yue and Huai operas that facilitated a multisensory consumption of the event. Many voluntarily created narratives by local stage troops or doctors in the hospital attested to the cultural enthusiasm to propagate the miracle while exhibiting a commitment to eulogization and ideological didacticism.[12]

The transmedia storytelling was bracketed within a self-reflexive search for the true "protagonist" (*zhujue* 主角) in the story, which strategically addressed official criticism that early news reports of the rescue inappropriately highlighted doctors as the main heroes and overlooked the "noble qualities of the working class."[13] The first to re-narrativize the rescue, "A Battle for Life" begins in medias res with cultural workers documenting "a battle in progress" at the hospital. When a filmmaker asks who should be written as the protagonist, a Party cadre answers, "everybody": "The Party connected our hearts together into one whole, and it was this community that saved our comrade."[14] Taking over this collectivist note, *Spring Reigns Everywhere,* which bookends the narrative fever, resets the conversation in the injured worker Ding Dagang and his fiancée Zhu Xiuyun's wedding at the end of the film. Surrounded by reporters, doctors, and factory workers—all participants in the rescue—the Party secretary Fang Qun jokingly asks not to be photographed since the protagonist is not her but society as a whole, which inadvertently echoes Kleinman's systemic view of medicine. Doctors noticeably recede from the spotlight yet remain part of the settings; they become integral to the healing community in a broader, more encompassing sense.

In the context of the Anti-Rightist Campaign (1957–1958), the search for the true protagonist externalized a fundamental question regarding medical expertise and its practitioners, which remained under heated debate throughout the socialist

11. Ba Jin, "Yichang wanjiu shengming de zhandou," *Renmin wenxue* no. 8 (1958): 107–12; Ma Xinde and Gu Meizhong, *Dang jiuhuo le ta* (Beijing: Shaonian ertong chubanshe, 1958); Chen Gongmin and Wang Lian, *Gongchanzhuyi de kaige* (Shanghai: Shanghai wenyi chubanshe, 1958); Xie Junfeng, et al., "*Shengming de kaige,*" *Zhongguo dianying* no. 1 (1959): 53–74. For a comparison of the narratives, see Qin Yi, "Yichang gonggong shijian de kuameiti chuangzuo: dui xianlipian *Chunman renjian* de kaocha," *Zhongwai yingshi* no. 2 (2020), 82–89.
12. Chen Shaochang, "Wo yu renyi de yidian yuanyuan," *Xinmin wanbao,* June 23, 2012.
13. Zuo Hua, "Women weishenme meiyou baodao hao Qiu Caikang," *Chuanmei pinglun* no. 10 (1958): 17, 23.
14. Ba Jin, "Yichang wanjiu shengming de zhandou," 107.

era.[15] The campaign started as a backlash against those who criticized the CCP when Mao encouraged critique from below during the Hundred Flower Movement (1956). One common complaint in science and medicine was that the CCP, a "paraprofessional" (*waihang* 外行), meddled with fields that only professionals (*neihang* 內行) understood. Soon, the Anti-Rightist Campaign condemned those who spoke up as rightists and subjected them to reeducation and even persecution. Amidst harsh attacks against technocratic elitism as a "superstitious" belief in the unchallenged authority of experts, the masses were elevated as primary agents and their practices as the only means of knowledge production.[16]

To reiterate the orthodoxy that "paraprofessionals can lead professionals," the aforementioned narratives deploy an episodic structure, where doctors learn from the patient, the masses, and CCP cadres how to apply Marxist–Maoist dialectics to medical practices.[17] A thought-reform episode, which features prominently in all narratives but is most elaborate in *Spring Reigns Everywhere*, offers a case in point. At a joint consultation, doctors all despair because the burns are over 70 percent, which, according to medical experts in the film, the "Evans statistics" from the United States identify to be indicative of 100 percent mortality. A top expert, Professor White, insists that statistical numbers reflect objective laws and cannot be altered by political enthusiasm—a view shared by a skillful yet conservative Director Fan.[18] The film's mise-en-scène spatializes the professional gap between doctors clustering at the center and workers from Ding Dagang's factory at the margin. This hierarchy is inverted when factory worker Liang Shichang, who is saved from fire by Ding, "opens up" the conversation controlled by a small clique. Drawing on his experience from the pre-1949 old society, where he was expelled from the factory and refused treatment in hospitals after injury, Liang questions why workers continue to be denied treatment in the new society. The chasm between doctors' professionalism and indifference toward patients is subtly highlighted with the mounted photo of the

15. Christos Lynteris, *The Spirit of Selflessness in Maoist China: Socialist Medicine and the New Man* (London: Palgrave Macmillan, 2012).
16. Sigrid Schmalzer, "Red and Expert," in *Afterlives of Chinese Communism: Political Concepts from Mao to Xi*, ed. Christian Sorace, Ivan Franceschini, and Nicholas Loubere (Canberra: ANU Press, 2019), 215–20. In the 1950s, the meaning of superstition expanded from pseudoscientific beliefs to be expelled by science to beliefs in expert knowledge to be redressed by Marxism. See Kunnze Rui and Marc Matten, *Knowledge Production in Mao-Era China: Learning from the Masses* (Lanham: Lexington Books, 2021), 1–29.
17. "Paraprofessionals can lead professionals" appeared in Guangci Hospital's work summary of the rescue circulated on newspapers, medical journals, and propaganda pamphlets. *Zhongguo gongchandang Shanghai dier yixueyuan weiyuanhui, "Guanyu qiangjiu tangshang gongren Qiu Caikang tongzhi de gongzuo zongjie," Shangyi xuebao* no. 2 (1958): 83–89.
18. "White and expert" (*baizhuan* 白專) was a derogatory term in the Anti-Rightist Campaign for reactionary and self-interested experts with an apolitical view of science, as opposed to the ideal of "red and expert" (*you hong you zhuan* 又紅又專).

Canadian doctor Norman Bethune "rescuing the dying and healing the wounded" (*jiusi fushang* 救死扶傷) on a makeshift operating table in wartime China.[19]

Turning the consultation into a "speaking-bitterness" (*suku* 訴苦) meeting—a form of political mobilization where individual sufferings were publicly narrated—Liang's words reinforce and feed into the CCP secretary Fang's class analysis. Later in the sequence, Fang mediates a debate between Director Fan and a progressive young doctor who criticizes Fan's "superstition" in foreign literature. Extrapolating Liang's experience in the Marxist view that all knowledge is class-based, Fang deconstructs the objectivity of the Evans statistics as a product of the exploitative Western society, where injured workers receive neither compensation nor treatment from capitalists and hospitals. Conversely, a socialist society can overcome the statistical limit because it cares for workers' lives and can mobilize resources to save them. These words, so fundamental to the mindset transformation of the bourgeoise doctors, are reproduced nearly verbatim from other narratives. Pinpointing the source of Fang's Marxist class analysis in the worker's lived experiences, the film underscores the mass line (*qunzhong luxian* 群眾路線) that incorporates the masses' practices, perspectives, and needs in knowledge production. Reshaping the doctors' cognitive knowledge about medical statistics helps to channel a new affective bond with the working class: unlike statistics generated within the context of capitalist sociopolitical systems that justify the dispensability of workers' lives, socialist medicine forges a caring doctor–patient relationship in the spirit of "serving the patient wholeheartedly" (*quanxin quanyi wei shangbingyuan fuwu* 全心全意為傷病員服務).[20]

Resonating with the mass line, Qiu Caikang's avatars undergo multiple recreations in the transmedia reiteration. While early works focus on hospital scenes, a prelude depicting the factory worker's skills in steel production was added to the spoken drama *A Communist Song of Victory* and retained in the two film adaptations, interpolating a form of the worker's expertise as equal to the doctor's medical knowledge. The positive characterization is enhanced by the reason for the injury, which shifts from an accident to the worker's self-sacrificial protection of his comrades and the public property of the factory. A more subtle revision lies in the meaning of physical pain that comes to be expressed as "intrinsically emotional/affective" and

19. Bethune came to support the CCP's wartime medicine in 1938 and died of fatal infection the next year. Valorized by Mao's memorial essay, Bethune embodied the spirit of sacrifice and humanitarianism in wartime and socialist China. Xiaoning Lu, "In the Name of Internationalism: The Cinematic Memorialization of Norman Bethune in Socialist China," in *The Oxford Handbook of Communist Visual Cultures*, ed. Aga Skrodzka, Xiaoning Lu, and Katarzyna Marciniak (Oxford: Oxford University Press), 341–63.

20. Fu Lianzhang, "Yiwu gongzuozhe he bingren zhijian," *Huli zazhi* no. 5 (1959): 137–39. For the revolutionized doctor–patient relationship, see Shao Dan, "Red Star over Medicine: Redefining Doctor–Patient Relationship in Early CPC History (1930s–1960s)," *East Asian Science, Technology and Society: An International Journal* 14 (2022): 1–31.

sublimated to a source of revolutionary spirit.[21] While "A Battle for Life" offers direct portrayals of physical suffering, where Qiu "grinds his teeth to suppress his groans" and evokes the spiritual healing of Chairman Mao, such stark depictions gradually phase out in subsequent narratives.[22] The educational film *A Song of Victory for Life* processes the inevitable pain in a debate over anesthesia, where the CCP cadre criticizes the doctors' suggestion of using general anesthesia as a lack of confidence in "the working class's strong willpower."[23] Equating pain with tenacity helps to displace corporeal vulnerability to a test of revolutionary virtues. Still, a scene in *Spring Reigns Everywhere* briefly captures the patient's agony before switching to the doctors and nurses who are experiencing the pain vicariously. The film suggests the transformative power of viewing another's pain, as the Party secretary Fang, visibly touched by witnessing the pain, is determined to save the worker's life in the following scene of the joint consultation. Increasingly fictionalized through reproductions, Qiu becomes the ideal type (*dianxing* 典型) of socialist realist aesthetics. This metamorphosis resonates with Mao's 1942 "Talks at the Yan'an Forum on Literature and Art," that "raw materials" from the life of the people should be refined and elevated "into the ideological form of literature and art serving the masses of the people."[24] Along with the remaking of the mind (expertise), spirit (self-sacrifice), and body (physical pain), Qiu transitions from being merely a patient to a multifaceted personality—a skillful laborer, selfless hero, and brave and tenacious warrior—which is not only a utopian model to be emulated by the audience but also a point of contrast to the self-centered and politically conservative intellectuals.[25]

The worker-patient ideal type possesses diagnostic and curative power. Evidently to echo the Anti-Rightist Campaign rhetoric, at the end of "A Battle for Life" the narrator compares Qiu's injury to "an illness encroaching the mind of the intellectuals for a long time"—a metaphor that is reinforced in *Spring Reigns Everywhere* through Director Fan thanking Ding for curing his illness.[26] In Western medicine, wherein the biomedical doctor's access to exclusive expertise and technology often grants

21. Rob Boddice, "Introduction: Hurt Feelings?" in *Pain and Emotion in Modern History*, ed. Rob Boddice (Basingstoke: Palgrave Macmillan, 2014), 2–3.
22. Ba Jin, "Yichang wanjiu shengming de zhandou," 111.
23. Xie Junfeng, et al., "Shengming de kaige," 60.
24. Mao Tse-tung, "Talks at the Yenan Forum on Literature and Art," in *Selected Works of Mao Tse-tung*, vol. 3 (Beijing: Foreign Languages Press, 1965), 84.
25. The process also foreshadows the production and transmission of an emulation culture during the Cultural Revolution, in which a model (*mofan* 模範) figure or institution in reality was established as the exemplar of revolutionary virtues, while a model (*yangban* 樣板) character or cultural product was an idealized fictional creation. These real and constructed models needed multiple copies to carry on their cultural and political valences. Laikwan Pang, *The Art of Cloning: Creative Production During China's Cultural Revolution* (London: Verso, 2017).
26. Ba Jin, "Yichang wanjiu shengming de zhandou," 112.

authority over the patient, such a reciprocal cure revolutionizes the hierarchical doctor–patient relationship by empowering an active and agential patient.[27] Yet, the film and other narratives also speak explicitly of an ultra-doctor—the CCP that cures the doctors' bourgeoise ideology and harnesses their expertise in the wholehearted service of the people. The treating procedure wherein ideological shortcomings are exposed to light, criticized, and cured through persuasion and education is captured in the slogan "to cure the illness and save the patient" (*zhibing jiuren* 治病救人).[28] First articulated by Mao in the 1942 Yan'an rectification campaign, in the socialist era the guiding principle stressed leniency and tolerance when handling solvable issues such as ideological deviance of Party cadres and the people. The triangulated CCP–doctor–patient dynamics, featuring a twofold cure that cloaks the doctor's transformation under the apparent physiological treatment, implicates a judgment of who is treatable. While in the rescue of Qiu Caikang, the question of treatability necessitates a critical reassessment of medical statistics that is revealed to be deeply political, the Maoist slogan medicalizes the political issue of who can be reintegrated to the ranks of the people. Socialist medicine identifies, recognizes, and produces a treatable subject, both the doctor and the patient.

An Ecological Cure

In the reportage literature "A Battle for Life," the conversation crediting society as a whole for saving Qiu's life is adjoined by the narrator's introduction of phage therapy, creating a textual affinity between the political message and the medical treatment. The narrator reports that Qiu is at a critical stage, as the *pyocyaneus* bacilli on his leg have begun resisting the antibiotic Polymyxin B, and everyone is waiting for the new medicine of bacteriophages to kick in. Phage therapy—the therapeutic use of bacteriophages to treat pathogenic bacterial infections—is extolled in the rescue and its narratives as an exemplar of the collaborative spirit of socialist medicine: it unites a bacteriologist's innovative treatment proposal, medical students' sample collection in sewage water and experiments with isolating virulent bacteriophages, and a research institute's assistance in producing sufficient doses.[29] Phage therapy is said to promptly contain the infection and save the worker's leg from the amputation

27. For the perfectly passive patient required by modern Western science, see Lei Hsiang-lin, "Fuzeren de yisheng yu you xinyang de bingren: Zhongxiyi lunzheng yu yibing guanxi zai minguo shiqi de zhuanbian," *Xinshixue* 14, no. 1 (2003): 45–96.

28. The complete slogan is "learn from past mistakes and avoid future ones; cure the illness and save the patient" (*chengqian bihou, zhibing jiuren* 懲前毖後，治病救人). Mao Tse-tung, "Rectify the Party's Style of Work," in *Selected Works of Mao Tse-tung*, vol. 3 (Beijing: Foreign Languages Press, 1965), 35–51.

29. Yi Jun, "Gongchanzhuyi sixiang de kaige: kan yingpian *Chunman renjian*," *Dianying yishu* no. 2 (1960): 59–61.

recommended by bourgeoise doctors, who believe antibiotics to be the only cure for bacterial infection. The competition between bacteriophages and antibiotics here symbolizes yet another "struggle between the socialist and capitalist treatment methods."[30] Examining the discourse around bacteriophages and phage therapy in socialist China, this section argues that, besides the literal level, phage therapy offers a medical metaphor and narrative structure of socialist medicine.

Competition with antibiotics signifies the rise and fall of phage therapy. The challenge of antimicrobial resistance that has raised global concerns and recently called attention back to phage therapy was prophetically foreshadowed in the 1950s Qiu Caikang rescue. Phage therapy was invented in the 1910s by the Pasteur Institute bacteriologist Felix d'Herelle, who was credited with the discovery of bacteriophages (literally "bacteria-eaters") separate from earlier findings by Frederick Twort of Britain. Interested in the potentials of bacterial viruses that could infect and dissolve their hosts, d'Herelle isolated phages from bacteria, cultured them to become more virulent, and experimented with them on infected patients. By the 1930s, phage therapy had traveled with d'Herelle and his collaborators to Japan, Egypt, Brazil, the United States, and Georgia of the USSR through a "Pasteur's Empire."[31] However, mass-producible antibiotics soon replaced phage therapy in most parts of the world in the late 1940s, since antibiotics were more stable compounds and could target a wider array of bacterial strains than mutant and selective bacteriophages, which were harder to produce, preserve, and prescribe.[32] It was during this period that the liaison between phage therapy and the Soviet Union was cemented. Soviet scientists either missed or intentionally overlooked phage therapy's decline on the other side of the Iron Curtain, due to halted medical exchange between the newly formed socialist and capitalist camps.[33] America's economic embargo created a lacuna of antibiotics in both the Soviet Union and the PRC, which also served phage therapy.[34]

---

30. *Zhongguo gongchandang Shanghai dier yixueyuan weiyuanhui, "Guanyu qiangjiu tangshang gongren Qiu Caikang tongzhi de gongzuo zongjie,"* 83.
31. Aro Velmet, *Pasteur's Empire: Bacteriology and Politics in France, Its Colonies, and the World* (Oxford: Oxford University Press, 2020). For the transnational routes of phage therapy, see William Summers, *Félix d'Herelle and the Origins of Molecular Biology* (New Haven, CT: Yale University Press, 1999), 125–72; Akihito Suzuki, "Public Health, Laboratory Experiment, and Asymptomatic Carriers in Japan, ca. 1920–1950," *East Asian Science, Technology, and Society: An International Journal* 13 (2019): 39–55.
32. Charlotte Brives and Jessica Pourraz, "Phage Therapy as a Potential Solution in the Fight Against AMR: Obstacles and Possible Futures," *Palgrave Communication* 100 (2020): 1–11.
33. Dmitriy Myelnikov, "An Alternative Cure: The Adoption and Survival of Bacteriophage Therapy in the USSR, 1922–1955," *Journal of the History of Medicine and Allied Sciences* 73, no. 4 (2018): 388.
34. Phage therapy promoted under Soviet assistance was never widely administered in the PRC and withdrew from the medical scene in the 1960s, losing its battlefield once again to antibiotics, whose efficacy was well-established during the War of Resistance against Japan (1937–1945). An Rui, "Shijunti zhiliao de qianshi, jinsheng, yu weilai," *Kexue tongbao* no. 23 (2017): 2577–80.

Phage therapy was packaged as a Soviet medicine when introduced to the PRC amid the "Learn from the Soviet Union" movement in the early 1950s. The Soviet label, lexicon, and practices provided an ideological shield at a time when the class nature of all knowledge, especially biological sciences, was under scrutiny. Chinese science writings about phage therapy credited the Russian physician Nikolay Gamaleya for discovering the phenomenon of bacteriophage lysis two decades earlier than Félix d'Hérelle. More important, the PRC inherited from the Soviet Union an ecological view of perceiving infection and recovery as interactions between different biological agents and their environment.[35] The ecological view informed two issues in phage research in the PRC: the relationship between bacteriophages and the human body in treatment, and between bacteriophages and the ecology in epidemic prevention.[36] Under the theoretical framework, the Soviet infrastructure raised phages against local bacterial strains using samples in situ from rivers, ditch drains, and patient stool. The modus operandi, reflected in the collection of sewage water and feces samples in the Qiu Caikang narratives, was adopted in the PRC when the regime was restructuring its pharmaceutical industry to better utilize indigenous resources and promote self-sufficiency in the face of a drug shortage.[37]

Drawing on the ecological model, bacteriologist Yu He 余賀 (a student of the bacteriologist Hans Zinsser at Harvard University and the prototype of the professor who proposed phage therapy in the rescue) explained the efficacy of phage therapy in terms of the interaction between therapeutic agent and pathogen, which once existed symbiotically.[38] Artificially injected phages must first unite with and multiply within bacteria before lysis could start, but the process was sometimes interrupted by the immune system, which (mis)recognized phages as harmful foreign bodies and absorbed them.[39] Hence, for phage therapy to take effect, a double alienation was prerequisite: first, the disengagement of bacteriophages from host bacteria; then a temporary inhibition of the immune system from cleaning the phages. The healing process of introducing, detecting, and eventually *integrating* the alterity complicates what Carlos Rojas calls "homesickness," a condition where "a node of alterity is structurally *expelled* from an individual or collective body in order to symbolically

35. The ecological model was first envisioned by Félix d'Hérelle but was significantly developed in the Soviet Union, especially in the George Eliava Institute in Tbilisi, Georgia. See William Summers, *Félix d'Herelle and the Origins of Molecular Biology*; Dmitriy Myelnikov, "An Alternative Cure."

36. Si Chengdong and Yu Zhili, "Liji shanghan ji fushanghanyi shijunti fenli fangfa de yanjiu," *Weishengwu xuebao* 2 (1955): 145–50; Chen Shu, ed., *Sulian chuanranbing yufang zhidao* (Shanghai: Huadong yiwu shenghuo chubanshe, 1952), 101–3.

37. Liz P. Y. Chee, *Mao's Bestiary: Medical Animals and Modern China* (Durham, NC: Duke University Press, 2021), 53–70.

38. "Guangci yiyuan qiangjiu Qiu Caikang bingshi dang'an xuanzai," *Dang'an zhencang* no. 4 (1998): 52–58.

39. Yu He, *Xijunxue* (Beijing: Renmin weisheng chubanshe, 1956), 48–53.

reaffirm the perceived coherence of that same body" (my emphasis).[40] Rojas argues that in the tumultuous modern Chinese history, differentiating and extricating internal alterity presented avenues to negotiate the boundary of the body, individuality, and political community, and to propel national transformation. Due to the liminality of bacteriophages as viruses stemming from the very bacteria they target, distinctions between infection and treatment, between the self and alterity, were less than clear-cut. Phage therapy, in this light, helped reimagine a biosocial ecology where phages, host bacteria, body organism, and the immune system coexist in coordination and interdependence.

The new conceptualization of an organically interconnected community, informed by phage therapy's ecological cure, is echoed in the Qiu Caikang rescue, where all social sectors contribute to the healing of Qiu's physical body and the reintegration of his renewed self into social production. The narratives are saturated with actions of care from the masses that complement the doctors' cure: pharmacies seek antibiotics and research institutes produce phage doses during drug shortages; chefs of local restaurants design menus to boost Qiu's appetite; factory technicians customize a bed that allows easy turnover without damaging the wound; and the large amount of blood, plasma, and skin necessary to remake Qiu's body come from the masses' donations.[41] These vignettes demonstrate a "circuit of care relations," wherein the need for care is identified, recognized, encoded, and decoded between multiple givers and receivers.[42]

Omitting most of the interludes, *Spring Reigns Everywhere* portrays the circuit of care beyond the hospital as enabled by a nexus of media technology and information dissemination. The film opens with a radio journalist's on-site reporting of a productivity competition between Ding Dagang and Liang Shichang. While speaking into his tape recorder, the journalist's occasional glance at the camera shows his awareness of an audience beyond the auditory. Broadcast through a Great Leap Forward radio program, the sound wave of the reporting accompanies a montage of domestic (living room), production (printing house and bicycle factory workshop), and consumption (bookstore and department store) spaces. A vibrant and orderly socialist urban life boasting material affluence provides the basis of the all-inclusive rescue. A similar montage reappears later, connecting workers, peasants, and soldiers practicing collective listening to radio news about the hospital's bold leap forward in

40. Carlos Rojas, *Homesickness: Culture, Contagion, and National Transformation in Modern China* (Cambridge, MA: Harvard University Press, 2015), vii.

41. Ba Jin, "Yichang wanjiu shengming de zhandou," 110–11; Ma and Gu, *Dang jiuhuo le ta*, 21–27, 30–32; Chen and Wang, *Gongchanzhuyi de kaige*, 48–61.

42. Amy Holdsworth, Karen Lury, and Hannah Tweed, introduction to *Discourses of Care: Media Practices and Cultures* (London: Bloomsbury Academic, 2020), 7.

overcoming doctors' superstition. The seemingly random listeners would reconvene at the hospital to donate skin for Ding Dagang.

Between scenes of the on-site reporting and the interview at the wedding that bookend the film, the rescue unfolds as a media event, as key treatment steps are either facilitated by communication media such as telephone calls and letters, or publicized through local and national media. The film is keen on showing the routes and nodes of communicative exchanges. Officially sanctioned news, amplified by close-ups of the radio station's tape player, radio receiver, and newspaper article, intersect with information circulating at the local level through a big-character-poster or in bus passengers' conversations. Early on, Ding's treatment faces an acute shortage of antibiotics. Right after domestic Polymyxin B finally becomes available and is transported via airplane from Kunming to Shanghai, a big-character-poster bulletin in the hospital courtyard announces the good news to a small group of readers, among whom the radio journalist and newspaper reporters continue to carry the information to a larger audience.

As the treatment progresses, a more intimate form of social relations infiltrates the biological realm to remake Ding Dagang's body. After Ding's infection is temporarily controlled, a call for skin donation attracts waves of donors from the holy worker-peasant-soldier alliance, intellectuals, and, beyond the PRC territorial border, an overseas-worker-turned-student. The standard for qualified donors, which excludes "people whose productive work might be impacted, who are not robust or with skin diseases, and women," is concretized by these young, strong male laborers contributing to socialist construction.[43] In a hospital hallway, where the donors compete to be selected, a deep sense of class feeling (*jieji ganqing* 階級感情) bonds the donors, who are motivated not just by elemental instincts of altruism but also by restructured social relations. As observed in an audience response, in the film, "communism establishes a deepest, perfect, and unprecedented interpersonal relationship."[44] Ending the skin grafting treatment abruptly with this convivial scene, the narrative insinuates a collectivist treatment that a small patch of skin is taken from each donor to shorten the recovery period and avoid slowing down social production. The film omits the fact that, due to the body's immunological reaction, homologous skin would fall off or disappear days after grafting and is only

43. The exclusion of female donors is based on the consideration that skin grafting would leave a scar on the body. In other narratives, the gender aspect is not mentioned, and skin from a just deceased person happens to be available right before the masses' donation.

44. Nanda zhongwenxi yingpingzu, "Renlei lishi de xinchun: xikan *Chunman renjian*," *Baihua* 11 (1960): 9. The donation of blood and organs in Chinese history is often motivated by patriotism or economic incentives. A case in point is blood donation in the Republican era, see Wayne Soon, "Blood, Soy Milk, and Vitality: The Wartime Origins of Blood Banking in China, 1943–45," *Bulletin of the History of Medicine* 90, no. 3 (2016): 424–54.

an expedient to preventing infection when autologous skin from the patient is not ready—as documented by Joshua Horn, a British medical expert in socialist China.[45] By fictionally suppressing Ding Dagang's immune system, which might recognize and clear homologous skin, the film inadvertently enhances the ecological mechanism of phage therapy. Ding's symbolically charged body is a collective work, which, segment by segment, absorbs biological differences among the people. Instead of fragmenting the body as an aggregate of replaceable parts, the transplantation recreates an integral yet interpersonal body—an ultimate purpose of socialist medicine.

While the circuit of care and collective skin donation reconstitutes Ding Dagang's physical body, the ecological cure of phage therapy also elucidates a broader understanding of the social body as an engaged member of social production. As mentioned above, phage therapy comes to the rescue when the patient's leg is about to be amputated due to life-threatening septic infection. In *Spring Reigns Everywhere,* Director Fan's insistence on amputation is grounded in the medical stance that prioritizes the preservation of life, but the Party cadre Fang reminds him that the patient should not merely survive but "live well." Fang says that a "doctor's responsibility is not just life and death, but to care about the people's happiness and ideals," which, for a socialist worker, means the freedom and right to participate in labor and contribute to social production. The social body, transcending biological existence and physical completeness, extends to the ability to fulfil social roles. Socialist medicine thus redefines recovery, measured not only by the disappearance of injury-related symptoms but by the patient's return to socialist construction.

Bio-ideological Discourses of Bacteriophages

Having discussed how phage therapy provides a narrative form for the rescue, the last section examines the evolving discourse of bacteriophages in socialist China that uncannily paralleled, commented on, and engaged with ideological discourses of the time to reconsider the CCP–doctor/intellectual relationship. Bacteriophage's promiscuous relationship with ideological debates must be contextualized within the turbulent transformation of biology in socialist China. A notorious case was the monopolization of Michurinism, which proposed that a change of environment could manipulate heredity and that acquired traits were hereditary. In response, Chinese biology had to revamp itself into this transformist model, at the great cost of denouncing and banning the so-called reactionary Mendalian-Morgan

45. Joshua Horn, *Away with All Pests: An English Surgeon in People's China, 1954–1969* (New York: Monthly Review Press, 1969). Grappling with the immunological reaction is hinted at in *A Communist Song of Victory,* in which skin grafting is compared to "experimental plots" (*zhong shiyantian* 種試驗田) that take repeated trials and errors. Chen and Wang, *Gongchan zhuyi de kaige,* 54.

genetic theories.[46] In microbiology, Michurinism was best represented by Olga Lepeshinskaia's postulation of noncellular "vital substance" that could develop into cells under external forces, and Gevork Bosh'ian's new conception of bacteriophages as a "phenomenon of decomposition, disintegration of the bacterial cell into particles" that could reassemble into bacteria.[47] How to interpret Bosh'ian's phasic view posed a challenge for Chinese biologists, who adopted a wide array of terms on the spectrum of animacy: ultramicrobial living cell, bacterial enzyme, bacterial virus, filtrable form of bacteria, composite of bacteria, and noncellular form of bacteria—all relationally defining phages through bacteria. Bosh'ian's bold claim of bacteriophages' liminal status between life and non-life was incorporated into textbooks and celebrated in mass media in the 1950s. In particular, the Marxist philosophy of science cited it to validate Friedrich Engels' idea of life as protein in the constant self-renewal of chemical constituents.[48]

Maoism constituted a localized contact zone between bacteriophages and ideology. In the early 1950s, professional and popular science writings alike introduced the bacteriophage with the sentence "Where there is a bacterium, there is its bacteriophage," to account for its ubiquity and diversity. In *Spring Reigns Everywhere,* the simple saying is repeatedly uttered by the bacteriology professor on the darkest eve of Ding's recovery to reassure the Party cadre that there must exist a natural antidote to *pyocyaneus* bacilli. That all pathogens had its antagonistic structure aligned perfectly with Mao's dialectical theory of contradiction, formulated during the War of Resistance against Japan, through which Mao articulated the universality and absoluteness of contradiction as "unity in opposites."[49]

When Mao refined his theory in the 1957 speech "On the Correct Handling of Contradictions among the People," the biological discourse of bacteriophages was accordingly updated. In the speech, Mao famously differentiated antagonistic contradiction between the people and the enemy from nonantagonistic and reconcilable contradiction among the people, and pointed out that in the concrete condition of China, the former could be transformed to the latter if handled properly.[50] Appropriating Mao's theory, Yu He distinguished the "antagonistic contradiction," where virulent phages lysed bacteria, from the "non-antagonistic contradiction," where moderate "prophages" coexisted with bacteria. The two types were also

46. Lawrence Schneider, *Biology and Revolution in Twentieth-Century China* (Lanham: Rowman and Littlefield, 2003).

47. Quoted in Dmitry Myelnikov, "Creature Features: The Lively Narratives of Bacteriophages in Soviet Biology and Medicine," *Notes and Records* 74 (2020): 589.

48. Liu Sizhi, "Shengming de qiyuan wenti," *Ziran bianzhengfa tongxun* no. 1 (1956): 60–61.

49. Mao Tse-tung, "On Contradiction," in *Selected Works of Mao Tse-tung,* vol. 1 (Beijing: Foreign Languages Press, 1965), 311–47.

50. Mao Tse-tung, "On the Correct Handling of Contradictions among the People," in *Selected Works of Mao Tse-tung,* vol. 5 (Beijing: Foreign Languages Press, 1965), 384–421.

interchangeable, argued Yu He. The DNA of an old virulent phage could enter a new bacterium as prophage that not only lived with the host but also immunized the host to its own lysis. However, since "the unity was conditional and relative and the struggle was absolute," when mutation occurred in certain conditions, the prophage would mature into a virulent phage once again and lyse the host bacteria, resulting in an endlessly cyclical struggle.[51]

Yu's analogy, at first sight a straightforward and even mechanical application of Mao's phrases to biology, unwittingly laid bare the unspoken subtext of the 1957 speech and commented on an inherent ambivalence of Maoism, which Carlos Rojas summarizes as the internal contradiction between "resolving" and permitting or even encouraging contradiction.[52] Mao's speech was first delivered in February 1957 to address recent changes to socialism at home and internationally, in particular the completion of the socialist transformation of agriculture, industry, and commerce in 1956. In the new context, Mao asserted that contradiction did not disappear but leaned towards the form of frictions and tensions among the people who supported socialism. Encouraging the ongoing Hundred Flowers Campaign was on Mao's mind; he attributed the people's critique of the CCP and Marxism as nonantagonistic and to be exempt from penalty. Confident that the Hundred Flowers Campaign was the correct way of handling contradiction among the people and that it would invigorate the Party, Mao assumed a linear change that turbulent class struggles abated to moderate and protracted struggles in the ideological realm.[53] The backward transformation from nonantagonistic to antagonistic contradiction, as the speech warned, only occurred because of improper handling or resistance. Such a view was implicitly countered in Yu He's bacteriophage analogy, which suggested that mutual transformation between the two contradictions was not only certain to happen but also constituted a driving force of evolution. In the same article, quoting Engel's definition of life as protein, Yu identified codependent interactions between parasitic agents such as viruses and phages and their hosts as the beginning of evolution, thus perpetuating mutual transformation of the two contradictions in a constant and continuous cycle.[54]

The cycle also ramified in the political realm. The general air of tolerance in the Hundred Flowers Campaign swerved to restriction when Mao sensed that criticisms of the Party started to get out of control. The heavily edited script of Mao's speech published in the *People's Daily* four months later shifted to a more solemn tone and added the threat of "right opportunists," who appeared to attack dogmatism and

51. Yu He, "Weishengwu yu jiti," *Zhexue yanjiu* no. 3 (1962): 23–28.
52. Carlos Rojas, "Contradiction," in *Afterlives of Chinese Communism*, 43–48.
53. Frederick C. Teiwes, *Politics and Purges in China: Rectification and the Decline of Party Norms, 1950–1965*, 2nd ed. (Armonk, NY: M. E. Sharpe, 1993), 233–82.
54. Yu He, "Weishengwu yu jiti."

bureaucratism, "but what they are really attacking is the quintessence of Marxism."[55] In the same month, the Anti-Rightist Campaign replaced "blooming and contending," reinterpreting what used to be a nonantagonistic critique from below as an antagonistic attack from the rightists. The speech by Mao witnessed the transformation it tried to forestall in the first place.

Written in 1962, Yu He's article could be read as a retrospective comment on the political context where the rescue of Qiu Caikang took place, packaged in the language of microbiology. Doctors in the rescue of Qiu Caikang, Yu included, were closer to witnesses than victims of the CCP's swerving policy, neither sent to the countryside for reeducation nor barred from medical practice. Rather, they received the treatment of "curing the illness and saving the patient," which Mao in the speech prescribed as the solution to contradiction among the people. As the endless struggle and mutual transformation continued, however, the Cultural Revolution would more radically revamp socialist medicine with the nationwide barefoot doctor program and a new wave of criticism against medical expertise and professional practitioners. Interestingly, Yu's 1962 article, written halfway between the rescue and the beginning of the Cultural Revolution, did not mention any therapeutic use of the antagonistic contradiction between virulent phages and bacteria, partly because phage therapy had already fallen from popularity. Phage therapy that required a temporary suspension of the immune system that would otherwise clear the phages also posed a subtle critique of the mechanism that thwarted the Hundred Flowers Campaign. To use Mao's own medical metaphor in the speech, the vision of "immunizing" the CCP and Marxism through "discussion, criticism, and reasoning" failed because critical voices that could have constructed a healthy body of political opposition were too swiftly recognized as foreign and harmful.[56]

55. Mao, "On the Correct Handling of Contradictions among the People," 411. For the textual revision from the speech to the publication, see Timothy Cheek, *Mao Zedong and China's Revolution: A Brief History with Documents* (Boston: Bedford/St. Martin's, 2002), 21–24.
56. Mao, "On the Correct Handling of Contradictions among the People," 410.

5

From Curing to Revolutionizing

The Politics of Disability in Chinese Socialist Medicine and Media

Chao Wang and Yuqian Yan

Disability poses a challenge to the socialist vision of revolution for improving the human condition. In the early People's Republic of China (PRC), the Chinese Communist Party (CCP) innovatively deployed medicine and media to demonstrate the curative and revolutionary potential of disabled bodies, countering the social stigma of being labeled "disabled and hence useless" (*canfei* 殘廢). Sarah Dauncey, in her examination of disability representation in PRC films, points out the significant absence of images of physically impaired individuals from 1949 to 1976, arguing that in Maoist China, only "picture-perfect" disabled figures, mostly the deaf-mute, testified to the socialist ideal of the "healthy body."[1] When disabled people were depicted in socialist media, they often underwent a transformation into "cured" individuals capable of contributing to socialist construction. And yet, such narratives of recovery from disability were far from homogenous, as they were shaped by the coevolution between Chinese medical practices and socialist politics. The treatment of the disabled body should not be readily equated with extracting labor potential for national development, nor does it imply a simplistic dismissal of people with incurable disabilities. Rather, the treatment of disabled bodies in socialist China accentuated access to medical resources as a form of political inclusion and a means of fostering revolutionary agency.

This chapter aims to scrutinize the socialist positioning of disability, specifically focusing on "deaf-muteness" (*longya* 聾啞), through the lens of its perceived

1. Sarah Dauncey, "Screening Disability in the PRC: The Politics of Looking Good," *China Information* 21, no. 3 (2007): 481–506. See also Sarah Dauncey, *Disability in Contemporary China: Citizenship, Identity and Culture* (Cambridge: Cambridge University Press, 2020), 56.

curability.[2] Our exploration reveals how media portrayals of what counted as a cure for the disabled intersected with shifting ideological legitimations of Chinese medicine and socialism. Socialist medicine and media framed physical impairment as contingent consequences influenced by diverse physical, social, and political factors, treating it as a matter of collective concern rather than individual liability.[3] Through our historically contextualized analysis, we illustrate how the medicalization of sensory impairments allowed the socialist state to manifest revolutionary objectives of overcoming social inequalities. We hope to reflect the way in which deaf-muteness becomes what Ian Hacking calls a "moving target," which encompasses diverse understandings of illness, social marginality, and political oppression.[4] The relatively stronger presence of deaf-mute people in media, as Dauncey noticed, was not simply because they "look good." Rather, the medicalization of deaf-muteness literally and metaphorically embodied the socialist rhetoric of "giving voices to people" as a critical step toward the ultimate realization of one's revolutionary agency.

The acupunctural treatment of deaf-muteness received significant media attention from the 1950s to the 1970s. Acupuncture-cured cases in media reports and representations generated an unlikely mutual transformation between the previously marginalized practice of acupuncture in Chinese medicine and the neglected role that disabled people played in the Communist Revolution.[5] By tracing the wartime development of Chinese medicine in Yan'an before 1949, we show how acupuncture had gained a foothold in the CCP's health politics by treating the "mass body" of soldiers and peasants. This path differed from the scientization of acupuncture to survive the competition with Western biomedicine in urban-based public health. After 1949, acupuncture became instrumental to the party-state's reformulation of socialist medicine from below. The new medical system aimed to ensure equal access to medical resources for previously underprivileged groups, among which the disabled was a representative group.

2. We use "deaf-muteness" to refer to hearing and speech disabilities in the realms of medicine and media. When deafness and muteness were discussed in the medical context of socialist China, the term "deaf-mutism" (*longya zheng* 聾啞症) was favored by doctors, as it indicates the medicalization of disability.
3. Originally created by disability activists in the UK, the "social model" negates the understanding of disability as an impairment and hence a medical problem of the individual. Rather, it views disability as socially constructed oppression, discrimination, and exclusion of people with impairments. See Michael Oliver, *The Politics of Disablement* (London: Palgrave Macmillan, 1990).
4. Ian Hacking, "Making Up People," in *Reconstructing Individualism: Autonomy, Individuality, and the Self in Western Thought*, ed. Thomas Heller et al. (Stanford, CA: Stanford University Press, 1986), 222–36.
5. A notable exception to the marginality of disabled groups in the revolutionary tradition of the CCP is blind artists, who had been effectively mobilized by the party to join the campaign to reform local folk culture in the 1940s. See Chang-tai Hung, "Reeducating a Blind Storyteller: Han Qixiang and the Chinese Communist Storytelling Campaign," *Modern China* 19, no. 4 (1993): 395–426.

Our use of "socialist medicine" refers to both the influence of the Soviet medical theory and the pragmatism devoted to addressing local problems with the combination of Chinese medicine and Western biomedicine.[6] Moreover, this hybrid approach to curability emphasizes the affinity between medical practices and political ideologies that reimagine the revolutionary agency of both the healers and those being healed. The relationship between disability and socialist medicine underwent significant changes in response to the shifting Sino-Soviet relations during the first two decades of the PRC. Driven by the alliance with the Soviet Union against capitalism during the early 1950s, Chinese medical doctors started to negotiate with the Republican-era legacy of scientific acupuncture by looking for alternative theoretical foundations in Soviet medical science. Their adoption of Pavlovian neuropathology in explaining the therapeutic effectiveness of needling facilitated a breakthrough in the conceptual legitimation of acupuncture. During the Cultural Revolution (1966–1976), the proclaimed healing of deaf-mute bodies was framed in Chairman Mao Zedong's political agenda of reforming urban-based public health to serve the masses. Getting access to medical treatment manifested a new politics of inclusion for the disabled.

This chapter begins by charting the pre-1949 effort of Chinese-medicine practitioners to reform acupuncture against the hegemony of Western biomedicine. The epistemic crisis not only gave birth to scientific acupuncture in the Nationalist public health; it also led to the Communist effort to draw from Soviet medical theory to revolutionize acupuncture for dealing with rural health problems and mass mobilization. We then move on to discuss the relationship between medical research and media representation of acupuncture-cured deaf-muteness in the 1950s. The appropriation of Soviet scientific methods to prove the miraculous effect of "making the mutes speak" valorized the status of acupuncture in socialist medicine. The last section turns to propaganda images, educational documentaries, and films to show the political transcendence of the cured deaf-mute people into revolutionaries with newly gained voices.

6. Some scholars viewed the post-1949 emulation of the Soviet model in the Chinese medical profession as a continuity of the "state medicine" model that originated in the 1930s, which paid special attention to the distribution of health care services in rural areas and the combination of grassroots health workers and Western-trained medical professionals. See AnElissa Lucas, "Changing Medical Models in China: Organizational Options or Obstacles?" *The China Quarterly* 83 (1980): 461–89; C. C. Chen, *Medicine in Rural China: A Personal Account* (Berkeley, CA: University of California Press, 1989).

Socialist Medicine before 1949: Acupuncture for the "Mass Body"

In the early twentieth century, Western medicine entered China through the expansion of foreign powers in the urbanizing treaty ports. In the context of semicolonialism, physicians of Western biomedicine and practitioners of traditional Chinese medicine clashed in perceptions of therapeutic efficacy, knowledge of disease, and the containment method. The Manchurian Plague of 1911 had installed a fear of germs on the post-imperial anxiety of national sovereignty, leading to the ascendency of biomedical power through replacing indigenous practices that were deemed "unscientific."[7] Take acupuncture as an example; practitioners of Western medicine noted that the lack of sterilization of acupuncture needles facilitated the spread of germs and infectious diseases, causing impairments due to the infections of smallpox, measles, and trachoma.[8] Since 1928, the Nationalist government in Nanjing prioritized biomedical treatments such as hypodermic injection in its urban-based public health campaigns against the spread of infectious diseases.[9] The lack of scientific validation further endangered the status of Chinese medicine in the state-sponsored national medicine (*guoyi* 國醫), causing a debate within Chinese medical circles over the abolishment of native medical practices based on speculative theories.

Responding to the marginalization and devaluation of Chinese medicine by Western doctors and Nationalist modernizers, two distinctive trends of reforming acupuncture could be observed in the Republican period (1912–1949). One is a theoretical endeavor by the reformers of Chinese medicine, who believed that this venerable tradition could only be saved by scientization. Cheng Dan'an, in particular, deployed Western anatomy in relocating acupuncture points (acupoints hereafter) and reclaiming their curative efficacy from the application of neurological

7. Sean Hsiang-Lin Lei, "Sovereignty and the Microscope: Constituting Notifiable Infectious Disease and Containing the Manchurian Plague (1910–11)," in *Health and Hygiene in Chinese East Asia: Policies and Publics in the Long Twentieth Century*, ed. Angela Ki-Che Leung and Charlotte Furth (Durham, NC: Duke University Press, 2010), 73–108.
8. From 1910 onward, Western physicians took special note of the "deadly acupuncture needles" and other instruments used in Chinese surgery that caused severe injuries and disabilities of the body. See W. Hamilton Jefferys and James L. Maxwell, *The Diseases of China, Including Formosa and Korea* (London: Bale and Danielson, 1910), 20–21.
9. Ruth Rogaski has documented the effort of the Nationalist Health Department to explain to citizens the danger of indigenous belief in acupuncture and scraping therapy as a means of legitimizing the connection between germ theory and the governmental capacity in managing epidemics. See Ruth Rogaski, *Hygienic Modernity: Meanings of Health and Disease in Treaty-Port China* (Berkeley, CA: University of California Press, 2004), 236–37.

theory.[10] The advocates of scientific acupuncture were based in Jiangsu and Zhejiang provinces. United in the Society of Reforming Chinese Medicine, they engaged in studying the clinical effectiveness of acupuncture in the treatment of sensory and neurological disorders and explaining the therapeutic action in terms of nervous stimulation.[11] The influence exerted by the community of medical reformers, however, did not fundamentally alter the marginal status of acupuncture in the Nationalist-led medical modernization. For example, the promotion of scientific acupuncture did not help practitioners of Chinese medicine to gain an equal professional status as those who earned a degree in biomedicine under the Nanjing government.[12] During the War of Resistance against Japan, the relocation of the Nationalist government had forced its biomedical personnel to adapt to a predominant Chinese-medicine marketplace in the southwest hinterland.[13] Despite this, the wartime regime's capacity to deliver health care for the military and civilians was heavily dependent on biomedical aid from the US and UK.[14]

In contrast, the CCP's medical modernization, developed in the rural base area of Yan'an, prioritized the treatment of the "mass body" with acupuncture as a way to overcome the domination of Western medicine in the name of science. Mao's call to mobilize all health resources for war resistance had created a space for a "new acupuncture" to emerge through the combination of Western anatomy and Soviet medical theory. The involvement of new acupuncture helped shape a revolutionary health politic that morphed into the socialist public health system in the 1950s.

After 1937, the CCP faced an even greater shortage of biomedical supply in Yan'an and other base areas due to the Japanese invasion and Nationalist blockade.

10. Bridie Andrews, *The Making of Modern Chinese Medicine, 1850–1960* (Vancouver: UBC Press, 2014), 198–205.
11. On blindness, see Xu Shichang, "Zhenci mumang zhi jingyan," *Yixue zazhi* 10 (1922): 101–3. On deafness, see Wei Zongdai, "Zhenci erlong ji shijuezheng zhi jingyan," *Yixiue zazhi* 35 (1927): 92–94. On paralysis, see Xu Shichang, "Banshen busui kouyan woxie cifa," *Yixue zazhi* 21 (1924): 103.
12. In 1929, the Ministry of Health revoked the professional licensing of Chinese medicine in an attempt to push such practitioners out of the field. See Sean Hsiang-lin Lei, *Neither Donkey nor Horse: Medicine in the Struggle Over China's Modernity* (Chicago: University of Chicago Press, 2014), 101–17.
13. In the wartime capital of Chongqing, the ratio of medical personnel between Chinese medicine doctors and biomedical physicians was about 2.5:1. Nicole Elizabeth Barnes, *Intimate Communities: Wartime Healthcare and the Birth of Modern China, 1937–1945* (Oakland, CA: University of California Press, 2018), 38.
14. From 1938 to 1940, the Red Cross Medical Relief Corps became a major funding and supply agency, connecting overseas Chinese and medical professionals with Chinese ties through organizations such as the ABMAC (American Bureau for Medical Aid to China) and the BFRDC (British Fund for the Relief of Distress in China). John R. Watt, *Saving Lives in Wartime China: How Medical Reformers Built Modern Healthcare Systems Amid War and Epidemics, 1928–1945* (Leiden: Brill, 2013), 129–37.

Promoting acupuncture was therefore a reasonable choice as it was cheap, portable, and effective in treating the military disease if conducted properly under sanitary conditions. A progressive view of Chinese medicine as a mass-oriented, useful technique with revolutionary potential was best illustrated in Mao's talk during a conference held in the Shan-Gan-Ning Border Region in 1944. Mao called on biomedical doctors to unite with Chinese medicine practitioners since the latter group was tied to the minds of local people. "If they (modern doctors) do not unite with thousands and more doctors and veterinarians of the old type," said Mao, "then they (traditional doctors) will actually be helping the witch doctors and showing indifference to the high human and animal mortality rates."[15] Despite the condescending tone, Mao's embrace of Chinese medicine in fighting quackery and superstition reflected a political strategy to cope with the insufficiency of biomedical resources without resorting to science as the common denominator for health recipients. The achievement of a united front of medical care for the masses was therefore not determined by the adoption of biomedicine. Rather, it relied on the Party's ability to harness the potential of Chinese medicine in treating the "mass body."

A major communist reformer of acupuncture was Zhu Lian 朱璉 (1909–1978), who was trained in biomedicine but later turned to Chinese medicine after joining the People's Liberation Army (PLA). Zhu was a leading figure in the experimentation of acupunctural therapies in Yan'an, and her book *New Acupuncture* was first published in 1951, two years after the Communists won the Civil War against the Nationalists. Zhu's major contribution was to theorize the therapeutic effects of acupoints with a combination of Western anatomy and Soviet medical theory, particularly the Russian physiologist Ivan Pavlov's theory of neuropathology. This theory holds that all pathological phenomena are caused by the stimuli of tissues (*zuzhi* 組織, which also means "organization" in Chinese), which is a key difference from the biomedical explanation of nervous stimulation as centered on individual cells. When used to interpret the working of acupuncture, according to Kim Taylor, the stimulation theory of tissue/organization satisfied the Communist strategy of wartime mobilization, as the medical terms carried military metaphors in the service of the Communist revolution.[16] In the new framework of revolutionized acupuncture, therapeutic effectiveness was no longer built on the basis of the Western stimulation theory that Cheng and other reformers had incorporated, which was "partial and fragmented" (*pianmian de, gelie de* 片面的, 割裂的), according to Zhu. Tissue

15. Mao Tse-tung, "The United Front in Cultural Work," in *Selected Works of Mao Tse-Tung*, vol. 3 (Peking: Foreign Languages Press, 1965), 235–37.
16. Kim Taylor, *Chinese Medicine in Early Communist China: 1945–1963* (London: Routledge, 2005), 26. It is worthy to note that in the draft of *New* Acupuncture completed in 1949, Zhu did not mention Pavlov in her credit to Soviet science. See note 118, in Taylor, *Chinese Medicine in Early Communist China*, 179.

stimulation provides an integral understanding of disease as controlled by advanced nervous function, namely the cerebral cortical control of nerve tissues through inhibition and excitation.[17] Pavlovian reflexology thus offered a theoretical foundation for the reconceptualization of acupuncture therapy as a way to trigger the repair of the nervous system beyond the acupoints surrounding a specific channel or skin area.

In Zhu Lian's new acupuncture, the incorporation of relevant acupoints located across anatomical sections had been key to treat illnesses by not directly intervening into a particular disease area. For example, when treating sensory disorders such as deafness, muteness, and blindness, new acupuncture combines the acupoints located in the anatomical sections of the ear, mouth, and eye with other related acupoints located in the head and neck section. This holistic approach allowed new acupuncture to move away from the medical reductionism of scientific acupuncture, which used cell pathology to explain the effectiveness of nervous stimulation.[18]

The gathering of acupoints into organizations of nervous stimulation carried political implications of mobilizing the maximum manpower for the rural Communist revolution. The CCP's recognition of a marginalized practice within the medical system of its political rival marked a major step in integrating acupuncture into socialist medicine. As we will show, revolutionary new acupuncture became a pillar of socialist medicine in the 1950s and redefined the curability of disability through the treatment of the "mass body."

Soviet Transformism, Socialist Medicine, and the Acupunctural Cure of Deaf-Muteness

After 1949, acupuncture was promoted by the CCP nationwide as an easy-to-learn, effective, and low-cost treatment for the masses. Besides the training of professional acupuncture practitioners, institutes of Western medicine also started to integrate acupuncture after Mao stated in 1954 that "the priority is to make Western medicine learn from Chinese medicine, not the other way around."[19] The wide application of acupuncture to treat popular diseases such as malaria, schistosomiasis, and

17. Zhu Lian, *Xin Zhenjiu Xue* (Beijing: Renmin weisheng chubanshe, 1954), 14.
18. For an exposition of the correspondence between nerves and disease cells in scientific acupuncture, see Cheng Dan'an, "Zhenci zhixiao zhi yanjiu," *Xinglin yixue yuebao*, vol. 47 (1933): 12–15. For a comparison with Soviet science in new acupuncture, see Taylor, *Chinese Medicine in Early Communist China*, 26–29.
19. Zhonggong zhongyang wenxianshi, *Mao Zedong nianpu* (Beijing: Zhongyang wenxian chubanshe, 1993).

appendicitis further secured its place in the socialist medical system.[20] The theoretical foundation that Zhu Lian laid out in her *New Acupuncture* remained influential in the early 1950s, when the nascent socialist regime adopted the "leaning to one side" foreign policy of the Cold War and placed medical science under the tutelage of Soviet science. In particular, the CCP valorized Ivan Pavlov's theory of conditional reflex in the treatment of sensory and neurological disorders. This was inherited from the ideology of Soviet transformism, which, according to Claire Shaw, originated in the 1920s as a strand of behavioral psychology that portrayed individual deficiencies as changeable through interactions with the social environment. Turning the deaf-mute into speaking subjects had been a key model of inclusion in the Soviet ideological landscape.[21] In the 1950s, Soviet transformism continued to be an inspiration for Chinese medicine to fashion a "cure" for the disabled in China. The acupunctural treatment of disability, and deaf-muteness in particular, provides a telling example of the "miraculous" transformation of the previously marginalized disabled group into capable and respectable socialist citizens. In the rhetoric of socialist medicine, such a "miracle" was reliant on scientific research and the participation of deaf bodies in the revolutionary politics of transformism.

Since 1950, clinical experiments on the acupunctural treatment of hearing disorders have been undertaken by a host of medical institutions, including medical schools, research institutes, and hospitals. In 1952, Ren Yizun, son of the famous Yan'an-era acupuncturist Ren Zuotian, successfully cured a deaf-mute patient. This led to the publication of a series of clinical reports on the effect of acupuncture in treating "deaf-mutism" (*longya zheng* 聾啞症), a term indicating the etiology of deaf-muteness as a disease. Ren was later assigned to work at the medical department of the Bureau of Industrial Machinery in Shenyang, together with two other practitioners of acupuncture, Wu Zhisheng and Zhang Zhixue. In 1953, the three of them conducted a clinical experiment with the treatment of deaf-mutism of four main types, including congenital deafness, and deaf-mutism caused by infectious diseases, external injury, and psychoneurological shock. According to their reports, among the 155 patients being treated with acupuncture therapy, thirty-seven (23.8 percent) regained hearing and speech functions. The measurement of curability also extended to those who obtained normal hearing in one ear (12.2 percent) or could hear partial sound (21 percent).[22] The experiment continued for another year with

20. For the role of acupuncture in medical campaigns against epidemics over the first seventeen years of the PRC, see Xiao Xiong, *Xinzhongguo shiqinian zhenjiu tuiguang yudong yanjiu* (PhD Dissertation, Guangzhou zhongyiyao daxue, 2021).
21. Claire L. Shaw, *Deaf in USSR: Marginality, Community, and Soviet Identity* (Ithaca, NY: Cornell University Press, 2017), 33.
22. A list of biomedical diseases is shown in the survey indicating the various curability rates. These include typhoid fever (13.5 percent), measles (12.2 percent), smallpox (0.64 percent), meningitis

an enlarged patient group of 355 and reported a similar rate of effectiveness (*youxiao lu* 有效率) as 54 percent.[23]

These clinical treatments of deaf-muteness primarily focused on enhancing the neurological effect of needling a set of traditional acupoints located in the ear section, such as *tinghui* 聽會 and *yifeng* 翳風, as well as *yamen* 啞門 of the neck section, until the patient feels sore and numb. This was intended to stimulate the receptor of the auditory nerve and cause the reflex of the brain to restore hearing and speech functions.[24] Research in 1956 showed that the majority of the cases of deaf-muteness occurred in the damage of the inner ear, which includes the disorders of the auditory receptor, the auditory nerve, and certain parts in the central regions of the auricle. Hence, the therapeutic method was focused primarily on the restoration of the auricular functions by acupunctural stimulation. These studies acknowledged that the method applied was particularly effective in the treatment of neurotic hearing and speech loss and less effective in restoring congenital and organic defects.[25] Such findings led to more selective inclusion of sample patients, resulting in higher reported rates of effectiveness in other regions, such as Shaanxi and Jiangsu provinces.[26]

One of the major problems in the definition of *effectiveness* was due to the lack of a uniform standard in clinical recordings and evaluations between doctors of Chinese and Western medicine. In fact, Wu Zhisheng mentioned as early as 1954 that Chinese acupuncturists lacked adequate knowledge and equipment to perform medical inspection, which led to the failure to identify those with incurable congenital deformities.[27] A team of physicians at the Beijing Hospital of Otolaryngology found that acupunctural treatment could not be successful in restoring the perpetual damage of the inner ear, and the general phenomenon regarding the improvement

---

(3.8 percent), cerebral concussion (3.2 percent), tympanites (1.9 percent), and throat diseases (3.2 percent). Wu Zhisheng, Zhang Zhixue, "Zhenjiu liaofa zhiliao longya zheng de jige bing'an," *Beijing zhongyi* 3, no. 5 (1953): 20.

23. The acupuncture-cured cases include 78 completely cured, 42 half-cured and 72 partial-cured. Shenyang zhongyi xuehui, "Guanyu zhenjiu liaofa duiyu zhiliao longya zheng de jiaoliu jingyan zuotanhui zongjie," *Beijing zhongyi* 3, no. 2 (1954): 31.
24. Wu Zhisheng, Zhang Zhixue, "Shenjingxing longya zhifa chubu jieshao," *Zhongyi zazhi*, no. 1 (1955): 32.
25. Wu Zhisheng, Zhang Zhixue, "Shenjingxing longya zhifa chubu jieshao," 35. For acupuncture-cured cases of neurotic deafness and mutism, see Wang Qiming, "Guanyu longya zhenjiu zhiliao qingkuang jieshao," *Zhongyi zazhi*, no. 1 (1956): 36–37.
26. Published reports by hospitals in Xi'an and Nantong in 1956 showed the rates of effectiveness for neurotic deaf-mutism as 73.8 percent and 78.43 percent, respectively. See Shaanxi sheng zhongyi jinxiu xuexiao fushe menzhenbu, "Zhenjiu shizhi longya 42 li de baogao," *Zhongyi zazhi*, no. 1 (1956): 31; Yuan Mingdong, Chen Xinyuan, "Zhenjiu zhiliao longya 153 li de jingyan xiaojie," *Zhongyi zazhi*, no. 12 (1956): 647.
27. Shenyang zhongyi xuehui, "Guanyu zhenjiu liaofa duiyu zhiliao longya zheng de jiaoliu jingyan zuotanhui zongjie," 31–32.

of hearing in most deaf-mute cases ended in regression after discontinuing the treatment.[28] The audiologist Deng Yuancheng conducted an investigation of twenty-eight patients who had been treated by acupuncture for a year. With the assistance of the electric audiometer, Deng found that only 3.6 percent had a distinct effect.[29] This finding contradicted the result obtained from treating neurotic deaf-mutism and revealed the lack of differentiation between effective and ineffective treatments.

During the Great Leap Forward (GLF), the framing of acupuncture-cured deaf-mutism as a political achievement not only further boosted the rate of effectiveness but also initiated the media portrayal of such treatment results as miracles. *People's Daily*'s report on the 11th Affiliated Hospital of Shanghai Chinese Medicine School in 1958 presented both statistics and detailed cases of cured individuals.[30] At the following national medical conference, the hospital representative gave a talk entitled "Acupuncture Creates Miracles," which included a tape recording of cured deaf-mutes cheering "Socialism is great" and "Long live the Chinese communist party."[31] The tape recording not only served as convincing proof of the result but more importantly turned the attendees into witnesses of miracles. By July 1959, the deputy minister of the health department announced that the effectiveness rate of selected hospitals had reached 85 percent.[32]

The miraculous effect of acupuncture was also highlighted in the publicity materials of the science and education documentary *Treating Deaf-muteness with Acupuncture*: "In the Mao era, deaf people can hear and mutes can talk. It is by no means an exaggeration, but a vivid reflection of our great times."[33] Produced by the Shanghai Science and Education Film Studio in 1959, the film features a young girl, Xiaoping, who loses hearing and speech due to an infection that damages the cochlear and acoustic nerves. Luckily, she receives proper education at a special school for the deaf-mute, thanks to the Party, and is eventually cured by Doctor Zhao through deep and prolonged needling, a method that is "inspired by the theory of Western medicine," as the film puts it. Different from the common perception of

---

28. Liu Ruihua, Liu Qian, Li Lin, Deng Yuancheng, and Tan Huizhen, "A Statistical Study of 560 Case of the Deaf in Peking," *Chinese Medical Journal* 75, no. 9 (1957): 753–63.
29. Deng Yuancheng, et al., "Longya zheng," *Zhongji yikan*, no. 9 (1956): 28–31.
30. Zhao Zhifang, "Zhenjiu zhi longya," *Renmin ribao*, August 27, 1958, 7.
31. Shanghai zhongyi xueyuan fushu dishiyi renmin yiyuan, "Zhenci chuangzao qiji: longzi ting daole zongluxian xuanchuan; yaba kaikou huijiang shehui zhuyi hao," in *Quanguo yiliao weisheng jishu geminig jingyan jiaoliu dahui huikan*, ed. Quanguo yiliiao weisheng jishu geminig jingyan jiaoliu dahui mishuchu (Beijing: Renmin weisheng chubanshe, 1958), 246–47.
32. Qian Xinzhong, "Zhongxiyi qinmi hezuo renzhen de zhengli yanjiu zuguo yixue," in *Quanguo zhongyi jingluo zhenjiu xueshu zuotanhui ziliao xuanbian*, ed. Quanguo zhongyi jingluo zhenjiu xueshu zuotanhui mishuchu (Beijing: renmin weisheng chubanshe, 1959), 3.
33. "Zhenjiu zhi longya," *Shangying huabao*, no. 8 (1959): 23. The film is currently unavailable for public access.

documentaries as recording or recollecting real-life stories, Xiaoping and Doctor Zhao were prototypes that represented a typical case of their times, showcasing a scientific miracle made possible by the advantageous socialist system of health care.

The character of Doctor Zhao was likely to be modeled on Yang Fuzhi, whose experiment with deep needling caught public attention through extensive reports by the *People's Daily* on December 10, 1958. Yang used to work in a local health station in Hubei province. After successfully curing several deaf-mute patients with acupunctural therapy, he was recruited into the county hospital and became a specialist in the field. According to the reports, Yang used his knowledge of Pavlovian physiology and anatomy to challenge the conventional understanding of *yamen* as a forbidden acupoint. He conducted experiments on his own body and applied controlled trials to prove the safety and effectiveness of deep needling at *yamen*.[34] As a physician trained in Western medicine but integrated with Chinese medical practice, Yang was praised for his achievement in uniting the two and for his anti-establishment spirit promoted during the GLF.

The use of scientific measurement to validate acupunctural treatments of deaf-muteness in the 1950s culminated in the extremely high rate of effectiveness (93.8 percent) that Yang allegedly reported. Sponsored by the state, socialist acupuncture no longer faced the threat of abolishment as it did in the Republican period, and yet it still relied on scientific explanation and statistics to prove its effects, even though the lack of uniform standards in measuring curability made many truth claims sound dubious today. Increasing media exposure toward the end of the 1950s popularized scientific methods and measurement into narratives of miracle making, highlighting the revolutionary spirits of both doctors and patients. This tendency would find its most manifest expression in the 1970s, as we shall show in the next section. Mere figures would no longer be sufficient to demonstrate effective curing, which became almost inseparable from a more profound transformation of the deaf-mute. As communist doctors were encouraged to overcome the barriers created by traditional and bourgeois authorities, deaf-mute bodies in the media also became active agents that could acquire, in the revolutionary language and voice, their passion for the nation and hence a sense of fulfillment.

Vocalizing Revolutionary Passion: Reimagining Deaf-Mute Bodies in the 1960s and 1970s

In the changing political context of the 1960s and 1970s, especially after Mao's major speech on the directive of health work in 1965, equal distribution of medical

34. Zhang Wei, "Rang yaba shuohua de ren"; "Yixiang zhongyao de chengjiu"; "Yunyong jiepouxue tupo zhenjiu jinxue," *Renmin ribao*, December 10, 1958, 6.

resources became the central focus of socialist medicine. Both acupuncture and deaf-mute people gained new significance in this period, as the former facilitated the spread of medical personnel from urban hospitals to doctors dispatched to the countryside, while the latter represented a renewed wave of ideological mobilization against "bourgeois medical authorities" (*zichan jieji yixue quanwei* 資產階級醫學權威), who were accused for depriving the right of marginalized groups to health care and to vocally express their revolutionary passion to the party. The mutual transformation of the doctors and the disabled into revolutionary agents centered on media promotion and representations of treating deaf-mutism, which redefined "cure" as a collective form of social and political inclusion.

The political agenda of Mao's medical reform and the validation of acupuncture in curing deaf-mutism during the Cultural Revolution are manifested in a color documentary film entitled *Relying on Mao Zedong Thought to Open the Forbidden Zone of Deaf-mutes* (1971), produced by the Central Studio of Newsreels Production.[35] In the currently circulating six-minute, black-and-white clip, we see a Mao Zedong Thought Medical Team from Troop 3125 going to Fu County in Liaoning Province to extend free medical treatment for rural people in the spring of 1968.[36] During their two-month stay at a local school for deaf-mutes, the medical team successfully restored hearing for all 105 students and helped the majority of them regain speech. Still, according to a contemporary film review, the film focuses on the team from Troop 3016 in Liaoyuan, Jilin Province. Both medical teams received significant media exposure in the late 1960s and shared almost identical stories of how they found the most effective method of deep needling at *yamen* by studying *Mao Zedong Thoughts* and conducting bold experiments on their own bodies.[37]

A decade after Yang Fuzhi's experiment with the acupoint *yamen*, the method was reinvented in media with a specific emphasis on the use of the acupuncturist's own body, demonstrating the doctors' revolutionary spirit of self-sacrifice, audacity to confront the establishment, and a rather personal relationship with patients. In particular, the "spirit of selflessness," an idiom drawn from Mao's memorial to the Canadian doctor Norman Bethune for his wartime service to the Red Army, played

35. The full version of the film is not available for public access. A six-minute, black-and-white clip can be accessed via the link: https://www.youtube.com/watch?v=-IiNo-TKwJM&t=58s.

36. Meng Qingyu, Wang Guizhen, "Qiannian tieshu kai le hua: zan caise jilu dianying *Kao Mao Zedong sixiang dakai longya jinqu*," *Renmin ribao*, November 12, 1971, 4.

37. Shi Liu, Si Qi, "Kao Mao Zedong sixiang dakai le longya 'jinqu': 3016 budui weishengke Mao Zedong sixiang yiliao xuanchuangdui zai Liaoyuan Longya Xuexiao zhiliao longyabing de shiji," *Renmin ribao*, October 30, 1968, 4; Anonymous, "Mao zhuxi wuchan jieji luxian de shengli kage: Ji renmin jiefangjun 3125 budui Mao Zedong sixiang weisheng gongzuodui kaichuang zhiliao longyabing de xinluzi," *Renmin ribao*, December 16, 1968, 3; Anonymous, "Mao Zedong sixiang shi zhenjiu liaofa huode xinde shengming: Shengyang budui kaizhan xin zhenjiu liaofa de diaocha baogao," *Renmin ribao*, September 16, 1969, 2.

a key role in defining what it meant to be a good doctor of socialist medicine.[38] But this seemingly practice-based method is, in fact, far from being scientific proof of medical effectiveness. It serves more as a narrative device to reinforce an almost mythical resonation among people with shared revolutionary passion.[39] Aligned with Maoism, the film defines deaf-mutism as a fairly common disorder among working-class people, portraying the children's loss of hearing and speech as a result of medical elites' divorce from the masses, especially the rural poor. Similarly, the health workers in the documentary, as well as in other popular media cases, were mostly soldiers with no preexisting medical background.[40] They were both mobilized to the forefront in Mao's war against the bourgeois medical authorities. Christos Lynteris argues that the ideological reform of medical experts was crucial to "construct a comprehensive bio-political apparatus that could render China's vast population scientifically intelligible and politically manageable."[41] Underlying such a biopolitical apparatus was a bodily and emotional bond between doctors and patients. Media narratives helped envision a deep unification among them to crack open the "forbidden zone" that barred deaf-mutes from equal access to medical resources and social participation.

Newly regained voices became deaf-mute people's most powerful weapon to fight. Like most documentary films of the period, the soundtrack is primarily dominated by voice-over narration, but the children's voices, from word-to-word uttering of "Long live Chairman Mao" to cheerful shouting of the whole sentence and eventually singing revolutionary songs, mark the attraction of the film. The slogan "Long live Chairman Mao" here is not only a default test for the evaluation of treatment effectiveness but also stands for the innermost feeling that deaf-mute people are most eager to vocalize. By speaking the same language as millions of other Chinese people at the time, the children were successfully transformed into a revolutionary mass, as indicated in the school's new name: the Revolutionary Committee of School No. 626. A crowd of cured children wave the Little Red Book

38. The cult of Bethune was linked to the cult of Mao during the Cultural Revolution period; it held that bourgeois self-interest ought to be negated and abolished in the medical field through emulation and self-criticism. See Christos Lynteris, *The Spirit of Selflessness in Maoist China: Socialist Medicine and the New Man* (London: Palgrave Macmillan, 2012), 101–7.

39. It is interesting to note that reports on acupuncture-cured deaf-mute cases conducted in other third world countries rarely employed the same narrative. The only mention of a doctor's self-needling is to demonstrate the safety of acupuncture to African patients. See Zhongguo yiliao dui, "Zhongguo yisheng ba ta de bing zhihao le: zhongguo yiliaodui zai Yemen zhiliao longya bingren de shiji," *Remini ribao*, November 15, 1969, 5.

40. The most well-known soldier-turned-acupuncturist in treating deaf-mutism during the Cultural Revolution was Zhao Puyu, who was also featured in this documentary. His articles "Wuxian zhongyu Mao zhuxi chuangzao qiji" and "Kao Mao Zedong sixiang dakai longya jinqu" respectively appeared in *Remin ribao*, May 19, 1969, 5 and October 24, 1969, 4.

41. Christos Lynteris, *The Spirit of Selflessness in Maoist China*, 16.

of *Mao Zedong Thought*, voicing their political loyalty before Mao's photo. Singing in the documentary renders more miraculous and emotionally arousing effects. In a film review written by two barefoot doctors, the authors noted that when the Deaf-mute Performance Team appeared on screen, they could not help singing along to "A Thousand-Year-Old Iron Tree Blooms" (*Qiannian de Tieshu Kaile Hua* 千年的鐵樹開了花) with them.[42] Even after the film ended, the Children's collective singing of *The East is Red* (*Dongfanghong* 東方紅) lingered with them.[43]

"Letting the people speak" was a distinct strategy of socialist mobilization, as evident in the practice of "speaking bitterness" (*suku* 訴苦) and in the political struggle sections. The cure of deaf-mutes literally embodied such a process, imbuing the medical practice with a layer of symbolic meaning that was inherently revolutionary. Being cured was not an end but a means to be involved in revolutionary endeavors. If the documentary showcased a collective image of the successful transformation of deaf-mute children into "junior red guards," Director Xie Jin's 1977 feature film *Youth* (*Qingchun* 青春) provides a vivid example of how a deaf-mute girl, *Yamei* (homophone of "mute sister"), exceeds her own limits and becomes a telephone operator with the help of a doctor.[44] Voice plays a central role throughout the film, turning from a conspicuous absence to a critical device through which the protagonist achieves her revolutionary dream.

The film opens with the voice-over narration of Yamei, announcing her determination to see Chairman Mao in Beijing against her grandfather's will. Her disability is soon revealed through her use of sign language and then confirmed in her voice-over: "My friends were singing when they departed, but I couldn't hear. I wanted to shout, but I could not. Because back then, I was still a deaf-mute." With an ironic emphasis on her lack of hearing and speech, the retrospective voice restores her agency by narrating the story from a first-person perspective. However, the real suffering from her disability is beyond any personal verbal articulation. When she is overwhelmed by the revolutionary ecstasy in Tiananmen Square, where Mao receives the Red Guards, she finds herself utterly powerless without the ability to cheer "Long Live Chairman Mao" like all others. Intercut with archival footage of

42. Given the fact that the song was written in 1971 and the documentary portrayed events in 1968, the footage is likely to be a reenactment shot in 1971.

43. Meng Qingyu, Wang Guizhen, "Qiannian tieshu kai le hua: zan caise jilu dianying *Kao Mao Zedong sixiang dakai longya jinqu*," 4.

44. Sarah Dauncey categorizes *Youth* as a post-Mao example of cinematic representations of disabled people since it was released in 1977, but its subject matter and source of inspiration were based on materials from the Cultural Revolution. For this reason, we discuss the film as a case from the Maoist era. Prior to *Youth*, Xie Jin directed *Spring Sprouts* (*Chunmiao* 春苗, 1975), which presents the practice of barefoot doctors during the Cultural Revolution. Ban Wang's chapter in this collection gives detailed analysis of this film. In 1991, Xie also focused on the theme of mentally disabled children in *Morning Star* (*Qiming Xing* 啟明星).

the crowd and Mao's image, the close-up of Yamei's face in slow motion amplifies her unspeakable suffering caused by the lack of voice at such a historic moment.

The shot is immediately followed by the singing of "A Thousand-Year-Old Iron Tree Blooms"—the same song that appeared in the aforementioned documentary. The high pitch of the female voice here is punctuated by waves crashing on the rocks, symbolizing the surging emotion that Yamei could no longer hold inside herself. The name of the song "A Thousand-Year-Old Iron Tree Blooms" was borrowed from the commonly used phrase that stressed the miraculous curing of deaf-mutism through acupuncture under the guidance of Chairman Mao.[45] Written in 1971 and popularized through radio broadcasting in 1973, it was the only officially approved song for coloratura soprano during the Cultural Revolution, although not used in this film. The lyrics assume the first-person voice of the recovered deaf-mutes, but the highly skillful singing style was not an obvious choice for those with a compromised vocal ability. Echoing the conspicuous choice of singing style, the film also explicitly expressed the extraordinary quality of the "regained voice" of the revolutionary deaf-mute.

After Yamei is cured, she insists on joining the army as a telecommunicator to serve the revolution with her newly gained hearing and speech. Incredible as it may seem, the plot was in fact based on the real story of Zong Jinguang 宗金廣, a student at the No. 3 School for the Deaf-Mute in Beijing who was cured by a PLA medical team after a treatment period of eleven weeks.[46] Zong was lucky enough to receive Premier Zhou Enlai's visit, who recommended that the young man work in marine telecommunication to improve his hearing and speech abilities.[47] The reportage of Zong's story caught the eye of director Xie Jin and became the inspiration of *Youth*. In his personal notes, Xie wrote that Zhou once told him, "(the portrayal of) the revolutionary spirit should not only focus on the cure of deaf-mutes but manifest in the will to move forward, fear no difficulty, and perpetuate revolution."[48] Quoting Chairman Mao, the film emphasizes the superability of a telecommunicator as "the scientific eye and ear that receives information from thousands of miles afar." Assisted by modern technology, Yamei's hearing and voice eventually overcome the limits of space, connecting the front with Beijing.

The medical narrative is concluded twenty minutes into the film, but Yamei's relationship with Doctor Xiang remains central to the storyline. By the time the

---

45. This expression was also used to describe the general condition of the liberation of the repressed groups, such as prostitutes in *Zizimeimei zhanqilai* (1951).
46. "Mao Zhuxi geile wo zuida xingfu: ji longya xuesheng Zong Jinguang canjun," *Xinhua she xinwen gao*, no. 811 (1971): 7–8.
47. Zhongguo renmin jiefangjun no. 1806 budui zhengzhibu, "Beijingshi Disan Longern Xuexiao shisheng huansong Zong Jinguang ruwu," *Renmin huabao* (June 1971): 44.
48. Song Xiaobin, *Jiali jiawai hua xiejin* (Beijing: Zhongguo shehui chubanshe, 2013), 82.

film was made, acupuncture had already been established as a standard treatment of deaf-muteness. Xie Jin employed the familiar narrative device of self-needling and two brief montage sequences to illustrate the treatment and vocal-training process. The challenge was not so much to convince the audience that Yamei could be cured as it was to portray her subsequent transformation under the help and guidance of Doctor Xiang. The importance of the medical narrative is further deconstructed by the fact that Yamei refuses to join the medical department, insisting on serving the Party with what the Party gives her. For Yamei, what cures her is not just the technique of socialist medicine but the mass politics that brings Doctor Xiang to her. This signifies a radical comprehension of the individual body as an integral component of the political collective—the "mass body" that socialist medicine has dedicated itself to since its inception within the CCP's revolutionary tradition. Only by "restoring" voice to the Party and the people can the deaf body achieve a deeper sense of self, enabling medical solutions to be fully integrated into mass politics.

Characters are interconnected physically and spiritually in the revolutionary narrative that blurs the boundaries between the healer and the healed, and between disabled and able-bodied individuals. A soldier during wartime, Xiang suffers from severe injuries and illness but keeps postponing her treatment for the sake of her patients. As Xiang claims, it is her revolutionary passion—and finding revolutionary passion in the younger generation, like Yamei—that sustains her youth. The subplot of the film, which appears in sporadic flashbacks, reveals that during the Long March, Xiang was saved by a deaf soldier, Old Geng, who sacrificed his life to steal penicillin for her. This story not only paves the way for Yamei's participation in new waves of revolution but also adds a layer of emotional complication to Xiang's feelings toward Yamei. As the spirit of Old Geng lives through Xiang, the latter's cure, care, and guidance for Yamei ensures the passing of the revolutionary legacy to the younger generation. The film ends with a symbolic image of Yamei wearing a headphone set in front of a switchboard. She signs to her friends outside the window that she has just been connected to Doctor Xiang. The interesting combination of headphones and sign language indicates both her ability to harness the technology of telecommunication and her past disability. The smile on her face seems to suggest that, disabled or not, people with revolutionary passion are all connected.

Conclusion

The miraculous cure of deaf-muteness toward the end of the Cultural Revolution signifies yet another breakthrough in the medicalization of disability that had been formulated in acupuncture's struggle with Western science and Chinese politics for more than half a century. The mobilization of socialist health agents ranging from clinicians, doctors, and paramedics sent down from the army was crucial for people with disabilities to enter revolutionary politics and become agents of their own fate. In socialist media, the search for a medical cure for the deaf-mute did not negate their disability as an undesired feature of revolutionary politics. Media portrayals of disability in the socialist body politic conveyed an important message for society to overcome the prejudice and stigma attached to disabled bodies and to bring about inclusion through relational becoming of the self and the other.

This is not to deny the fact that the medical construct of deaf-mutism as an illness also contributed to the erasure of deafness as an identity.[49] For sure, acupuncture-cured cases may not represent the identity shared by those who cannot be cured or those who insist on using sign languages to develop minority cultures. However, we argue throughout this chapter that disability, and deaf-muteness in particular, is a fluid concept revolving around the search for cures beyond the body proper. As we have shown, disability functioned as a vehicle through which the mutual transformation of acupuncture and deaf-mute bodies was made in the combination of Soviet science and socialist medicine. The medical construct of deaf-mutism since the 1950s generated new expressions of curability in the media and paved the way for the transformation of disabled figures into revolutionary agents.

The history of socialist medicine and its proclaimed objective to transform disabled bodies into revolutionary subjects is simultaneously a history mediated by images, sounds, and films. In their experimentation with acupuncture's curability of deaf-mute patients, medical doctors, PLA health agents, and filmmakers creatively exploited the advantage of acupuncture in the revolutionary tradition of healing and human transformism embedded in Soviet science and Cold War politics. The fact that acupuncture remained an imperfect technique of healing deaf-mutism, as illustrated by the lack of uniform measurement for effective cure and the intrusiveness it caused to the bodies of both doctors and patients in deep needling, opened new possibilities for documentary makers and film directors to utilize sound recording and visual symbolism for constructing curative metaphors on the screen. Although deaf-mute bodies and characters are presented in a binary and oftentimes dramatic contrast between total disablement and full recovery, the media representations of curability and the transformative effect it entails transcend the dichotomous relationship between the doctor and patient, disabled and able-bodied, and individual and collective. It was the revolutionary cause for socialist medicine to bring about inclusion of marginal subjects that defines the politics of disability.

49. Today members of the deaf community tend to distinguish "Deafness" (with a capital D) from the audiological condition of "deafness" (with a lower-case d), and they consider the former as a cultural difference in human experience rather than a disability or disease. Paddy Ladd, *Understanding Deaf Culture: In Search of Deafhood* (Clevedon, UK: Multilingual Matters, 2003), xvii.

6

The Mass Biopolitics of Medicine in Socialist Chinese Films

Ban Wang

One of the incentives to investigate medicine in humanistic and sociopolitical terms is the recognition of the limit of the biological or biomedical paradigm. As a discourse and practice dominating the medical landscape in the West since the Cold War, the "biological approach alone," as Mikael Leiman and Anna Maria Viljanen point out, "cannot address the various human phenomonna that physicians encounter in their everyday medicine."[1] This approach reduces patients to diseases and bodies and ignores persons in concrete contexts and relations—the multilayered social and political contexts that make for a whole living human person. Under the rubric of dehumanization, the biomedical approach is marked by "overspecialization," overprofessionalization, "insensitivity to personal and socio-cultural values; too narrow a construal of the doctor's role; too much science; . . . not enough liberal arts; too much economic incentives; . . . insensitivity to the poor and socially disadvantaged; overmedication of everday life."[2] To Barbara Rothman, these sins of overmedication became aggravated during the COVID-19 pandemic. Under the rubric of "biomedical empire," Rothman examines how the empire—driven by the neoliberal, technocratic and profit imperatives—has damaged rather than protected the social body from the virus, widening the gulfs of race, gender, and class and weaponizing the deadly virus for partisan gains.[3]

Drawing on Michel Foucault's notion of biopolitics, Rothman reveals how modern states regulate their subjects through "an explosion of numerous and diverse

1. Quoted in Thomas R. Cole et al., *Medical Humanities: An Introduction* (Cambridge: Cambridge University Press, 2015), 8.
2. Cole et al., *Medical Humanities*, 6.
3. Barbara Katz Rothman, *The Biomedical Empire: Lessons Learned from the COVID-19 Pandemic* (Stanford: Stanford University Press, 2021).

techniques for achieving the subjugation of bodies and the control of populations."[4] The concept of biopolitics tells us how the modern state's mechanisms of security are "installed around the random element inherent in a population so as to optimize a state of life." Biopolitical measures aim "to take control of life and the biological processes of man-as-species and of ensuring they are not disciplined but regulated."[5] Against this top-down control, Michael Hardt and Antonio Negri posit a bottom-up resurgence of social and biological power. They critique Foucault's biopower as a "power over life"—a power to "administer and produce life," which functions through the governance of populations and management of reproductive capacities, social health, and labor.[6] Under the military and industrial regime, such power "not only threatens us with death but also rules over life." "Biopower stands above society, transcendent, as a sovereign authority and imposes its order."[7] In search of alternative forms of power, Hardt and Negri point to the social and popular basis for biopower under the rubric of "biopolitical production." Biopolitical production keeps faith with the desire and capacity of masses of people for social change, shifting from the "power over life" to a recognition of the groundswell potentials immanent to productive social bodies as political subjects. By creating social relations and collaborative labor, biopolitical production proposes a "power of life" that resists the dominant power and strives to "determine an alternative production of subjectivity."[8] Mass biopolitics arise from the production of socioeconomic life, as working people engage in the reproduction of biological and social life. This perspective captures productive efforts and everyday experiences of laborers, families, and communities in reproducing life and connecting with one another. In addition to life necessities, the social strata also produce "immaterial goods," such as ideas, subjectivities, affects, knowledge, forms of communication, and relationships. Invoking the mass-line tradition in the Chinese Revolution, Hardt and Negri consider the third world and Chinese peasantry to be an example of vibrant political subjectivity and valorize their collaborative labor and power for social transformation. The struggles of the peasants are not merely oriented toward "the defense of the soil" in land reform but also strive to transform social life in its entirety. In their own "cultural revolution," the peasants overcome their traditional passivity and isolation and become "communicative, cooperative, and articulate as an active collective subject."[9]

4. Rothman, *The Biomedical Empire*, 24.
5. Michel Foucault, *Society Must be Defended* (New York: Picador, 2003), 246–47.
6. Michael Hardt and Antonio Negri, *Commonwealth* (Cambridge, MA: Harvard University Press, 2009), 57.
7. Michael Hardt and Antonio Negri, *Multitude: War and Democracy in the Age of Empire* (New York: The Penguin Press, 2004), 94.
8. Hardt and Negri, *Commonwealth*, 57.
9. Hardt and Negris, *Multitude*, 124.

The reference to the Chinese Revolution and its popular power brings up the revolutionary movements during the Cold War. In resisting colonizing empires and related biomedical domination, underdeveloped third world countries waged political and medical revolutions. In the transformation of health care systems, the newly independent nations strove to resist capitalist medical power and profit-driven pharmecertical industries, and newly independent people built their own health care systems and ran decentralized and communal health care to mutual care.[10] China's health care reform during Mao's era was part of this decolonizing trend. The communal health care and barefoot doctor practices were an inspiring symbol of popular and communical medicine in Latin American countries. By examining films made in the socialist era, this chapter seeks to articulate social medicine and health care reform fueled by biopolitical and biomedical production by working people. Rather than a technique, power, or status wielded by doctors, technocrats, and medical industry, health care is decentralized and medical knowledge is acquired and practiced among the masses. The distinction between the medical establishment and popular medicine reflects the divide between the "red" and "expert" orientations that are threaded throughout socialist China. "Red" denotes health care workers' commitment to public well-being as citizens, whereas "expert" refers to the monopoly and elitism of the medical profession and establishment.

Zhen Junli's film *Spring Comes to a Withered Tree* (*Kumu fengchun* 枯木逢春, 1961) tells the story of how public health campaigns reject the biomedical approach of professional elites, mobilize peasants to battle schistosomiasis, treat patients through the combined use of Western and traditional Chinese medicine, and ensure the biological continuity of families and community. The tension between "red" and "expert" escalates in Xie Jin's film *Spring Sprouts* (*Chunmiao* 春苗, 1975). The film upholds the barefoot doctor as an emergent symbol of mass health movement and grassroots responses to the elitist medical profession. As a symbol of socialist modernity, the barefoot doctor epitomizes a faith in the creativity of the ordinary people and a rejection of domination by an administrative or technical elite under the aegis of the Western and Soviet models of modernization. The films examined in this chapter demonstrate that although medicine is a biochemical process subject to the scientific criteria of truth, a politics of masses and mobilization always intervenes and inheres at its core. When a mobilized population strives to adjust and regulate biomedical relations between humans and nonhuman worlds, a mass politics of medicine is born.

Social relations, emotion, and subjectivities are visceral and embodied experiences vital to health care, as manifested in "affective labor." By fostering emotion, sympathy, and compassion, health care workers perform affective labor through kin

10. Howard Waitzkin, *Medicine and Public Health at the End of Empire* (New York: Routledge, 2016).

work, healing, nursing, maternal care, and health service. Affective labor addresses "affect" of pain and sickness and engages body and mind, highlighting the "social flesh" that parallels ecological relations.[11] In socialist China's anti-epidemic campaigns, affective bonds forged a collective solidarity against nature's blind forces and diseases by building an "iron wall." The public health campaign was an effort to tame nature by "conjuring into being 'the people' as a collective force," writes Tina Chen. The people's power "rested on the welding of bodies to one another to create a collective force of history."[12] Like water, air, earth, and fire, the social flesh denotes "an unformed life force" and an "element of social being, aimed at the fullness of life."[13]

Mass Mobilization in *Spring Comes to a Withered Tree*

"All disease," Ivan Illich asserted, "is a socially created reality."[14] Diseases originate in and remain endemic to a social and political ecology. Articulating the "political genesis" of disease, Illich noted the modern Chinese perception of disease as a "political problem" rather than a biomedical one.[15] David Lampton viewed this politics-medicine nexus as a legacy of traditional Chinese medicine. The ancient doctrine views disease as stemming from a cosmic, ecological, and ethicopolitical horizon. The purpose of medicine is not just to keep the biological body fit, but to protect the health of the whole political community. "The keystone of the Chinese medical tradition is the art of maintaining health, not curing diseases."[16] Mao's "emphasis on preventive medicine is perfectly consistent with this legacy."[17] Political structure, moral values, cultural sentiments, and medicine are deeply imbricated and interlocked. *The Yellow Emperor Classics of Internal Medicine* goes way beyond a conversation of medicine to become "a treatise on general ethics and regimen of life," as well as religious beliefs, political advice, and ecological wisdom.[18] As Ilza Veith noted, ancient thinkers regarded medicine as the responsibility of the state: the function of the various organs of the human body "is compared to that of various

11. Hardt and Negri, *Multitude*, 108.
12. Tina Mai Chen, "The Human-Machine Continuum in Maoism: The Intersection of Soviet Socialist Realism, Japanese Theoretical Physics, and Chinese Revolutionary Theory," *Cultural Critique*, no. 80 (2012): 163.
13. Hardt and Negri, *Multitude*, 192.
14. Ivan Illich, *Medical Nemesis* (London: Marion Boyars, 2010), 166.
15. Illich, *Medical Nemesis*, 168.
16. David M. Lampton, *The Politics of Medicine in China: The Policy Process, 1949–1977* (London: Routledge, 1977), 11.
17. Lampton, *Politics of Medicine*, 3.
18. *The Yellow Emperor Classics of Internal Medicine*, trans. Ilza Veith (Berkeley, CA: University of California Press, 1975), 10.

officials in an empire."[19] The human body is deemed analogous to the body politic: the heart is metaphoric, for instance, of the minister with insightful advice; the liver is compared to the military capable of strategic defense. Rather than a realm removed from medicine, politics remains immanent within biological and biomedical processes.

The medicine-politics nexus persisted during the Chinese Revolution. In the wars against the nationalists and the Japanese invasion, medicine was inextricably part of the military operation that required a robust force of the political body. "Red Army medicine" came into being when the revolutionaries "had to adapt to manpower and resources scarcities" in the attempt to treat the wounded and prevent contagious diseases. They developed strategies that involved "the use of paramedics with little formal training" and mass mobilization of everyone in a war against diseases.[20] Examining stories of epidemic prevention in Yan'an, Wang Yu has shown that, faced with deaths and damage due to the spread of typhoid and other diseases, the local organizations and governments launched a mass campaign to popularize hygienic habits while treating the sick. The narratives of revolutionary medicine portray the anti-epidemic activities as integral components of the general political, economic, cultural, and military activities waged by nationwide movements of land reform, the Anti-Japanese War, and the formation of a health care infrastructure.[21] This practice was carried over to Mao's China, whose touchstone of health care and medicine was a mass politics that mobilized social bodies and forged intracorporeal bonds. Many health campaigns strove to empower the people to exercise their sovereignty to engage in collaborative labor, to dismantle old ideas and superstitions, and to maintain an ecological balance between humans and nature.

After 1949, public health care was immediately on the agenda of national politics. New China was, as David Lampton put it, "a truly unhealthy society." The poor and sick were mired in a condition "arising from pervasive infection, malnutrition, inadequate education, and poor environmental hygiene."[22] The situation was especially dire in rural areas, where modern health care and medicine were nonexistent, and hospital facilities were out of reach of rural populations. Between the cities and the countryside, inequality of health care and medical service were abysmal. The peasants lived and suffered in the total absence of medicine and were constantly plagued by infectious epidemics. Even in the cities, only the privileged stratum had access to medical services and resources.

19. Ilza Veith, introduction to *The Yellow Emperor Classics of Internal Medicine*, 28.
20. Lampton, *Politics of Medicine*, 11.
21. Wang Yu, "Yan'an wenxue zhong de yiliaoweisheng xushi," *Xueshu yuekan* (2017): 132–40.
22. Lampton, *Politics of Medicine*, 13.

The new state quickly placed medicine as a key element in the general socioeconomic development. Throughout the socialist era, the health care system did not run smoothly, and incessant contestation raged over the distribution and appropriation of financial and medical resources. While the state had the decision-making power, the conflict over the nature, direction, and beneficiaries of the medical system never ceased within the CCP and the government. Escalating to pitched battles in the Great Leap Forward and the Cultural Revolution, the conflict centered on this stark reality: medical resources were concentrated in the cities, and the rural population bore the brunt of many epidemics without treatment. It boiled down to the tension between a technocratic medical bureaucracy and a mass-based medicine serving the needs of rural areas.

The controversy, both political and cultural, finds a dramatic expression in *Spring Comes to a Withered Tree*. The film tells the story of how the mobilized peasants of a village battle schistosomiasis, treat the patients, and ensure the health and productivity of the family and community. The campaign against schistosomiasis was frequent in the first two decades of socialist China and "stands as one of the most famous public campaigns in the history of the People's Republic of China."[23] Built into the fabric of the unsanitary environment of rice farming, the epidemic threatened and wrought havoc. In the Yangtze River Basin, the disease easily transmitted from snails to humans and affected millions, ravaging the land and causing debilitating infection and catastrophic death. It had claimed an estimated 10.5 million victims in the early 1950s.[24] Although China's Ministry of Health Care took measures to deal with the disease, the emphasis leaned toward research and development rather than a cure. Frustrated with the medical bureaucracy's agenda, the Party Central Committee sent a task force to run the antiparasitic campaign outside the Ministry of Health Care and medical professions. The fight against schistosomiasis became a focal point for launching mass movements aimed at prevention, cure, and the reform of the technocratic profession, provoking political controversy over the direction of medicine across the urban-rural divide.

Spring Comes to a Withered Tree draws much inspiration from Mao's well-known poem about the campaigns against schistosomiasis. In 1955, deeply concerned about the ravages of the epidemic, Mao issued a call that "we must eliminate schistosomiasis!" On June 30, 1958, the Chairman read a *People's Daily* report about the elimination of schistosomiasis in Yujiang county, Jiangxi province. Linking this the event to the Chinese Revolution and anti-colonialist wars, Mao noted that the epidemic had destroyed millions of lives in China—more than all the casualties at

23. Miriam Gross, *Farewell to the God of Plague: Chairman Mao's Campaign to Deworm China* (Oakland, CA: University of California Press, 2016), 1.
24. Lampton, *Politics of Medicine*, 14.

the hand of imperialist and colonial aggression since the late nineteenth century. And 100 million people were still suffering. The victory of Yujiang's anti-epidemic campaign was nothing less than a victory over a formidable enemy. With the mind churned with thoughts and unable to sleep, Mao wrote a poem, "Farewell to the God of Plague" ("Song wenshen" 送瘟神), to celebrate the victory. The key to the success, Mao pointed out, is a political combination of "leaders, experts, and the masses." For a long time, doctors and researchers had been rather pessimistic, but in recent years, "new hopes arise as the Party took the lead and mobilized masses on a large scale in the anti-epidemic campaign. The party organizations of all levels, scientists and doctors, and masses of the people joined hands, driving out the God of Plague."[25]

The film presents a multileveled mass campaign against the epidemic, where social bodies emerge from obscurity and are mobilized to meet the challenge. The story begins with a pandemic crisis in the pre-Liberation era, when the family of Ku Meizi (Sister Ku)—literarily "bitter sister"—has suffered from schistosomiasis for generations and is fleeing their plagued home village in South China. With her sick father dead on the road and chased by the Guomindang soldiers, Sister Ku loses touch with her fiancé and would-be mother-in-law. In the new era under socialism, the film presents sunny and vibrant scenes of agricultural production. But the plague persists. Although Sister Ku marries and has a new family, schistosomiasis strikes down her husband and makes her gravely sick. Soon her lost fiancé comes to work in the village and meets her, rekindling the hope to rebuild the family. In a diagnosis of her condition, Dr. Liu from Shanghai declares her illness terminal. But the station leader Luo Shunde tries to treat her. A leader in disease prevention and treatment, Luo involves doctors of Western medicine and traditional herbalists. In contrast, Dr. Liu, though part of the team of cure and prevention, is more interested in his own medical research and prestige. Engrossed in seeking fame and professional advancement, Liu forgets to secure the crucial herbs to save Sister Ku's life. In the nick of time, Luo acquires the lifesaving herbs and a treatment based on combined Chinese and Western medicine and cures Sister Ku. In the end, she marries her former fiancé and gives birth to twins.

The film portrays the pre-1949 spread of schistosomiasis not merely as a health threat but as signs of the political collapse of the Guomindang regime. Mao's poem opens with a pristine landscape ravaged by the disease and left to rot by an uncaring government, where "hundreds of villages choked with weeds, men wasted away; Thousands of homes deserted, ghosts chanted mournfully."[26] The film intensifies

25. Wang Jianxin, "Zaidu Mao Zedong 'Qilü ershou songwenshen'," February 24, 2020, http://dangshi.people.com.cn/n1/2020/0224/c85037-31601095.html.

26. Ma, Wen-yee, *Snow Glistens on the Great Wall: A New Translation of the Complete Collection of Mao Tse-tung's Poetry* (Santa Barbara, CA: Santa Barbara Press, 1986), 34.

the atmosphere of desolation with grey lighting, and its theme song intones "bitter waters," "barren hills," "poverty and sickness." Epidemic refugees flee the plagued areas, only to find themselves stranded in another disaster zone. In the socialist era, we see a lush and spring-like rural landscape and fields, where peasants engage in farming and harvesting. But the disease continues to harm their bodies and threatens their new life. The need for prevention and treatment in rural areas is critical and urgent. In response, the leadership and medical institutions send doctors and epidemiologists to the countryside on a mission to educate and mobilize the peasants to set up health clinics.

The film evolves around two contrary approaches to the epidemic. As a well-trained epidemiologist, Dr. Liu comes to the village along with his sister, their express task being to provide treatment and conduct field research. But Liu deals with the epidemic not in the interest of rural patients and their well-being but with the ambition of advancing his career and gaining professional status. His sister, a medical student, evinces signs of the integrated "red-expert" in her growing empathy with the peasants and care for their medical needs. Against her brother's advice for her to secure a position in a medical school equipped with modern libraries and resources, she resolves to settle and work in the village.

The local leader Luo Shunde exemplifies the grassroots, mass-based approach. His work taps into the energy and wisdom of peasants, local resources, herbal medicine, and preventive measures suited to the local biosphere. Luo criticizes Dr. Liu for his indifference toward the patients and their families. The latter disparages the herbs and exults in experts and advanced medicine. Brandishing a volume on epidemiology written by his professor, he claims that killing snails with chemicals is the key to prevention. Though on the team for Sister Ku's treatment, Dr Liu breaks off to a conference at the critical moment. At the conference, his professor acknowledges Liu's rural field work as an important tribute to his own authority and prestige, turning the data into intellectual capital and professional credit, completely oblivious to the suffering on the ground. Liu's pursuit of status is an indifference toward the pain of patients and the deadly severity of the epidemic. Epidemiologically, Liu treats human beings as identical to snails—merely one link in the chain of transmission. Countering that, Luo Shunde insists that human beings are the most precious force in building a new society. The old society robs people of their health and lives; the new society must reclaim and restore their health and vitality. Instead of a mere biomedical and technical matter, Luo values and encourages the political participation of the peasantry in maintaining the biological body and body politic.

Dr. Liu's arrogance and elitism epitomized a technocratic and bureaucratic trend in China's modernization and in the medical system. This trend valorized technoscience development as an engineering process supervised by experts and scientists. This Cold War model, often aligned with Soviet revisionism, came under fire in the late 1950s and during the Cultural Revolution. Critics charged that medical bureaucrats and professionals were entrenched in elitism and relied heavily on experts, advanced techniques, and highly trained doctors. Medical resources and hospitals were concentrated in the major cities and served mainly the urban and privileged strata. With a lopsided emphasis on research, careerism, and prestige, the professionals monopolized the transmission of medical knowledge and expertise. Dr. Liu embodies a medical profession that was increasingly out of touch with the needs of ordinary people and rural populations.

Luo Shunde represents the opposite. He implements the mass-line health policy and engages in mass politics. Hailing from a peasant family in the same area and empathetic to locals, he places full trust on the masses to run anti-epidemic activities by relying on their initiatives, energy, experience, and collaborative labor. Although he opposes Liu's technocratic elitism, he believes that the mobilization of the populace's energy, "combined with professional skill, can overcome problems that would remain unresolved if total reliance was placed upon professionals and formal government institutions."[27] Woven into the fabric of agricultural production, the community, and the biosphere, schistosomiasis is a menace but also calls for enhanced practical skills and medical knowledge. By modifying their lifeways and farming methods, by acquiring modern medicine combined with herbs, and by clearing up the disease-prone environment, the peasants prove capable of overcoming the plague and meeting their pharmaceutical demands.

The film dramatizes the link between politics and medicine in an emotional, corporeal, and quasi-religious episode. One night, Chairman Mao arrives in the county and meets the local leaders to discuss the disease and the needs of the peasants. A series of montages creates an ambiance of the leader as having deep compassion for the peasants. One window after another opens, and the peasants look out from their homes in unison, straining their eyes to catch a glimmer of light from the building where Mao converses with local cadres—as if the building were within the visual reach of each. Back in the village, Luo tells the gathering how he has talked and shaken hands with Mao, happily passing on Mao's personal grace by shaking the hands of community members. Some villagers are concerned that Mao stays up late; the leader's response, conveyed by Luo, is "I cannot sleep" when people are suffering. The remark moves all to tears. Critics with Cold War perspectives may balk at the blind worship of Mao. But I contend the episode illustrates a politics of emotional and bodily bonds.

In a defense of the Mao cult, French philosopher Alain Badiou suggests that what looks like top-down leadership can be seen as stirrings of popular democracy,

27. David Lampton, "Development and a Health Care: Is China's Medical Program Exportable?" *World Development* 6 (1978): 624.

which is an instance of biopolitical production. The power over life should be read as a power of life. By exulting in the people's excitement and emotion, the charismatic display of the leader functions to galvanize and empower the masses. Instead of blind and passive followers, the masses become the "Prometheans" embued with political agency in making social change.[28] Badiou invokes "The Foolish Old Man Who Removes the Mountains" ("Yugong yishan" 愚公移山), a 1945 speech that Mao delivered at the 7th National Congress of the Chinese Communist Party in Yan'an. In it, Mao recalled the Taoist fable of an indefatigable old man, who urged and led his sons in an impossible mission: digging away two mountains that block their view and communication with the outside world. This undertaking moved the gods in heaven, who sent fairies to remove the mountains. Confronted with the Japanese invasion and the impending Civil War, Mao says, "Today, two big mountains lie like a dead weight on the Chinese people. One is imperialism, and other is feudalism. The Communist Party has long made up its mind to dig them up. We must persevere and work unceasingly, and we, too, will touch God's heart. Our God is none other than the masses of the Chinese people. If they stand up and dig together with us, why can't these two mountains be cleared away?"[29]

Deemed able to match the gods, the people are capable of overcoming challenges and prevailing over adversity. Yugong figures as an impetus to the masses, inspiring and energizing them to overcome obstacles and diseases. Christian Sorace cautions that this "religious" aspect may elevate the leader above the masses, widening "the religious divide" between Mao and the people.[30] But as the engine of mobilization, Yugong sutures the gap between heaven and earth, placing leader and led in a symbiotic and reciprocal relation. The people will touch the gods, and the gods of the socialist world are none other than the Chinese people. With mass bioproduction intertwined with mythology, the Yugong image puts the leader back among the led and renders the masses into their own leaders—as masters of a new social and biopolitical order.

Significantly, the given name of Luo Shunde literally means "the virtue of Shun." Shun, along with Yao, are the legendary kings of Chinese antiquity and are mentioned together in Mao's poem. Shunde invokes the Confucian ideal of the benevolent governance of society and compassionate care for the welfare of ordinary people. In the context of public health, the concept of virtue underscores the state's responsibility for disease prevention and making health care universally available for all people, communities, and regions. In the past, such virtue resided

28. Alain Badiou, *Théorie du sujet* (Paris: Éditions du seul, 1982), 340–41.
29. Mao Tse-tung, "The Foolish Old Man Who Removes the Mountains," in *Selected Works of Mao Tse-tung* (Beijing: Foreign Languages Press, 1965), 321–22.
30. Christian Sorace, "Saint Mao," *Telos*, no. 151 (2010): 176.

in the expectation, often illusory and unrealistic, of a benevolent king. But the mass biopolitics of medicine inverts the ancient virtue from the bottom up. "Six hundred millions people are all Yaos and Shuns," Mao proclaims. As the Yugongs of the new age, the masses develop new virtues of empathy and compassion for families and communities, taking charge of their own medical needs and health care. As the peasants triumph over the epidemic, the "magic landscape" (*shenzhou* 神州) is restored to its green health, enveloped in a divine aura and cleansed of schistosomiasis, attesting to an artwork crafted by working people. The honor is due everyone who participates in the health campaign. The working people are taking over and are transforming the sky and changing the earth:

> With our silver hoes
> We till the five majestic peaks that pierce the clouds;
> With our arms of iron/We shape the three mighty rivers that flow across the land.[31]
>
> 天連五嶺銀鋤落
> 地動三河鐵臂搖

The people are now leaders of themselves, organizing their labor, meeting challenges, and changing the world.

The film highlights the motif of the masses as masters of a new society, the theme of self-salvation and self-reliance, and the patients as their own doctors. After Mao's visit, the film launches into an extension of the anti-epidemic combat on a broader scale. Truckloads of medical graduates come to the village to help; the villagers work in unison in public works that modify and change the landscape, rivers, and fields, creating an environmentally hygienic habitat. Local herbs and doctors of traditional Chinese medicine are enlisted in the treatment of patients. Emotional mobilization, indeed, is not limited to medical affairs but exemplifies the political culture of a socialist society constituted by working-class people.

The Barefoot Doctor in Biopolitical Production

The tension between medical technocracy and mass health care came to a head during the Cultural Revolution. By upholding the barefoot doctor as a symbol of mass health care, the film *Spring Sprouts* critiques the top-heavy and elitist medical profession. Backed up by the medical bureaucracy, the medical profession and resources were skewed in favor of elites and urbanites. Although a system of socialized health care was taking shape during the first two decades after 1949, urban hospitals and clinics increasingly became the privileged enclave for bureaucrats, cadres, and urbanites. Victor Sidel, American physician and Nobel Laurate for public health,

31. These lines are translated by Ma, *Snow Glistens on the Great Wall,* 111.

visited China in 1971 and observed situations of health care and medicine in the cities and countryside. He complained that the first-rate doctors in the urban centers "were divorced from proletarian politics, from workers, peasants, and soldiers," and they devoted attention, energy, and resources to the treatment of rare disease and difficult cases, oblivious to common diseases affecting ordinary working people.[32]

The barefoot doctor emerged as a grassroots and low-cost health care initiative in the late 1950s. A campaign to train a large cadre of paramedical workers, the program began during the Great Leap Forward and—in response to Mao's June 25, 1965 directive "in medical and health work, put stress on the rural area"—came to national and global eminence during the Cultural Revolution.[33] The new health care agent refers a peasant or factory worker who, having acquired basic medical knowledge and skills, is able to treat coworkers with common ailments. The barefoot doctors, reported Victor Li in 1975, represented the "most innovative and far-reaching efforts to provide better health care for the entire population." In contrast with the Western model centered around highly trained professionals, advanced technology, elaborate equipment, and expensive drugs, barefoot medicine signaled an alternative health care that was inexpensive, mass-based, egalitarian, ecological, and beneficial to rural communities.

Inequality in health care marks the opening scene of *Spring Sprouts*. A doctor of the commune clinic, engrossed in a phone chat with an official about longevity, delays urgent care to a village girl, causing the latter's death. In today's China, commercialization and privatization of medicine in the last three decades has exacerbated the gap in health care between the haves and have-nots, the privileged and disadvantaged. This makes this 1975 film all the more poignant and compelling. Outraged by this incident, the protagonist Tian Chunmiao, a robust girl of socialist labor, becomes involved in the training program for barefoot doctors. Guided by the new policy and recommended by the village's leadership and community, she enrolls in the barefoot doctor program taught by professionals. Overcoming barriers set by the technocrats, she learns medical knowledge and basic skills, and dedicates herself to serving rural patients. The dramatic conflict builds toward the confrontation of two diametrically opposed lines in health care, raising the questions: What is a public health-care system that refuses to deliver medical care to ordinary people? Public health for which public?

The rise of the barefoot doctor was a radical response to the growing tensions between socialist and technocratic paths in China's modernization. In contrast with

32. Victor W. Sidel, "The Barefoot Doctors of the People's Republic of China," *New England Journal of Medicine* 286, no. 24 (1972): 1294.

33. Victor H. Li, "Politics and Health Care in China: The Barefoot Doctors." *Stanford Law Review* 27, no. 3 (Feb. 1975): 827.

the Western-style developmental paradigm premised on technocratic rationality and the military industrial complex, the socialist modernizers strove to attain an all-around development of equality and prosperity by overcoming the divides between the city and the countryside, industry and agriculture, and intellectual and manual work. Touted as a program to improve living standards in underdeveloped countries, the Western developmental model was, in Sigrid Schmalzer's words, "a strategy for preventing ideologies opposed by the U.S." and neutralizing revolutionary mass politics.[34] The technocratic approach relied on "technical experts to provide technological fixes for social and political problems."[35] Socialist modernizers were constantly vigilant of the technocratic pitfalls that China was slipping into. In the two decades after Liberation, a technocratic elite was looming and the gulf was widening between urbanites and peasants, cities and the countryside. As "the cadres of a revolutionary party became administrators and bureaucratic functionaries," wrote Maurice Meisner, the ideal image of the red-and-expert cadres turned to mere experts and administrators, governing the masses from their office desks.[36] The techno-bureaucratic model fostered a fetish in the expertise and power of experts and specialists, recreating a pattern of inequality and hierarchy at the expense of the revolutionary spirit and the ethos of equality.

In *Spring Sprouts,* the conflict between medical bureaucracy and grassroots medicine is rendered into a class struggle. The medical establishment holds authority, power, and resources and is unconcerned about the needs and suffering of the peasant population. Mr. Du, the director of the commune's health center, is in league with Doctor Qian, a residual figure of the arrogant medical profession of the past. They sideline the barefoot doctors, withhold pharmaceutical resources, deny their training, and pay no heed to the sick and the spread of disease. In opposition to this dominant class, the collective health care initiatives, led by Tian Chunmiao and the sympathetic doctors, push back and strive to learn skills and deliver health care to the peasant population and treat regional diseases.

The notion of class is vital to mass politics in medicine and health care. It is well-known that class struggle frequently degenerated into abusive estrangement, classification, and persecution of innocent people. While the abuse was real and destructive, I contend that class analysis needs to be historicized: the concept takes on different meanings and serves different polemics and political expediency. The class category allows us to identify a grounded subject position and force in social movement. Class analysis illuminates forgotten features of socialist modernity

34. Sigrid Schmalzer, *Red Revolution, Green Revolution: Scientific Farming in Socialist China* (Chicago: University of Chicago Press, 2016), 3.
35. Schmalzer, *Red Revolution, Green Revolution,* 3.
36. Maurice Meisner, *Mao's China and After* (New York: Free Press, 1999), 114.

and biopolitical production. Marked by "a heavy reliance on the creativity of the Chinese people, particularly the peasantry," and a "rejection of domination by an administrative or technical elite operating through a centralized bureaucracy," class analysis gives primacy to "popular participation, decentralization and community power."[37] As one of the three linked movements of China's socialist modernization, "class struggle" was aligned with the other two fronts: the struggles for production and scientific experiment. The triple movement aimed to avoid the traps of capitalist modernity so that China would be free "from bureaucracy and immune against revisionism and dogmatism."[38] In the mass politics of medicine, class analysis works to critique bureaucratic entrenchment and the rising technocratic elite, enabling a recognition of the agency and power of medically disadvantaged classes. As Carl Riskin has shown, as "administrative state planning had combined political and economic power in the hands of a bureaucracy aloof from the masses," class barriers and disparity became aggravated, favoring "the cities over the countryside, workers over peasants."[39] Social and medical reforms challenged class barriers "through administrative decentralization and mass mobilization."[40] Mass mobilization addressed the contradiction between an all-around development and elitist privileges and arrogance. The decentralization sought to energize the masses in the grassroots, give full play to their initiatives, and bring them into political and economic processes.

Class divides were most glaring in terms of unequal access to medical care and resources, manifest in the gulf between the privileged urbanites and the deprived peasants with urgent but unmet medical needs. The biopolitical notion of class comes into play here, pointing to the action and aspiration to bridge the class divide and to forge solidarity across different classes and strata. Class is a focal point for mobilizing energy, common purposes, solidarity, and corporeal connectivity. Class unity across social spectrums explains why medicine and health care should be grasped by ordinary men and women to serve the well-being of the broad masses.

Spring Sprouts puts a class stamp on the peasantry by highlighting the generational sufferings of rural victims and their deprivation in the past and present. The peasants share histories, memories, and experiences as a poor and alienated class, even though they are supposed to have been "liberated" from the old society. They live in the shadow of a smoldering trauma related to their collective suffering due to contagious diseases, illness, and the deprivation of health care. On the other hand, an awareness of belonging and attachment to the soil and the regional biosphere marks

37. Mark Selden, *The Yenan Way in Revolutionary China* (Cambridge, MA: Harvard University Press, 1974), 210.
38. Schmalzer, *Red Revolution, Green Revolution*, 4.
39. Carl Riskin, *China's Political Economy: The Quest for Development since 1949* (New York: Oxford University Press, 1988), 184.
40. Riskin, *China's Political Economy*, 184.

the peasantry as a stratum grounded in human-nature interdependence and imbued with corporeal, emotional, and ecological ties. Chunmiao identifies with her village and the peasant class and exhibits intimate corporeal bonds with her coworkers and community, as well as organic rootedness in the field. Her work weaves her kin, neighbors, coworker, and village community into a tightly knit family. The "doctor-patient" relationship in barefoot care goes way beyond clinical, medical, and professional concerns and is fleshed out in class and ethical bonds expressed in kinship ties and in bodily touches in nursing. She feels the pain of the sick intimately and acutely and relates to patients as coworkers, neighbors, kinfolk—bonded together in the ethical sense of bodily connectivity.

The name Tian Chunmiao—literally "plants sprouting in springtime"—captures barefoot medicine's organic embeddedness in the rural community and soil. The image is animistic and ecological, signaling interdependence and intimacy between humans and nature, between the individual and community. Both healer and laborer, Chunmiao does manual labor in the field and treats patients during and after work. As Victor Li noted, since barefoot medicine is inseparable from farm labor, it is unlikely for barefoot doctors to develop the arrogant and elitist attitude due to their growing medical knowledge and skills. They must develop "greater understanding of local and individual illness, hygienic issues, environment, and resources."[41] Working the field and nursing the bodies of coworkers bear the same ecological meanings of intersubjectivity and inter-corporeality.

The organic connection to community and nature is illustrated in the designation of the barefoot doctor as "soiled foot" (*nituizi* 泥腿子), signifying a human person fully planted in the fields and walking the earth. A related expression, *tu yisheng* 土醫生, means "earthy" or "indigenous," as well as "nonprofessional" healer. The naming signals the literal sense of barefoot medicine intertwined with cultivating the soil and crops. As the lyrics of the film's theme song declare: "the fragrance of herbal medicine mingles with the scent of the soil" (*yaoxiang banzhe nitu xiang* 藥香伴著泥土香), and "Spring shoots sprouts out of the earth" (*chunmiao chutu* 春苗出土). Chummiao is "implanted in the hearts of community members; and the sun nurtures her strong growth." Going door to door to serve the villagers, "she leaves her footprint in every home." She regards and treats the sick son of a neighbor as her own flesh and blood. In one treatment with herbs, she regards Uncle Shuichang, an elderly neighbor with back pains, as her own father. She risks her own health and life by running a trial with a higher dose of herbs on herself to be sure it is safe for the patient.

41. Victor H. Li, "Politics and Health Care in China: The Barefoot Doctors," *Stanford Law Review* 27, no. 3 (1975): 837.

While the peasants strive to acquire knowledge and skill of medicine and run their own health care, the bureaucrats and professionals monopolize knowledge and resources and hold on to their class privilege and power. Clinging to the age-old doctrine of class distinction that "those who work with their brains rule; those who work with their hands are ruled" (*laoxinzhe zhiren, laolizhe zhiyuren* 勞心者治人，勞力者治於人), they disparage the peasants and barefoot doctors. Du claims that Chunmiao, a farmer wielding a hoe, cannot handle a syringe" (*na chutou de buneng na zhentou* 拿鋤頭的不能拿針頭). In retort, she shows that peasants have used their hands to cultivate the land and sustain life for countless generations. They have used their hands in dismantling the three mountains of the old society and changing heaven and earth.[42] A powerful revolutionary force, the peasants are capable of becoming masters of the new society as well as masters of the syringe.

The organic image challenges the traditional distinction between intellectual and manual labor and asserts the potential of the uneducated peasants in tapping into modern medical knowledge and indigenous medical traditions. Despite the clampdown on the self-education of barefoot doctors, Chunmiao and her peers engage in training seminars taught by well-trained and committed doctors, learn from folk healers, practice their skills on themselves and on each other, and make strides in medical expertise.

The film's critique of technocratic medicine should not, however, be equated with the anti-intellectual, anti-science rejection of medical knowledge and professional skills. Rather, the barefoot doctors embrace both modern medical sciences and traditional Chinese medicine, passionately striving to become more knowledgeable and skilled in their work. In the spirit of the red-and-expert, their study program combines theory with practice and integrates learning with labor in a variety of half work, half study programs. This practice rests on the conviction that barefoot doctors, by merging socialist consciousness with medical expertise, will become masters of medical science and technology. The self-education epitomizes, according to Maurice Meisner, the socialist ideal that "the masses must make themselves masters of culture and science." Breaking the technocratic elite's monopoly of knowledge and meeting the needs of the masses, the red and expert agenda not only serves as "a means to integrate the professional elite of experts and the political elite of reds but also narrow the gap between both elites and the common people."[43] The barefoot doctors' grasp of knowledge and skills exemplifies a revolutionary movement to make useful and available specialized medical knowledge for the masses.

---

42. The "three mountains" refer to the targets to be overcome by the Chinese revolution: imperialism, feudalism, and bureaucratic capitalism. The last denotes the colonial nationalist rule of the Guomindang regime.
43. Maurice Meisner, *Marxism, Maoism, and Utopianism* (Madison: University of Wisconsin Press, 1982), 127.

In *Spring Sprouts* and *Spring Comes to a Withered Tree*, the most effective cures come about through joint efforts of amateurish doctors working with well-trained professionals. Ivan Illich, socialist philosopher and critic of the corporate monopoly of medicine, captures the barefoot doctor's "vernacular" and revolutionary spirit of mass science: "the time has come to take the syringe out of the hand of the doctor as the pen was taken out of the hand the scribe during the Reformation in Europe."[44] The mass science reenacts the revolutionary idea of "put theory into practice," and the call for intellectuals to integrate with the workers and peasants. This agenda represents the mass-based effort to gain advanced knowledge of modern medicine while avoiding the negative aspects of elitism, professionalism, and bureaucracy.

Conclusion

By examining two Chinese films, this chapter argues that medicine and health care in socialist China can be seen as events of biopolitical production, testifying to the politics-medicine nexus. The transformation of medicine and public health care is fueled by a mass biopolitical production, a dynamic social movement derived from the mass-line mobilization in the revolutionary tradition. The films represent the tensions between a technocratic path of development and socialist mass biopolitical production. Depicting mass health initiatives and barefoot doctors, they critique the medical establishment and profession and the arrogant technocratic class, which became distant and divorced from the health needs of the peasants. They register the growing gap between the city and the countryside, the privileged and the deprived. The anti-epidemic campaign against schistosomiasis demonstrates a symbiotic relationship between leader and the led, the solidarity among the masses, and the deep potential of the people in making social and medical change. The barefoot doctor symbolizes a community-based, ecological, and corporeal reciprocity in the peasant class, the integration of Chinese and Western medicine, and a stringent critique of class disparity in health care.

44. Ivan Illich, *Tools for Conviviality* (New York: Harper and Row, 1973), 48.

Section III

Precarious Ecology and the Body

7

Ecological Crisis and Pathologies of Modernity in the South Korean Films *Crowded* and *Zero Woman*

Max Balhorn

This chapter examines the South Korean films *Crowded* (*Manwŏn*, 1977), directed by Chŏn Cho-myŏng, and *Zero Woman* (*Yŏngnyŏ*, 1979), directed by Pyŏn Chang-ho, which were produced in the late 1970s during a period of heightened public anxiety over the destructive effects of Park Chung-hee's heavy and chemical industrialization drive on the environment and public health. After taking power in a coup in 1961, Park initiated an aggressive industrialization campaign that promised to "modernize the fatherland" while bringing prosperity to all for the price of accepting extreme curtailments to democratic rights. Beginning in the late 1960s, the construction of industrial complexes and manufacturing districts began along South Korea's south-eastern coast. Industrial complexes were located in close proximity to Korea's largest rivers, causing ecological harm to waterways, nearby seas, earth, and air. By 1977, the cultivation of the *tongil* rice variety (meaning "unification rice") had enabled South Korea to achieve self-sufficient rice production.[1] However, the chemical fertilizers and pesticides necessary for guaranteeing high rice yields brought devastating side effects. Chŏng Yŏnghong writes that the enforcement of compulsory, top-down policies severely damaged the fertility of cropland, endangered the health of farmers, and polluted surrounding ecosystems to the degree that plant and animal species were greatly reduced.[2] In industrializing cities such as Ulsan, Onsan, Busan, Masan, and Gwangyang, people living in proximity to factories experienced a variety of eye, respiratory, and skin problems.[3]

1. Mun Man-yong, "Ijung ŭi noksaek hyŏkmyŏng: Park Chung-hee sidae sikryang chŭngsan kwa sallim nok'wa," *Chŏnbuk Sahak* 36 (2010): 164.
2. Chŏng Yŏng-hong, *Chayŏn ŭi haebang kwa minjung ŭi soyo han'guk ŭi hwan'gyŏng munje e taehan kwan'gyeronjŏk chŏpkŭn* (P'aju: Hanul ak'ademi, 2008), 101–27.
3. Han'guk konghae munje yŏn'guso, *Han'guk ŭi konghae chido* (Seoul: Irwŏlsŏgak, 1985), 75–77.

In 1970s South Korea, pollution was omnipresent and constituted a real threat to residents' lives. As Ko T'ae-u writes, "In the mid- to late 1970s, environmental pollution surpassed a critical threshold, with 'pollution diseases' appearing in both human and non-human organisms alike," and as a result, an "undeniable crisis of pollution spread throughout Korean society."[4] However, despite increasingly visible signs of ecological disaster—such as deformed fish caught in the Han River, mass deaths of migratory birds, and highly publicized incidents of mercury poisoning—the Park administration regularly downplayed or outright denied harm caused by pollution, instead choosing to protect the interests of capital and maintain business confidence.[5] Korean intelligence services also intimidated and threatened academics who spoke out about systemic sources of pollution, as such speech was regarded as an attack on state economic policy.[6]

In this context, the two films discussed in this chapter are notable among 1970s South Korean films for placing the issues of pollution and public health at the center of their narratives. Indeed, both *Crowded* and *Zero Woman* conveyed a sense of crisis that reflected real social anxieties over urban pollution, industrial waste, and pesticide toxicity in 1970s South Korea. *Crowded* is set in 1970s Seoul against the backdrop of overflowing landfills, overcrowded city buses, and smog-covered skies. The narrative follows female protagonist Yun, a young newspaper reporter preparing an exposé on the deleterious effects of the "population bomb" on South Korean society. Drawing heavily on neo-Malthusian discourse, the film depicts Seoul as a crowded, dirty, and morally depraved urban jungle that has exceeded its carrying capacity—resulting in worrying implications for the physical, mental, and spiritual health of the population. Reporter Yun visits various medical professionals to obtain information for her article before finally retiring to the countryside to educate villagers about the importance of family planning. In *Zero Woman*, protagonist Chŏng-hŭi, the wife of an overzealous "pollution scientist," suffers repeated bouts of "neurosis" triggered by environmental pollution and loneliness. Her husband's obsession with population statistics leads her to develop an increasingly intense fear of toxic contamination, causing her anxiety to devolve into a state of delusional psychosis. Ultimately, she murders her husband and his young female assistant.

Despite being released by commercial film studios, both films were, in fact, produced with the direct assistance of government health agencies, medical experts, and prominent scientists. *Crowded* received logistical support from the Ministry of Health and Social Affairs, and the studio sought consultations with representatives

4. Ko T'ae-u, "1970–nyŏndae Han'guk ŭi konghae sanghwang kwa chaenan insik," *Kaenyŏm kwa sot'ong* 28 (2021): 14.
5. Ko, "1970–nyŏndae Han'guk ŭi konghae," 23–26, 29–30.
6. Yun Che-yong, "Nugu rŭl wihan hwan'gyŏng chŏngch'aek in'ga," in *Salminya chukŭminya*, ed. Chŏng Ho-kyŏng and Kim Chi-ha (Seoul: Hyŏngsŏngsa, 1985), 101.

from the Economic Planning Board, the Office of Maternal and Child Health, and the National Assembly.[7] Similarly, for *Zero Woman*, Kwŏn Suk-p'yo, director of the Pollution Problem Research Center at Yonsei University, served as an advisor.[8] The involvement of experts from the government and academia is explained by the fact that both films were produced with the explicit objective of being designated as "outstanding films" by the government under a system intended to coerce film studios into producing propaganda films by rewarding them with foreign film importation credits, which were an essential source of revenue for South Korean film studios during this period. As Cho Chun-hyŏng explains, in 1976, the share of foreign film importation credits to be awarded for "outstanding films" increased considerably. In addition, until 1976, the state-run Film Promotion Agency had overseen the production of so-called "policy films" meant to popularize government policies. In 1977, however, the Film Promotion Agency ceased production of policy films, and ten additional foreign film importation credits were allotted for "policy films" produced by commercial studios. As Cho emphasizes, by 1977, nearly all foreign film importation credits were reserved for films deemed "outstanding," which was a determination made by the government.[9] The profits that could be earned from importing foreign films were substantial. As one journalist put it in 1977, earning a foreign film importation credit was a matter of "life and death" for film studios during this time.[10] Although the government did not stipulate the criteria for "outstanding films," it was clearly understood what was expected. For example, director Kim Ho-sŏn commented, "The sickness plaguing Korean Film is the impetus to make films quickly on small budgets that fit the policies of the government in order to earn foreign film importation credits. It is no exaggeration to say that there are no true film producers or filmmakers [in South Korea]."[11]

7. During the preproduction phase of *Crowded*, Union Pictures wrote to the Family Planning Research Institute requesting guidance and logistical support. The institute in turn contacted the Ministry of Health and Social Affairs asking for their cooperation while endorsing *Crowded* as a "family planning film" and "public health film." The ministry responded that it had reviewed the content of *Crowded* and that the film, if distributed widely, would contribute to family planning efforts. The ministry, therefore, committed to providing any needed support for the film's production. See the following documents held in the Korean Film Archive's digital archives: Family Planning Research Institute, "Chemyŏng 'Manwŏn' yŏnghwa chejak e taehan t'ongbo," June 8, 1977, Reference number RK03154004; Ministry of Health and Social Affairs, "Kajok kyehoek yŏnghwa chejak hyŏpcho," June 27, 1977, Refence number RK03154005.
8. See digital database entry for *Zero Woman* at the Korean Movie Database, kmdb.or.kr. The extent of Kwŏn Suk-p'yo's contributions to the film is unclear.
9. Cho Chun-hyŏng, "Kukka ka shijangŭl chibae haessŭl ttae: 1970–nyŏndae chunghuban usu yŏnghwa-oehwa suip k'wŏt'ŏ k'ŏneksyŏn kwa han'guk yŏnghwa," *Yŏnghwa yŏn'gu* 96 (2023): 17.
10. *Chosŏn Ilbo*, "Ch'iyŏlhan kyŏngjeng, usu yŏnghwa sŏnjŏng," August 28, 1977.
11. *Chosŏn Ilbo*, "'Munhwa 77' ŭi ŏlgul (6) yŏnghwa," December 17, 1977.

Crowded and *Zero Woman,* however, are unique among other "outstanding films" from the 1970s. Whereas most of these films centered on themes such as the threat of the communist North, the modernization and industrialization of the "fatherland," and national identity, these two films deal with pollution and environmental degradation—issues that, depending on their treatment, could threaten to delegitimize Park's "growth-first" ideology.[12] As public concern over the effects of pollution on health and the environment grew in late 1970s South Korea, the government could no longer ignore growing discontent, and the state became increasingly active in producing its own counter-discourse to redefine common understandings of the relationship between humans and the environment. For example, Wŏn Chu-yŏng documents how mass mobilization projects led by the state that sought to extract voluntary labor from citizens increasingly placed the responsibility for urban pollution on citizens themselves, with most of the blame reserved for poor urban migrants living in shanty towns without proper plumbing or sewage systems. Wŏn states that urban pollution was reframed as a result of the moral decay that accompanied substandard urban living environments, with authorities arguing that urban problems derived from a lack of concern for one's neighbors, which amounted to a "pathological condition" that required treatment.[13]

As Wŏn demonstrates, as the ecological costs of largely unregulated industrialization proliferated, government agencies and experts in positions of authority began promulgating a new vocabulary for thinking and talking about pollution. While maintaining a similar focus on the pathologizing of pollution, this chapter explores the contribution of medical discourse to popular discussions of pollution and the environment by examining how *Crowded* and *Zero Woman* construct the medicalized body as a crucial mediator that regulates the metabolic relationship between nature and society in 1970s South Korea. I articulate how the narratives of *Crowded* and *Zero Woman* draw on the language of family planning, physical and mental health, and social pathology to reshape common sense understandings of humans' relationship with the environment during a period when the natural ecology was undergoing violent and rapid transformations. Ultimately, this chapter demonstrates how medical knowledge reframed growing tensions between industry and ecology in terms of the individual's responsibility to care for their physical and mental health as a form of active participation in the "spiritual revolution" necessary

12. *Zero Woman* and *Crowded* were not the only Korean films of the late 1970s to dramatize fears over pollution and ecological destruction. Indeed, despite having been taboo subjects for most of the 1960s and 1970s, pollution and the environment became the narrative focus of several films produced at the end of the 1970s, including *Leoh Island* (*Iŏdo*, 1977), *Best Friend* (*Tantchak*, 1979), and *A Monstrous Corpse* (*Koeshi*, 1980).

13. Wŏn Chu-yŏng, "Ŭishik kaesŏnŭl t'onghan hwan'gyŏng kwalli: 1970–nyŏndae ch'o toshi ŭi hwan'gyŏng munje wa toshi saemaŭl undong," *Han'guk kwahaksa hakhoeji* 45, no. 1 (2023): 64.

to propel South Korea along its road of development. Nevertheless, my analysis also recognizes that the studios and directors responsible for *Crowded* and *Zero Woman* were not simply agents of the state. The late 1970s marked a particular moment in Korean film history during which private film studios were increasingly experimenting with combining the genre conventions of narrative cinema with the didactic messaging mandated for the production of "outstanding films." Therefore, in my analysis, I analyze both the narrative structure and thematic content of the films, revealing how these directors manipulated the "outstanding film" genre to negotiate between propaganda and popular appeal.[14]

Sexual Self-Mastery and the "Scientification of the Nation" in *Crowded*

Crowded is composed of one main storyline, as well as several thematically related independent vignettes and musical montages that transport viewers across Seoul to witness scenes of car accidents, petty crimes, sexual promiscuity, congested city streets, and polluted waterways, portraying Seoul as a Malthusian dystopia exceeding its carrying capacity. During one musical interlude, the singer asks, "How did it get this way? Is everyone crazy? Compassion is dying, people are dying, everyone is dying together. How did things get this way? Everyone has become strange. Trees are dying, the air is dying, everything is dying together." Sequences of tightly packed houses and apartments are juxtaposed with beehives and extreme close-ups of disembodied mouths devouring food to convey the "*feel* of overpopulation" and construct abstract humanity as the culprit of pollution.[15]

In the opening sequence of the film, Yun leaves her neatly landscaped, upper-class home in Seoul and arrives at the newsroom, where she learns that she will be doing a story on the world's fastest chicken sexer. Before the interview begins, the man laments that, to his dismay, his pregnant wife has just given birth to another baby girl. Although the man can sex fifty to sixty baby chicks a minute, he is, ironically, powerless to influence the sex of his unborn child. In subsequent scenes, reporter Yun travels around Seoul seeking out knowledge from a gynecologist, family planning educator, and social scientist as she writes her exposé on South Korea's "population explosion." These scenes of Yun traveling around Seoul are interspersed with the exposition of her tragic backstory: unable to become pregnant, Yun and her husband consult a fertility doctor. However, her husband's sperm is not the problem.

14. For a discussion on this negotation between government pressure and popular tastes, see Lee Sun-jin, "Taean yŏnghwa eso sŏnjŏn yŏnghwa kkaji: Han'guk munhwa yŏnghwa ŭi yŏksa wa chaengjŏm," in *Chiwŏjin Han'guk yŏnghwasa: Munhwa yŏnghwa ŭi an kwa pakk*, ed. Lee Byŏng-hun (Seoul: Han'guk yŏngsang charyowŏn, 2014), 14–18.

15. Paul Ehrlich, *The Population Bomb* (New York: Ballantine Books, 1968), 16.

Rather, Yun is told she has "a body that is unable to get pregnant." After divorcing her husband out of shame, she visits a Buddhist temple and a fortune teller, where she seeks advice on how she can reverse her fate and become pregnant with a baby boy.

Interspersed among Yun's fact-finding missions and the exposition of her failed marriage are short, loosely connected vignettes. In one subplot, a short, shifty-eyed man stops a tall, virile-looking man on the street. Following a covert conversation at a café, the two men visit a clinic, where the stranger is given a vial in which to ejaculate. After handing the vial containing his semen to a nurse, the stranger meets the same man in the waiting room, where he is given an envelope of cash. The shifty-eyed man reveals that the semen is for a male friend who is infertile. This sequence is crosscut with scenes of Yun's now ex-husband, who works as a farm veterinarian. Juxtaposed with the scenes of the man at the clinic ejaculating into a vial, Yun's husband is shown collecting semen from a bull. Next, Yun's husband observes the bull semen under a microscope and asks the farmer whether he would like the impregnated egg to become female or male. Here, the narrative strays into the realm of biomedical science fiction, as bovine sperm sexing technology was not developed until the 1980s.[16] In another sequence, a young woman lies in a hospital bed after having given birth as a surrogate mother. An angry older woman tells her that she will only be paid 30,000 won for having carried her son's baby and that she must keep the baby herself, as it turned out to be a girl. In downtown Seoul, a young teenage couple stumbles down a bustling city street after spending the night at a dance club and hotel. Once caught by their parents, they show no shame and talk back. In another display of sexual deviance, a married man out drinking takes a young woman back to a hotel. When his wife questions him the next day, he asks her if she really was a virgin when they married. In a flashback, a mother and embarrassed-looking daughter stand in a doctor's office. The mother asks the doctor to perform a hymenoplasty on her daughter so that she can find a husband. The doctor rebukes her request, asking how her daughter would ever be able to repair the damage to her conscience. In another vignette, a high school sexual education teacher lectures an embarrassed and overexcited class of high school students on human fertilization. In the following scene, she walks in on her own son masturbating in his room. She explains to him that he shouldn't be ashamed: "For humans, sexuality is a rational energy. It's like nuclear energy. Use it correctly, and it is a good thing; use it incorrectly, and it is harmful. What you have done isn't bad."

The narration of *Crowded* vacillates between moral and immoral uses of sex and reproductive technologies. That is, there are disciplined, rational, and intentional applications of sex to facilitate both animal and human reproduction in ways that

16. D. L. Garner and G. E. Sidel Jr., "History of commercializing sexed semen for cattle," *Theriogenology* 69, no. 7 (2008): 886–95.

serve the developmentalist objectives of the state, as well as commoditized and self-serving uses of sex and, quite literally, seminal fluids. In line with Park's "total mobilization of society," in these two films, sex and reproduction are reimagined as calculable, manageable activities performed under the guidance of medical authorities. Sang-hyun Kim writes that under Park's developmentalist regime, state discourse compelled individuals to "transform themselves into national subjects of a new type"—or, as Park Chung-hee stated, "national subjects practicing science." As Kim relates, Park's spearheading of heavy and chemical industrialization in 1973 was supported by the "scientification of the all-nation" movement, which called for the promotion of science and technology as well as the application of scientific thinking for the "rationalization of everyday life."[17] The experimental, omnibus structure of the film depicts a confusing new world where sex and intimacy have been subordinated to a new economic logic enabled by the increased penetration of reproductive technologies and biological markets.[18] The subplots emphasize that in a modern industrial society oriented around efficiency and productivity, sex and reproduction—both animal and human—become subject to the logic of scientific planning and capitalist market exchange. That is, the "scientification" of everyday life removes sex and reproduction from their place in traditional society as unplanned activities of pleasure and subjects them to the logic of economic planning.

On the one hand, this medicalized control over biological reproduction has the potential to unleash the productive capacity of the economy, as demonstrated by the benefits of chick and cattle sperm sexing for agriculture. Yet, on the other hand, it also makes society equally vulnerable to debased and immoral applications of sexual energy that threaten to undo the economic progress of Park's industrialization policies. In this context, this film activates Park's "spiritual revolution," which sought to cure Korean people of the social pathologies that accompanied industrialization and "Westernization" and required individuals to remain vigilant against the potential for sex to be used immorally for deception, individual gain, and pleasure. That is, the didactic message of the film is that when sexuality is treated as a "rational energy"—as represented by the scientific exactness of the farm veterinarian—the negative ramifications of modernization can be mitigated. Likewise, citizens were also repeatedly warned against immoral and degenerate uses of sexuality and medical

17. Sang-hyun Kim, "Science, Technology, and the Imaginaries of Development in South Korea," *Development and Society* 46, no. 2 (2017): 331–32. The Park Chung-hee qoutation is also quoted from this source.

18. The first successful human in vitro fertilization occurred in 1978, a year after *Crowded* was produced. As Se-Kwon Jeong documents, beginning in the early 1970s, the Korean press began actively reporting on the medical innovations in reproductive technology that led to the first human in vitro fertilization. See Jŏng Sae-kwŏn, "Shihŏmgwan agi esŏ ch'eoe sujŏng ŭro? 1970–80-nyŏndae saeroun kwahak kisul e taehan ŏllon podo pyŏnhwa," *Yŏksa pip'yŏng* 136 (2021): 466.

technologies, as symbolized by the semen broker, the parents who hire a surrogate, and the mother seeking a hymenoplasty for her daughter.

For viewers, *Crowded* likely felt suspiciously similar to state-produced newsreels and so-called "culture films" produced in support of family planning initiatives. Indeed, the Family Planning Association and the Ministry of Health and Social Affairs, in collaboration with the National Film Production Company, produced culture films about family planning throughout the 1960s and 1970s, and many of the themes present in *Crowded* can be found in these films.[19] Unsurprisingly, it appears that the film never premiered in Seoul, and perhaps nowhere in the country.[20] A newspaper article from 1979 summarizing the career of actress Lee Kyŏng-sil, who played Reporter Yun, neglects to even mention *Crowded,* despite Lee having played the leading role in the film.[21] This implies that the film may have never been released commercially and that even if it was, its reach was minimal. That said, archival documents at the Korean Film Archive show that Union Pictures filed for screening extension approvals for various provinces up until 1980, suggesting that the film perhaps was screened after all. Nevertheless, the film was selected by the Ministry of Culture and Information as an "outstanding film" in the newly created "policy film" category, granting the studio a foreign film importation credit.[22]

However, as a film produced by a commercial studio, the narrative also contains elements that exist in excess of the edifying function of the film. For example, under the pretext of delivering educational messages about sexual health, *Crowded* grants viewers voyeuristic access to sexual education classrooms, gynecologists' offices, couples' bedrooms, and late-night hotel rooms. This access is most literal in the final sequence of the film, which begins with a finger poking a hole in a paper screen door. The camera then steals a look through the hole, revealing a married couple on their wedding night dressed in traditional *hanbok*. As the groom begins to slowly undress the bride, more fingers poke holes in the screen door, and more watching eyes appear. The giggling of spectators gets louder as the villagers fight over the holes in the screen. Finally, the groom leans over and blows out the candle, and the screen goes black.

---

19. Byŏn Chae-ran, "Taehan nyusŭ, munhwa yŏnghwa, kŭndaejŏk kihoek ŭrosŏŭi 'kajok kyehoek'," *Yŏnghwa yŏngu* 52 (2012): 215–19.
20. Although the Korean Movie Database states that the film premiered in Dongdaemun on January 15, 1978, the Korea Box Office Information System has no records of ticket sales for the film. In his study of outstanding films, Cho Chun-hyŏng also lists *Crowded* as having never premiered in Seoul. See Cho, "Kukka ka shijangŭl chibae haessŭl ttae," 47.
21. *Kyŏnghyang Sinmun,* "Yŏnghwa Osakka ŭi byŏl chuyŏn ŭro: T'aellŏnt'ŭ 4-nyŏn choyŏn tan'gol, Lee Kyŏng-sil yang," July 28, 1979.
22. *Donga Ilbo,* "Munye, silhwa yŏnghwa kakgwang," September 19, 1977; *Chosŏn Ilbo,* "Kongshik palp'yo ŏpshi hwakchŏng doen haban'gi usu yŏnghwa," October 2, 1977.

Perhaps most interesting is the character of Reporter Yun. By the end of the film, she has overcome her shame regarding her infertility and has dedicated her life to spreading family planning knowledge in the countryside. Ironically, in a film meant to normalize the nuclear family as the ideal modern family structure, Yun finds meaning outside of marriage as a single woman who determines her own fate. Indeed, in the context of the social panic over absent housewives and the larger misogynistic backlash against women's growing demands to receive higher education and be recognized as full members of society in the 1970s, the character of Yun is a rather progressive portrayal of a single woman.[23] The film also portrays contraception as a decision to be made independently by wives, not their husbands, and depicts men and parents who reduce their wives and daughters-in-law to their reproductive capacity as backward. Interestingly, around the same period that the film was being produced, the actress who plays Yun, Lee Kyŏng-sil, was involved in a stage production titled *Wall of Love*,[24] which was put on to commemorate the opening of the Women's Baekin Hall by the Korean Legal Aid Center for Family Relations, a progressive organization that sought to revise the hetero-patriarchal Family Law and "enable women to enjoy their rights as full individuals."[25] Although completely speculative, Lee Kyŏng-sil's involvement in the *Wall of Love* suggests a possible connection between the production of *Crowded* and progressive women's organizations. This is not a completely unlikely scenario because, as Kim Hye-kyŏng relates, by 1970, the nascent women's movement had seized on population politics as a useful rhetoric for advancing the rights of women. In particular, women's groups argued that to undo the social preference for male sons, which was seen as the primary motivator for having large families, it was necessary to revise the Family Law to remove articles that vested most legal rights in the male heads of households.[26]

Pollution-Induced Neurosis and Pesticide Hysteria in *Zero Woman*

In contrast to *Crowded*, director Pyŏn Chang-ho's *Zero Woman* conforms to both the stylistic and formal conventions of narrative cinema while disguising its social messaging in intrigue, drama, and suspense. Although the film was made just two years after *Crowded*, the system for compensating outstanding films with foreign film importation credits had undergone significant changes in the intervening two

23. Kim Hye-kyŏng, "Park Chung-hee ch'eje ha 'haekkajok' tamron ŭi byŏnhwa kwajŏng kwai wŏn kujo yŏngu: 'Chosŏn ilbo' rŭl chungsim ŭro," *Sahak wa yŏksa* 82 (2009): 192.
24. *Chosŏn Ilbo*, "Sarang ŭi pyŏk," October 5, 1977.
25. So Hyŏn-suk, "1956–nyŏn kajŏng pŏpryul sangdamso sŏlrip kwa hojujae p'yeji rŭl hyanghan kinagin yŏjŏng," *Yŏksa pip'yŏng* 113 (2015): 73.
26. Kim, "Park Chung-hee ch'eje ha," 190.

years. As mentioned earlier, the system had been routinely criticized by film practitioners. It appears, however, that as the 1970s drew to a close, the government became increasingly aware of the limited reach of "outstanding films." Indeed, policy films and "outstanding films" more generally often failed at the box office, with some never even being released in theaters.[27] In March 1979, at a seminar organized by the Association of Korean Filmmakers titled Korean Film in Transition, Professor Ch'oe Chŏng-ho offered the following insight: "Because outstanding films are still films, they need to follow and respect the principles of commercial appeal and entertainment, which are the very essence of film. The educational, enlightening, and moral elements required for outstanding films should be hidden in the background. It is ideal for the educational, edifying, and moralizing elements to be wrapped in commercially appealing entertainment."[28] Ch'oe's opinion here is likely fairly representative of the dominant opinion of the time, as just one month later, he was appointed to the Performing Arts Ethics Committee,[29] a body composed of members from civilian society that, in 1979, replaced the Ministry of Cultural and Public Information as the body responsible for selecting outstanding films. With this change, the selection committee members now consisted of practitioners from the film industry for the first time in history.[30]

Perhaps anticipating this change in policy, Pyŏn significantly recalibrated the ratio of edifying content to entertainment in *Zero Woman*. When considering the star-studded cast, it appears likely that the studio was seeking to produce a film that could earn box office revenue while also securing a foreign film importation credit. Similar to *Crowded*, the production of *Zero Woman* also involved consultation with an expert in a position of authority. Yonsei University Pollution Problem Research Center Director Kwŏn Suk-p'yo, who had a background in pharmacology and public health, was an advisor for the film. Kwŏn was an interesting choice for a film intended to serve as state propaganda, as he often spoke frankly in public about the shortsightedness of ignoring industrial and urban pollution in the blind pursuit of economic growth. However, likely because he understood that his words could easily anger authorities, he often avoided singling out individual polluters or the government and evaded questions of power and the unequal distribution of environmental harms. Instead, he emphasized the need for consciousness-raising among the public and frugal living, while describing consumers and industry as

27. Oh Chin-gon, "1970–nyŏndae Han'guk 'usu yŏnghwa' ŭi sidaejŏk t'ŭksusŏng koch'al: Yusin chŏngkwŏn sigi chedo, naeyong, sanŏp, hŭrŭm chungsim ŭro," *Inmunhak yŏngu* 47 (2014): 643–44.
28. *Donga Ilbo*, "Usu yŏnghwa simsa munjae itda," March 21, 1979.
29. *Donga Ilbo*, "Yŏnghwa kŏmyŏl wiwŏn wich'ok," April 07, 1979.
30. *Donga Ilbo*, "P'ando tallajil usu ch'uch'ŏn yŏnghwa . . . Yesim wiwŏn chŏnwŏn i yŏnghwage chongsaja," October 27, 1979.

"accomplices" in the destruction of the environment.[31] In this way, Kwŏn's framing of environmental problems was not fundamentally incompatible with Park's modernization discourse, which emphasized that economic growth could only be achieved when individuals voluntarily remade themselves into rational, modern citizens who practiced frugality and diligence while putting the interests of one's family, and by extension, the nation, above one's own interests.[32]

Despite Kwŏn's involvement and the film's explicit focus on pollution as a social problem that threatens social stability, the Performing Arts Ethics Committee neglected to select *Zero Woman* as an outstanding film for 1979.[33] The film did, however, achieve relative success with audiences. The film sold 45,649 tickets in Seoul,[34] with one reviewer at the *Chosŏn Ilbo* commenting, "Byŏn Chang-ho's film *Zero Woman* continues to increase in popularity . . . Director Byŏn uses the narrative techniques of mystery to highlight the issue of mental pollution. The film reminds us that this tragedy of one professor's family could happen to any of us."[35] Another review in the *Kyŏnghyang Sinmun* highlights both the film's timely subject matter and engaging storytelling, writing that the film is a suspenseful and fast-paced "psychodrama" about a "protagonist suffering from sexual hysteria caused by a physical ailment resulting from air pollution, which sends her to a mental hospital."[36]

The plot of *Zero Woman* revolves around a love triangle involving pollution scientist Professor Kang, his wife, Chŏng-hŭi, and his young female assistant, Nami. Chŏng-hŭi first appears in the film wandering through heavy traffic in downtown Seoul. The scene is shot from both Chŏng-hŭi's perspective and that of the cars on the street. The scene is captured using a fish-eye lens and is accompanied by dark, foreboding music, establishing Chŏng-hŭi as a vulnerable yet potentially dangerous character driven mad by pollution. This sequence is crosscut with a scene of Professor Kang lecturing to his students, warning them, "The domination of nature has been the development of humankind. That has been the flow of history, and it continues to this day. Yet, this domination of nature has destroyed the cycle of the ecosystem. Consequently, pollution is an invisible murderer that is putting us all at risk." While pointing to a fishbowl containing deformed fish affected by industrial

---

31. Kwŏn Suk-p'yo, "Sobi rŭl churinŭn kil pak e," *Kyŏnghyang Sinmun*, July 1, 1975.
32. This is not to say that Kwŏn was an apologist for South Korean industry or the Park administration. Throughout the 1970s, he regularly stressed the need for stricter and more comprehensive pollution regulation, and on several occasions, he was interrogated by national intelligence authorities in retaliation for his outspoken position on the negative consequences of unregulated economic growth on the environment and public health. See Ku Cha-gŏn, "Oyŏm munje yŏmnyŏ hada koch'o 'hakcha yangshim' chik'yŏ naesyŏtchyo," *Han'gyŏre*, March 3, 2010.
33. *Kyŏnghyang Sinmun*, "Usu ch'uch'ŏn yŏnghwa simsa ssago yŏlpung," November 16, 1979.
34. Ticket sales data obtained from Korea Box-Office Information System, https://www.kobis.or.kr/.
35. *Chosŏn Ilbo*, "0-yŏ," September 9, 1979.
36. *Kyŏnghyang Sinmun*, "0-yŏ, konghae e tchidŭn ingan kŭryŏ," September 7, 1979.

waste, he warns his students that human babies can suffer similar fates. Similar to *Crowded*, the use of distorted perspectives, rapid cuts, close-ups, and car-mounted cameras all function to simulate the disorientation of urban life. While in his lab, Professor Kang receives a call from his housekeeper informing him that his wife, Chŏng-hŭi, has fled the house in a strange mental state. In the next scene, Professor Kang arrives at the psychiatric ward where Chŏng-hŭi has been admitted. The doctor explains that Chŏng-hŭi's illness has been caused by "malaise, anxiety, and nervousness." Next, the doctor takes Professor Kang on a tour of the ward where his wife and other female patients have been admitted. The patients are held in what looks like prison cells, and they reach out through the bars like zombies to grab passersby. The doctor explains, "Recently, we have had a large increase in these types of patients. Although it is unclear why, it seems that the cause may be various forms of pollution in their environments."

After Chŏng-hŭi's diagnosis, Nami comes to live at Professor Kang's home to help with housework while Chŏng-hŭi recovers. However, Chŏng-hŭi becomes jealous and repeatedly hallucinates visions of the two in intimate situations. It becomes clear that for years, Professor Kang has been engrossed in his pollution research and has neglected his marriage. Moreover, his obsession with pollution has caused his wife to develop an overwhelming fear of industrial toxins, pesticides, and radioactive fallout. Like Reporter Yun in *Crowded*, Chŏng-hŭi seeks out a medical doctor and a gynecologist. While examining her for hearing loss, the doctor tells her that traffic noise can impair the body's physiological processes and comments that chickens raised near airports have been shown to lay fewer eggs. Next, she visits a gynecologist and asks him to perform a tubal ligation on her because she is "consumed by the fear" that she will give birth to a deformed baby. When asked how she reached this conclusion, she relates the story of a family in New Mexico that had unknowingly fed grain sprayed with pesticide containing mercury to their pig and then ate the pig, causing serious disability in the unborn child of one of the family members—an obvious reference to an actual event that occurred in the United States in 1970 and was reported around the globe, including in Korea.[37]

As Chŏng-hŭi's jealousy over Nami intensifies, her actions become increasingly violent. In one scene, she grabs her husband's hunting rifle and begins shooting at her pet birds and even points the rifle at the housekeeper. In a later scene that resembles an erotic thriller, Chŏng-hŭi enters the bathroom while Nami is showering and offers to wash her back. Once in position, Chŏng-hŭi digs her ring into Nami's back, drawing blood. Shortly after, Chŏng-hŭi hallucinates Nami chasing her up the stairs and onto the rooftop. The scene uses horror genre conventions,

37. Martin Waldron, "Mercury in Food: A Family Tragedy," *The New York Times*, August 10, 1970; *Donga Ilbo*, "Pungmi hach'ŏn ŭi suŭn oyŏm," October 2, 1970.

such as low-key lighting and dissonant strings, heightening the suspense. Once on the roof, Nami strangles Chŏng-hŭi and throws her from the top of the apartment tower. In reality, however, Chŏng-hŭi is collapsed at the top of the stairs, drained by her hallucination. Bedridden and listless, Chŏng-hŭi laments that she has "lost all qualifications as a wife." Unlike Nami, who is an excellent cook and a disciplined and frugal housekeeper, Chŏng-hŭi is absent from the household and, in her own words, "fails to fulfill her duties as a woman to her husband."

In 1970s Korea, the increase in diagnoses of neurosis was interpreted as a sign of a general pathological sickness in Korean culture and society itself.[38] Moreover, particular attention was paid to married women, as doctors noted that rates of neurosis among married women had begun rising rapidly in the 1960s.[39] Academics also began drawing connections between urban pollution and increasing rates of mental illness. At an academic conference titled "Pollution and Neurosis" held in 1970 at the Young Women's Christian Association, Doctor Kim Jong-un from the psychiatric center at St. Mary's Hospital commented that although pollution is not sufficient to cause hysteria, noise and car exhaust, as well as other forms of pollution, contribute to the prevalence of "anxiety neurosis" among the population. One journalist summarized the content of Dr. Kim's presentation, relating, "Kim stated that in an environment like South Korea, where it is difficult to improve society, rather than asking how negative of an effect pollution will have on society, it is better to consider how to cultivate individuals who can withstand any and all pollution. He said that, for example, mothers should take responsibility for their children's mental health and take certain precautions beginning with prenatal education . . . and stated that a countermeasure against neurosis must involve raising individuals with strong mental fortitude that allows them to withstand shocks."[40] Meanwhile, at another symposium held in 1973, Professor Ŭn Chun-kwan argued that the "mental crisis" facing humankind in the modern age cannot be explained solely in terms of the dehumanizing effect of modernity on the inner life of the individual. Rather, he stated that "external changes, such as the environmental pollution spoken about by ecologists and the breakdown of human relationships in the sociological sense, are also primary causes." He continued, "We must see anxiety and pollution as an organic reality that exists in a mutually penetrating relationship."[41]

In *Zero Woman*, Chŏng-hŭi is not the only woman stricken by pollution-induced hysteria. As the jealousy and tension build between Nami and Chŏng-hŭi, Nami

38. Im Chi-yŏn, "1960–70-nyŏndae Han'guk chŏngsin ŭihak tam'ron yŏngu: Chŏngsin wisaenghak eso hyŏndae chŏngsin ŭihak ŭro," *Ŭisahak* 26, no. 2 (2017): 203.
39. Ch'oe U-yŏng, "1970–nyŏndae chubu tam'ron ŭi hwaksan kwa kŭ yŏnghyang: Chubu tŭlŭi chilbyŏng kwa 'talson' ŭl chungsim ŭro" (Master's thesis, Kookmin University, 2021), 18.
40. *Kyŏnghyang Sinmun*, "YWCA anbang semina konghae wa noirojae," June 18, 1970.
41. *Chosŏn Ilbo*, "Hyŏndae ŭi hwangyŏng: Jŏngsin ŭi pyehae, bulan kwa konghae," October 17, 1973.

reveals that she, too, suffers from an all-consuming fear of pollution. She relates that her father, who used to work at a pesticide plant, became severely disabled after falling ill from mercury poisoning. She is now terrified of marriage and pregnancy, as she worries that she also may have absorbed these toxins, which may result in her giving birth to a severely deformed baby. As Nami speaks, successive in utero images of developing fetuses reminiscent of the photographs of Lennart Nilsson fill the screen. For viewers in 1979, this anecdote would have been understood as a direct reference to a mercury poisoning incident that occurred in Damyang County in South Jeolla Province the year prior, which dominated the headlines.[42] Farmer Ko Ŭn-sŏk and his family began suffering from general paralysis and blindness in October 1977. Initially, the local physician in Gwangju concluded that they were suffering from mercury poisoning after spraying large amounts of pesticide.[43] As one of the first publicized cases of heavy metal poisoning, the event drew national attention. National health authorities became involved in early 1978. They collected hair, urine, and blood serum samples from the patients and sent them to the National Institute of Health for analysis.[44] The question of whether Ko and his family were suffering from mercury poisoning became a point of tension between the government and national health authorities on the one hand, and university researchers and the opposition party on the other. The New Democratic Party organized its own investigation team, and after finding evidence of mercury poisoning, they asserted that the authorities were attempting to cover up evidence.[45] After much anticipation, the government released its findings on April 10, 1978, claiming that no significant amount of mercury had been detected and that Ko and his family were not suffering from pesticide poisoning.[46] Under pressure, President Park intervened in the debate, suggesting that a joint research team including government health officials and academics should be formed.[47] However, this plan soon evaporated, as the Park government and ruling party politicians ultimately opposed the measure, stating that the results of the government survey were "scientifically valid" and that there was no need to cause further confusion among the public.[48]

In *Zero Woman*, Chŏng-hŭi's fears of pollution and pesticide poisoning are similarly doubted. Following one of Chŏng-hŭi's desperate visits to the hospital after her

42. The *Donga Ilbo* listed the incident as one of the top ten stories of the year. See *Donga Ilbo*, "Kyŏktong ŭi 78 ponsasŏnjŏng 10-tae nyusŭ," December 28, 1978.
43. *Chosŏn Ilbo*, "Ssal tŭng nongyak ppurin nongjangmul mŏkko ilga 6-myŏng mansŏng suŭn chungdok chŭngse," March 25, 1978.
44. *Chosŏn Ilbo*, "Tamyang ilga suŭn nongyak chungdok hwakshil handŭt," April 9, 1978.
45. *Kyŏnghyang Sinmun*, "Tamyang nongyak chungdok sagŏn sun chungdok yŏbu ŭigyŏn ŏtkallyŏ," March 30, 1978.
46. *Kyŏnghyang Sinmun*, "Ko ssi ilga suŭn chungdok anida," April 10, 1978.
47. *Donga Ilbo*, "Suŭn p'ihae animyŏn mwŏn'ga hakkye wa haptong chosa ŏttŏlchi," April 13, 1978.
48. *Chosŏn Ilbo*, "Tamyang kibyŏng ŭi chaejosa rŭl," April 16, 1978.

initial hospitalization, her doctor secretly calls Professor Kang, informing him that his wife is suffering from an acute case of "pollution paranoia." In the final third of *Zero Woman*, Professor Kang takes Chŏng-hŭi to the countryside to recuperate at a remote cabin on a lake far from the pollution of the city. For several weeks, she makes progress and begins to put her problems behind her. With the unexpected arrival of Nami, however, her paranoia returns. When Professor Kang departs for a lecture in Seoul, leaving the two women alone together, Chŏng-hŭi lures Nami into the basement, where she strangles her and leaves her for dead. When Professor Kang returns, Nami stumbles up from the basement, still alive. Chŏng-hŭi grabs her husband's hunting rifle and shoots and kills Nami and Professor Kang in a fit of manic ecstasy.

Although *Zero Woman* was produced in 1978 and released in September 1979, Donga Entertainment had initially submitted the film to authorities for pre-censorship approval in 1977. In November 1977, however, the studio retracted its initial submission. It resubmitted a new script in May 1978.[49] Therefore, it is possible to compare the 1977 script, which was written before the Damyang poisoning incident, with the 1978 script, which, having been submitted for pre-censorship screening in May 1978, was likely written during the months that the Damyang controversy reached its climax. The primary difference between the two scripts lies in the characterization of Chŏng-hŭi. In the 1977 script, Chŏng-hŭi's neurosis is primarily explained as a result of being neglected by her pollution-obsessed husband and the jealousy she feels towards Nami. The 1977 version lacks the scene where Chŏng-hŭi seeks out a gynecologist for a tubal ligation out of fear of giving birth to a deformed baby. Also missing is a scene where she screams hysterically at Professor Kang when he comes home wet from the rain, as she believes he has been contaminated by radioactive fallout. In the 1977 script, Chŏng-hŭi and Professor Kang also have a young son named Min, and Chŏng-hŭi does not directly express any anxious or paranoid thoughts about pollution. Moreover, whereas in the final film, Nami reveals her own fears of pesticides, the 1977 script makes no mention of this backstory. That is, in the new script, which was likely written during the Damyang incident, pollution anxiety is featured more prominently as the cause of Chŏng-hŭi's neurosis and Nami's hesitations about marriage. The most obvious difference, however, is the ending. In the 1977 script, the murder of Nami and Professor Kang by Chŏng-hŭi is simply another of Chŏng-hŭi's hallucinations. In the final scene, a rehabilitated Chŏng-hŭi is discharged from the hospital into the custody of Professor Kang, and the two decide

49. See the following documents held in the Korean Film Archive's digital archives: Korean Performing Arts Ethics Committee, "Kŭngnyŏnghwa shinario shimŭi kyŏlgwa pogo," September 13, 1977, Reference number RK03318001; Donga Entertainment, "Kŭngnyŏnghwa 'Yŏngnyŏ' chejak shin'go chajin ch'wiha," November 2, 1977, Reference number RK03318004; Donga Entertainment, "Yŏnghwa chejak shin'gosŏ," May 30, 1978, Reference number RK03318006.

to take a vacation to Jeju Island. As they depart, Professor Kang opines, "Worrying is what makes us sick. Worrying is a form of mental pollution that is scarier than industrial pollution. Got it, darling?" Chŏng-hŭi responds, "Yeah, that's right. If we simply live diligently, everything will work out." To this, Professor Kang replies, "Of course. As they say, it is an honor just to have been born. Life is joyous."

In both versions of the film, Chŏng-hŭi is depicted as both a sympathetic patient in need of compassionate psychiatric care and an unstable psychopath appropriate for a slasher film. After one of her hallucinations, Chŏng-hŭi is visited by a doctor. Resting in bed, she tells her husband that she is "consumed by overwhelming darkness." Her husband comforts her, stating, "Don't talk nonsense. In the era of pollution, all modern people are patients. Right now, your rest is paramount." As Im Chi-yŏn writes, beginning in the 1960s, mental illness began to be seen as an index of South Korea's economic development, with newspaper advertisements for new drugs meant to treat neurosis referring to the condition "an accessory of modern people,"[50] reflecting the increasing visibility of and familiarity with mental illness in everyday life. Concurrently, the post-liberation generation of psychiatrists argued that becoming a modern nation mandated treating people with mental illnesses as patients in need of love and support. This was particularly true in the context of recent highly publicized murders committed by mental health patients who did not receive proper care due to South Korea's insufficient mental health services.[51] Im Chi-yŏn writes that in the context of Park's Yushin ideology, which stressed the creation of a "cheerful" and "healthy" society, there was an imperative to treat mental health patients as individuals in need of scientific intervention and professional treatment.[52]

In this context, the changes made to Chŏng-hŭi's character may help explain why the film failed to receive outstanding film status. That is, the initial ending to the film frames Chŏng-hŭi's fear of pollution as a treatable phobia of modern people and emphasizes that the solution to pollution lies in the "diligence" of the individual receiving care. The final version of the film, however, jettisons this didactic story of redemption and rehabilitation and instead intensifies the action by emphasizing Chŏng-hŭi's mental instability and abnormality while relocating Chŏng-hŭi's violence from her dreams to the real world. In the context of the government's largely indifferent response to the Damyang incident, these changes likely reflect the studio's attempts to seize on growing public anxiety over the poorly understood risks of environmental pollution by shifting the focus of the narrative from pollution itself to mental illness as a pathological response to pollution anxiety. Nevertheless, the

50. Im, "1960–70-nyŏndae Han'guk," 201.
51. Im, "1960–70-nyŏndae Han'guk," 196.
52. Im, "1960–70-nyŏndae Han'guk," 199.

studio seems to have miscalculated the Performing Arts Ethics Council's tolerance for violence. Writing in 1979, a nameless commentator argued that although the transfer of censorship duties from the government to the civilian-run Performing Arts Ethics Committee was anticipated to result in more relaxed censorship and more artful and entertaining films, the undeveloped and immature state of the Korean film industry meant that this change may result in an overall lowering of standards because of "filmmakers who focus exclusively on sex scenes and shocking depictions of violence under the pretext that it is art."[53]

In the final scene of the film, one of Professor Kang's male students visits Chŏng-hŭi in the psychiatric ward, but she has lost her capacity for rational conversation and simply giggles uncontrollably. He walks out onto the street, where he stumbles on an anti-pollution rally. A troop of young male scouts led by an all-girl marching band holds a banner reading, "Let's create a cheerful society by expelling pollution." It is an overtly propagandistic image that uses the familiar rhetoric of official state discourse. The rally itself can be placed within the larger history of state-facilitated "environmental protection" campaigns that began in the late 1970s and included activities such as mass trash cleanups meant to mobilize citizens as part of Park's "spiritual revolution." The awkward insertion of this rather out-of-place final scene can be seen as an attempt to enforce ideological finality on a text that has strayed far from its edifying function as an aspiring "outstanding film."

Conclusion

In both *Crowded* and *Zero Woman*, medical discourses seeking to diagnose the social pathologies of industrializing South Korea reshape common sense notions of pollution and public health by drawing attention away from the widening metabolic rift between society and nature and instead framing pollution as a medical problem that requires individuals to manage their own physical and mental health. That is, under the authoritarian cultural politics of Park Chung-hee's Yushin regime, pollution was represented as an inevitable byproduct of modernization and industrialization that risked eroding the physical, mental, and moral health of the nation. Moreover, as both films demonstrate, medical professionals gained increasing authority over defining the proper attitude that the individual must take toward pollution. Likewise, the narratives of both films function to define normal and abnormal responses to pollution and ecological destruction.

In *Crowded*, for example, pollution is not conceived as a result of a disequilibrium between the natural environment and human society; rather, it is conceived as a *moral* problem of human behavior. In short, in *Crowded*, environmental pollution

53. *Kyŏnghyang Sinmun*, "Yŏnghwa kŏmyŏl ŭi min'gan iyang," March 24, 1979.

begins not in the factory but in the bedroom.[54] When Reporter Yun speaks with Doctor Kim in his hospital office, he tells her that the key to lowering population growth is eliminating sexual immorality, which is caused more generally by a loss of "humanity" and the continued increase of "inhuman" elements in society, including "arousal, pleasure, and empty attachment," as well as a loss of "individual dignity and responsibility." Back at her typewriter, Yun continues her article, writing, "Birth must be the product of love . . . However, these days, you can see everywhere births that are the result of a love mistake. This collapse of sexual morality is another factor contributing to population growth."

Despite having possibly jeopardized the film's chances of achieving "outstanding film" status, the changes to *Zero Woman* take on an additional political connotation in light of the Damyang incident. Following the hospitalization of the Ko family, health authorities repeatedly denied their claims of pesticide poisoning, arguing that if they were sick, it was the result of an as yet unidentified illness. After the incident, the government displayed a general indifference toward better understanding the extent of pesticide poisoning and failed to allocate sufficient resources for further epidemiological studies.[55] Similar to Doctor Kim Jong-un's emphasis on the cultivation of "individuals who can withstand any and all pollution" through "strong mental fortitude," responsibility for pesticide poisoning and other forms of pollution came to rest with the individual rather than the state. That is, medical responses to pollution in 1970s South Korea served to neutralize social anxieties and public anger over increasing disease caused by industrial pollution, deflecting attention away from questions of power and inequality and reframing pollution as a matter of consciousness.

---

54. Critiquing green populationism and its tendency to blame population growth rather than corporate abuses for environmental pollution, environmentalist Barry Commoner states, "Pollution begins not in the family bedroom, but in the corporate board-room." Quoted in Michael Egan and Robert Gottlieb, *Barry Commoner and the Science of Survival: The Remaking of American Environmentalism* (Cambridge, MA: The MIT Press, 2007), 130.
55. Yi Sŭl-gi, "Nongyak chungsim ŭro pon noksaek hyŏngmyŏng: 1970-nyŏndae chŭngsan kwa konghae e karyŏjin nongyak chungdok," *Han'guk kwahaksa hakhoeji* 43, no. 1 (2021): 230–31.

8

Beyond Locality

Ke Chin-yuan's Environmentalist Documentary and Cultural Nativism

Pao-chen Tang

The ending of the Taiwanese filmmaker Ke Chin-yuan's 2018 documentary, *The Age of Awakening* (*Qianjin* 前進), shows a group photograph (Figure 8.1) in which Ke stands next to Wang Zhi-zhang and Cai Ming-de—a reunion of three media workers who have been recording grassroots eco-activism since the dusk of Taiwan's martial law period (1949–1987) under the Kuomintang's (KMT) authoritarian rule.[1] Behind them stands Taiwan's Presidential Office Building, a conscious background selection as we hear Ke ask the photographer to confirm if this consummate symbol of political authority is included in the image. Given that the film conducts a critical survey of key environmental movements and their outcomes across Taiwan from the mid-1980s to the late 2010s, the ending strikes a somewhat defeatist tone, however smiley the three men might seem. After thirty years of eco-activism in Taiwan, media activists like Ke, Wang, and Cai are still physically and symbolically *outside*, even though their agendas have been supported by various political forces at different stages during their pursuit of power. Indeed, one of the film's central inquiries is how bottom-up environmentalism could ever find its way into the system, which always seems to privilege industrial development at the expense of ecological conservation and public health.

In terms of realpolitik, such a stalemate is hardly unsurprising. Since 1996, there have been three rounds of democratically elected alternations in power between the two major political parties, the KMT and the Democratic Progressive Party (DPP).

1. There are two versions of *The Age of Awakening*: a fifty-five-minute one and a 108-minute one. The difference in length is related to each version's target platform of exhibition. The former was first broadcast through Taiwan's Public Television Service, for which Ke had been working in the news division since 1998; the latter debuted at the 2018 Taiwan International Documentary Festival. My discussion of the film throughout this chapter refers to the latter since I believe its length affords a clearer articulation and contextualization of Ke's ideas and agendas.

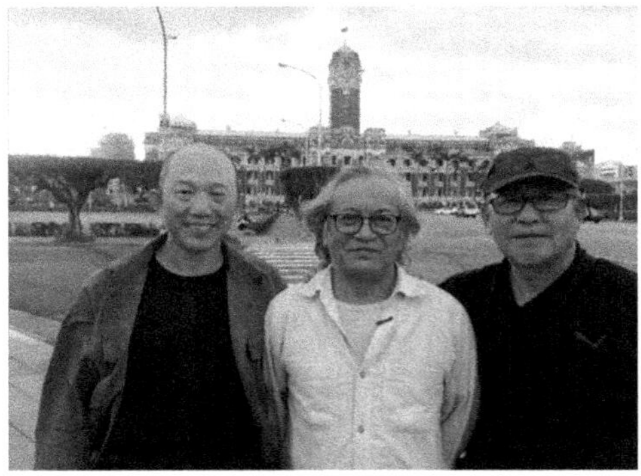

Figure 8.1: Three veteran media activists in front of the Presidential Office Building. Courtesy of Ke Chin-yuan.

During this period, there have been many instances of politicians' disavowals of their electoral promises of change once they ascend to power. As prominent writer, scholar, and activist Chen Yu-feng openly criticizes in his introductory speech at the premiere of *The Age of Awakening*:

> I have to say that the environmental condition in Taiwan has only deteriorated, especially after the DPP obtained both executive and legislative powers. Let's spell out the obvious: Why did those politicians who had promoted environmental protection to gain fame and credibility before May 20, 2016 [the new government inauguration date], once tainted by power, disappear during the campaign against the construction of the Shuangxi Reservoir? Or the destruction of algae reef? Or the construction of landfills in Matoushan and Longqi? Why didn't you stand out against the deceitful National Spatial Plan or Forward-Looking Infrastructure Plan? During all the air pollution protests, where have you been hiding?[2]

This is not to say that all environmental movements since the late 1980s have failed; several were successful, which the film acknowledges. However, as Wang mentions towards the end of the film, "although progressive social movements, initiated by the people for the people, have existed in Taiwan for more than thirty years, has the environmental condition really improved? One protest after another still takes place, with each fight getting more arduous and complex." Discrete cases of triumph have not led to structural change, despite media activists' ongoing attempts to shape an ecologically minded civic society, from which the two major parties have in turn gained the consent of the governed.

---

2. Chen Yu-feng, "Qianjin yu Aige: ke chin-yuan daoyan jilupian shouying yinyan," *Shanlin shuyuan*, May 12, 2018, http://slyfchen.blogspot.com/2018/05/blog-post_12.html. Unless otherwise indicated, all translations from Chinese to English are mine.

But beyond laying bare political hypocrisy that is hardly news for anyone, *The Age of Awakening* interrogates this impasse from an aesthetic perspective by self-reflexively examining the entangled relations among media production, activism, and the dominant cultural-political discourse. As the film reevaluates several major eco-activist events, it braids together old and new images from Ke's own filmmaking, archival news footage, segments of other documentaries, and interviews with activists young and veteran alike. In revisiting an array of aesthetic strategies and modes of representation that Ke and fellow activists have taken up in their collective mobilization of mass media, the film wonders why none of the strategies have been truly effective in enacting positive changes at the macro level of public policy.

This chapter studies the changing aesthetics across Ke's recent films, with the goal of using them as a paradigmatic case study to clarify how the political reality and the development of environmentalist documentary in Taiwan have mutually shaped each other. Taking a cue from Chen's stark critique of the DPP at the film's premiere, I am interested in exploring Ke's work in relation to the ideology of nativism (*bentu zhuyi* 本土主義), which nationalist social actors, including DPP affiliates, have frequently mobilized to construct a Taiwan-centric consciousness in the public sphere. Culturally, this ideology prioritizes localist rather than transregional concerns; politically, it tends to support a separatist project of establishing an independent, democratic Taiwanese statehood—both *de facto* and *de jure*—that counters the different interpretations of "one China" offered by the KMT and the Chinese Communist Party. An example of how this ideology operates, as demonstrated by Jeremy E. Taylor, is Taiwanese nativism's localization of sundry cultural and linguistic symbols by erasing their nonlocal mobility and history, such as the transregional topolect Hokkien, which has come to be appropriated by pro-independence social actors as "the preserve of Taiwanese nationalism."[3]

From the literary sphere in the 1960s to the film industry in the 1980s and beyond, numerous works of art have responded to this nativist ideology in diverse and dissonant forms. In their study of Taiwan New Cinema, for instance, Darrell William Davis and Emilie Yueh-yu Yeh identify how nativist ideology structures "a narrative and psychological resource" for people whose cultures, stories, and languages had been marginalized in the public sphere by the ruling KMT, given that they were considered "provincial and rural" in the officially endorsed Sinocentric cultural paradigm, which has privileged "things that preoccupied Chinese émigrés and the KMT: developments on the mainland, anticommunism, or patriotism."[4]

3. Jeremy E. Taylor, "From Transnationalism to Nativism? The Rise, Decline and Reinvention of a Regional Hokkien Entertainment Industry," *Inter-Asia Cultural Studies* 9, no. 1 (2008): 63.
4. Darrell William Davis, and Emilie Yueh-yu Yeh, *Taiwan Film Directors: A Treasure Island* (New York: Columbia University Press, 2005), 63.

While there is no single coherent "nativist style" specific to cinema, the antagonism between the official and the provincial frequently manifests itself through a range of thematic and stylistic tropes. Some examples are the urban-rural dichotomy, the celebration of non-Mandarin dialects (especially Hokkien), the formation of grass-roots communities and identities, and political liberation against the KMT.

Crucial to note here is that the nativist ideology is not to be conflated with these aesthetic practices that reflect on it, insofar as the politics of the abovementioned tropes do not inherently idealize locality or promote a specific set of political agendas. As Christopher Lupke reminds us, even if the label of nativism might be assigned to certain artworks that engage with the nativist ideology, not all artists necessarily embrace the term, nor do they unanimously reject the influence of Chinese culture or accept the separatist agenda. Many of them have offered profound critiques of the constructed nature of the Taiwan-centric consciousness and its conceptual dichotomies since the 1960s.[5] By studying Ke's recent documentaries in relation to nativism, therefore, my point is not to suggest the existence of a united front of nativist social actors (including politicians and artists) against which Ke is reacting. Nor am I interested in identifying the director's personal political or ideological inclination. Rather, I hope to explore how this dominant cultural discourse functions like a heuristic device, sharpening an edge through which Ke's tropes, filmed subjects, actions, and the relations among them might be interpreted and rendered available (or not) to social practices. The fact that Ke's films are meant to be viewed as documentaries does not conflict with their mobilization of nativist tropes. Indeed, some of his films have been described as, following Frederic Jameson's much-discussed take on third world literature, "national allegories" that offer "a down-to-earth geographical curriculum of nationalism, a geographical self-education for the Taiwanese."[6]

Ke's filmmaking, I would submit, once relied on the nativist discourse as an expedient tool to facilitate the channeling of political passion into environmental protection. Problems emerged, however, when it became clear that the convergence of these two kinds of loves—of the imagined nation and of the concrete land—was insufficient as a conceptual frame for mapping ground-level social reality. With a growing awareness of the drawback of idealizing locality as inherently environmental and anti-authoritarian, Ke's filmmaking embarked on a search for an alternative set of aesthetic devices that better served his eco-activist goals. In this process, he has experimented with various strategies of staging an image of Taiwan that more

5. Some famous examples include writers Huang Chun-ming and Chen Ying-zhen, and filmmakers Hou Hsiao-hsien and Wang Toon. Christopher Lupke, "Nativism and Localism in Taiwanese Literature," in *The Columbia Companion to Modern Chinese Literature*, ed. Kirk A. Denton (New York: Columbia University Press, 2016), 258–59, 263.

6. Chen Pen-juin, "Jilupian zuowei guozu yuyan: women de lingyitang dilike," *Xinwenxue yanjiu*, no. 129 (2016): 3, 13.

accurately captures the island's current role at both local and global levels: a major source of industrial pollutions and greenhouse gas emissions. As this chapter aims to demonstrate, these strategies indicate at once an eco-political stance and an aesthetic choice.

Considering Ke's prolificity (more than thirty documentaries to date), I can only selectively discuss the inner complexities of his still-expanding oeuvre. My focus will be on a group of films that effectively demonstrate his aesthetic transformation: *Formosa vs. Formosa* (*Fuermosha dui fuermosha* 福爾摩沙對福爾摩沙, 2010), *Ebb and Flow* (*Tuichao* 退潮, 2011), *Black* (*Hei* 黑, 2013), and *The Age of Awakening*. These films tackle such detrimental environmental impacts as the industrial pollution of air, water, and land, as well as the resulting long-term public health hazards. While industrial pollution is only one among many topics that Ke's filmmaking has addressed (other major concerns include nature conservation, animal welfare, high-altitude mountaineering, and Taiwan's military bases in the South China Sea), my decision to isolate these films is informed by their shared engagement with the nativist discourse. Additionally, social movements against industrial pollution themselves served as crucial channels through which political movements against the KMT took place in the 1980s. The decade witnessed, according to Ke himself, "heated debates over nativist culture and the emergence of reportage literature and reportage photography. This was also the time when the authoritarian governance was gradually collapsing and various social movements were rising. This was a burgeoning time for the environmental documentary, and the development of the genre started with two strands, documentation of people's protests and that of nature."[7] The topic of industrial pollution thereby offers a vantage point from which Ke reevaluates the potential and limitations of endowing a set of thematic and stylistic tropes with an inherent (eco)political stance.

My study of these films follows their chronology, insofar as they exemplify different stages in the trajectory of Ke's recent filmmaking. *Formosa vs. Formosa* and *Ebb and Flow* adhere to the nativist opposition between the governmental and the local, between the privileged and the subaltern. *Black* reworks this opposition by demystifying the romanticized depiction of "the local," especially rural subjects in areas troubled by industrial pollution. *The Age of Awakening* further rejects an essentialist account of Taiwanese subjectivity by remapping it from an ecological perspective, one that repositions Taiwan's imagined self from a localized victim of pollution to a neo-imperial hegemony, which produces and exports pollution at a transregional level.

---

7. Tsai Tsung-lung, Yu Li-ping, and Ke Chin-yuan, "A Glimpse at the Development of the Environmental Documentary in Taiwan," *Concentric: Literary and Cultural Studies* 39, no. 1 (2013): 173.

Formosa Then and Now

The opening of *Formosa vs. Formosa* edits together images of assorted sources and modes of production to clarify the two entities of the titular opposition: one comes from "Ilha Formosa" (beautiful island), a moniker of the main island of Taiwan dubbed by the Portuguese in the 16th century; the other refers to the establishment of Formosa Petrochemical Corporation under the support of the KMT and the United States' foreign aid in the mid-1950s. By depicting Taiwan as a site of beautiful, bountiful natural resources, the former foreshadows the incorporation of the island into an emerging global network of Western imperialism and colonialism. The second Formosa bears witness to the island's ultimate transformation from exotic Other into a developed and exploited site, driven by foreign investment into rapid infrastructural and industrial expansions facilitated by Cold War geopolitics. A relation between the local and the global is thus established, mapped onto which is a fraught tension between low and advanced stages of economic development.

Here, the global primarily entails a partnership between the KMT government and Pax Americana in postwar East Asia. The partnership is demonstrated in the film through the insertion of black-and-white archival news footage of the 1957 opening of a Formosa petrochemical plant in Kaohsiung, with the wife of Joseph Lancaster Brent, an American foreign aid official, being the guest of honor. The use of news footage from the 1950s and 1960s to contextualize the history of industrial development is a recurring move across Ke's oeuvre, typically serving as an attribution of the long-term cause of an environmental problem in present-day Taiwan to the developmentalist mentality that undergirds specific Cold War ideologies: in this case, the privatization of the petrochemical industry with American financial and technical assistance. Jumping ahead thirty years, the opening of *Formosa vs. Formosa* adds another layer to this local-global tension by juxtaposing the black-and-white footage with color TV footage of the 1987 debate between Wang Yung-ching, the founder of Formosa, and Chen Ding-nan, then elected Magistrate of Yilan County (who had no party affiliation at the time but later joined the DPP in 1993). The debate took place because Yilan was selected by Formosa as the site for its sixth naphtha cracker complex, which Chen opposed based on its potential environmental pollution. Another dichotomy is thus introduced, further qualifying the film's titular opposition as one between the KMT-backed enterprise and the democratically elected, non-KMT leader of the rural county.

This opening effectively endorses a confrontation that situates the ecological in relation to the local and the democratic, which is pitted against the industrial as associated with the global and the authoritarian. To illustrate the negative aspects of the latter, several animated sequences punctuate the film; they literally demonize Formosa Petrochemical Corporation as a Godzilla-like green monster.[8] Formed by the aggregation of industrial pollution, the monster devours land and water recourses before releasing toxic chemicals into the surroundings. Parts of its body explode at one point, mirroring the explosions of several Formosa factories in recent years. Collectively, these sequences restate the film's straightforward agenda. Indeed, on several public occasions, Ke expressed his intention to make the film's ecopolitics as transparent as possible. He especially took pride in receiving a letter from an elementary school teacher, which indicated that the animated sequences had made the film's message comprehensible to the students.

By welding the nativist dichotomy and Ke's environmentalist commitment, the film establishes "the local" and "the global" as not only cultural or political categories but attitudes toward developmentalism and its concomitant impacts on the ecosystem and public health. Released a year after *Formosa vs. Formosa*, *Ebb and Flow* further amplifies this discursive structure by staging a stronger reaction against industrial growth at the local level *tout court*, even if underdevelopment might prove equally if not more arduous for local livelihood. As such, however, *Ebb and Flow* is caught up in the impasse of romantic anti-capitalism frequently associated with a commonly seen form of ethnographic representation, not least due to its emphasis on the timelessness of locality.

A result of three years of filming, *Ebb and Flow* provides a concentrated portrayal of Fangyuan, a village adjacent to an intertidal wetland in rural Changhua County. The coastal area serves as the ground for the villagers' barely self-sustaining life. Most of them work in agriculture, fishing, and oyster farming. They ride their oxcarts daily to the wetland early in the morning and begin a day of physical labor against strong sea winds and general coldness. As the villagers till the intertidal land following the oceanic rhythm, animals such as oxen, migratory birds, and dogs travel in and out of the frame. Given the area's harsh conditions, rural exodus and population ageing have been irreversible; the only young worker seen in the film is a junior high school student who helps his grandfather with oyster farming during the school break for extra pocket money.

By no means does the film conceal the hardship of local livelihood. Several interviewed villagers openly express how laborious their jobs are, but few have

8. As some of the animated sequences show how several products by Formosa Petrochemical Corporation, including clothes and toys, are used by Taiwanese people in their daily lives, Chia-ju Chang suggests that the film hints at the company's benefits from both "government complicit backing and, more subtly and perhaps unwittingly, the complicity of the Taiwanese consumers." While *Formosa vs. Formosa* does not explicitly develop the latter, as the rest of this chapter will demonstrate, Ke's subsequent films adopt a bottom-up perspective to interrogate how such public complicity is formed in Taiwan. Chia-ju Chang, "Frankenstein's Migratory Subject: *Under the Dome* and *Formosa vs. Formosa*," *Journal of Modern Literature in Chinese* 15, no. 2 (2018): 226.

considered relocation or career change due to a clear awareness of the limited alternatives they might have elsewhere. Therefore, when the state-owned Kuokuang Petrochemical Technology Corporation selects the wetland as the site for a new petrochemical plant, a heated debate takes place in the village, eventually leading to a local referendum. The outcome is rather one-sided, with 389 votes for the construction versus 181 votes against. For many of the villagers, the petrochemical industry's potential threat to the environment and their personal health, in the face of an otherwise stagnant and gruesome reality, seems like a bearable price to pay. As one supporter of the construction puts it, "it's dead here anyway with or without the plant." Crucial to note, though, is that while the film interviews a couple of supporters, less than a minute of screen time is devoted to presenting these people's views or lives, unlike the rest of the fifty-nine-minute film, which stays with the villagers who prefer to maintain the status quo. Here emerges a representational conundrum that troubles *Ebb and Flow* in relation to the favorable connection between the local and the ecological in standard nativist discourse: How should it address the fact that almost seventy percent of the villagers have rejected the film's ecological ideal?

One common approach to dissolving the dichotomy between the local/natural and the modern in ethnographic filmmaking is to rework the cultural evolutionist notion of "local tradition" as something primitive that would be left behind in the developmentalist trajectory toward modernity. According to Salomé Aguilera Skvirsky, this move can be achieved via an acknowledgement of the intelligence, brilliance, or even artistic quality of the local labor in and of itself, frequently through a processual representation that shows "acts of making and altering *as* processes—that is, the steps that make up the process have been presented chronologically, and the process has a visibly identifiable beginning, middle, and end point."[9] Whether development/modernity is viewed positively or negatively, this form of ethnographic filmmaking rejects the cliched projection of tradition "back into the nether reaches of time as something static, unchanging, sclerotic—something to be contrasted with the movement, innovation, and dynamism of modernity"; and if a local tradition somehow persists, it is because it continues to be "the most effective" method of production after repeated trial and error.[10] Local subjects represented as such, therefore, "are treated as world makers. Their status as agents rather than photogenic objects of sympathy, or victims of the world's bad ideas."[11]

The processual form of labor representation, however, is not used in *Ebb and Flow* for the reasons mentioned above: to mobilize this powerful formal device in the

9. Salomé Aguilera Skvirsky, *The Process Genre: Cinema and the Aesthetic of Labor* (Durham, NC: Duke University Press, 2020), 16.
10. Skvirsky, *The Process Genre*, 190.
11. Skvirsky, *The Process Genre*, 192.

depiction of the locals' labor risks celebrating what several villagers have reluctantly taken up for lack of a better alternative. Imagine the conflicted implications of the film had it at once shown the oyster farmers' complaints about their job and devoted itself to capturing the intricate process of their labor, from spawning and fertilization to setting up the racks in the farm, from deploying specialized techniques of maturation and cultivation to the skillful harvesting and shucking by hand. As if to avoid the power of processual representation, the film only reveals *what* the locals do rather than *how* they do it. Indeed, to formally glorify local tradition based merely on the fact that it is nonindustrial (and thus relatively environmental-friendly) is to perform an uncritical anti-capitalist romanticization. The film seems to be aware of this limitation and tries to solve the contradiction between its own environmentalist agenda and the locals' desire to better their livelihood. Such a sense of contradiction is felt, too, in one of the film's final proposals for increasing local revenue: the transformation of the area into a site of eco-tourism. That said, the film does not reflect on the common critique of the eco-tourist industry's conceptualization of the environment, or local culture as a fantastical commodity for the alienated urban middle class's search of a sense of authenticity.

If the local is not necessarily the ecological, is it therefore incompatible with the democratic spirit emphasized in the nativist discourse? *Ebb and Flow* almost seems to indicate this by suggesting the illegitimacy of the referendum, though ultimately the film does not dwell on this aspect given that the critique of a democratically supported view based solely on its developmentalist inclination is itself anti-democratic. Right after the referendum starts, the film shows an exchange at the voting station between a public representative and a villager against the petrochemical plant. The latter openly criticizes the design of voter identity verification, which in her view favors those who support the construction, without clearly explaining exactly where the flaw lies. When the former assures her of the referendum's fairness, she resorts to a class-based critique of him as an "upper-class person" detached from working-class reality. To her critique, the representative intriguingly replies: "There is no such distinction. We all grew up in this land." Had the film amplified the villager's vague accusation of a faulty design, it would destabilize the positive correlation between the local and the democratic in the nativist discourse (itself mobilized in the public representative's rebuttal). After all, unlike the late 1980s presented in *Formosa vs. Formosa*, when vestiges of the KMT's pro-development authoritarian rule could still be identified as the obstacle against which a democratically elected local leader insists on his environmentalist agenda, the same dichotomy no longer holds water in 2010, when democracy has been the norm across all levels of Taiwanese politics. As the viewer is left unable to assess the legitimacy of the referendum, so the film shows that the will of most of the locals is pro-development, or at best unclear. Again, like the film's treatment of the locals' arduous labor, it is not that the film does not acknowledge the pro-development voters' desire; rather, it understands that this very desire to better their livelihood in relation to environmentalism can itself be conflictual and contradictory.

While there is no denying that one can be in favor of the democratic process but still denounce it when the process seems to be abused or misused, the real crux of the problem, as the villager points out, lies in income inequality. This issue cannot be magically fixed by political democracy, which is perfectly compatible with the ethos of global capitalism. In fact, accompanying democratization and a mounting Taiwan-centric consciousness in the post-martial law era is a full-on neoliberalization of the society, which has qualitatively transformed the relation between the public and private sectors. As Chiou Yen-bin points out, if under the KMT's authoritarian rule the relation between the government and the capitalists was still one of top-down clientelism, the rise of the localist regime split the party and resulted in this relationship's transmutation into a partnership from the early 1990s onward.[12] In the same way that democracy can be attuned to the needs of progressive anti-authoritarianism and neoliberal capitalism alike, the nativist claim, when appropriated on the political front for profit, can similarly cover up the dire consequence of economic (over)expansion at the local level. The public representative's response to the villager reflects the dominance of such an ideology, which denies inequality in the name of a shared locality-based identity.

Herein lies the inconsistency between the film's means and ends. On the one hand, it resorts to nativist tropes in the portrayal of Fangyuan to advance its environmentalist argument. On the other hand, neither could it glorify the local mode of living nor commit itself to challenging the legitimacy of the referendum—to do either is to fashion a screen world that the documentary cannot support with enough evidence, such as an inarguable abuse of power during the voting. What *Ebb and Flow* therefore exposes is the inadequacy of the nativist ideology by self-reflexively (even if inadvertently) suggesting that its own environmentalism can be unrealistic in the sense that it romanticizes locality; or, the very idea of environmental sustainability that the film sets out to promote turns out to be unsustainable considering the economic hardship of the area. Unless locality can be decoupled from the conceptual realm of nature and the material condition of underdevelopment and, instead, interrogated in relation to other crucial factors such as class, the complexities of the social reality in Fangyuan cannot be unpacked. As the following section demonstrates, these fissures motivate a shift in Ke's filmmaking, manifested in his subsequent films as a deeper reflection on the diverse forms that "the local" can take up beyond romanticized stereotypes.

12. Chiou Yen-bin, "Hengchang yu wuchang: lun Zhutianxin 'Gudou' zhong de kongjian, shenti yu zhengzhi jingjixue," *Zhongwai wenxue* 35, no. 4 (2006): 80–81.

The Local Reconsidered

The opening sequence of *Black* sees an animated figure undergo constant metamorphoses against a white background: from a seed to a small plant; from the corpses of the plant and other creatures in the same geological stratum to a high forest on the ground; and from a paddy field to an industrial plant and its polluted air, which falls on the surrounding environment. As the pollution spreads, one brushstroke of blackness after another swallows the frame until its entirety becomes a lump of blackness, flattening out any discernable figure-ground distinction. The definite but unstable figure that assumes the shape of potentially any entity recalls Sergei Eisenstein's famous account of Disney animation's "plasmatic" quality and hence anti-capitalist potential, except in this case industrial pollution likewise possesses such a power of transformation.[13] As Ursula K. Heise notes, the plasmaticness of animation is a resource available to all ideologies, open to the oppressor and the oppressed alike.[14] What the film's opening presents is not only the flexibility of animation and its potential contributions for viewers to reassess themselves as perpetual becomings in the constant flux of the world, but also the dark side of such a state. A comparison between this animated sequence with those in *Formosa vs. Formosa* further manifests an evident change in Ke's filmmaking. Unlike the clear-cut, fixed distinction between the monstrous Formosa, local residents, and natural environments in the latter, a new way of understanding their flexible interrelation emerges in *Black*, which examines how industrial pollution has contaminated rice fields via irrigation water across Taiwan. This change of animation style, I would argue, reflects Ke's loosening of his reliance on the nativist discourse.[15]

To be clear, *Black* still resorts to some conventional nativist tropes in establishing a provincial perspective that guides the viewer through its call to action against industrial pollution. Such a perspective, more precisely, is tied to Ke's first-person account, articulated through his own voice-over narration. This choice beckons, given its marked distinction from the disembodied female voice-overs in several of Ke's films, including *Formosa vs. Formosa*. The personal intimacy that characterizes this sound design in *Black* likewise motivates the unfolding of the film's visual track. Following the animated opening, the camera showcases the farmers and rice fields

---

13. Sergei Eisenstein, *Eisenstein on Disney*, ed. Jay Leyda, trans. Alan Upchurch (Calcutta: Seagull Books, 1986).
14. Ursula K. Heise, "Plasmatic Nature," *Public Culture* 26, no. 2 (2014): 312.
15. My reading echoes Tam Yee Lok's observation that Ke's documentaries of marine life conservation, such as *Remembering Coral* (2004) and *Squid Daddy's Delivery Room* (2007), similarly reject the binarism of the modern/development versus the native/conservation by presenting "a new, revised assemblage of aesthetics and mechanics of existence" featuring both human and nonhuman agents. Tam Yee Lok, "Colourful Screens: Water Imaginaries in Documentaries from China and Taiwan," *Interactions: Studies in Communication & Culture* 2, no. 2 (2010): 117–18.

in Ke's hometown in Changhua County. As Ke's narration introduces us to a ritual practiced by local farmers to pay homage to the gods of the land and crops before the harvest, a performative aspect of his voice-over stands out to anyone familiar with Mandarin: his accented delivery, which sounds nothing like the female voice-over in "standard" Mandarin in his other films, confirms his ties to the displayed location. The presentation of agricultural activities and folk religion, together with the sociolinguistic implication of Ke's marked accent, audiovisually imbue this opening scene with a strong sense of local color.

But just as one might expect *Black* to be another concentrated study of a rural area like *Ebb and Flow*, the rest of the film travels to other places in western Taiwan, including Taichung City, Taoyuan County, Hsinchu City, Kaohsiung City, Tainan City, and Miaoli County. This transregional coverage speaks to the wide scope of industrial pollution. Like the annihilating blackness in the animated sequence, the kind of pollution addressed in *Black* is not just a local concern, traceable to a monolithic, officially supported origin such as the Formosa complex or the Kuokuang plant. It is, rather, the sum of pollutions from numerous unregulated small factories, themselves constituents of a much larger industrial network within and beyond Taiwan. Given that the pervasiveness of this pollution structures a human-environment relation that cannot be simply defined in relation to the local culture or mode of living in any single area, the association between the local and the ecological needs to be rethought. If the nativist construct of the local as anti-capitalist in *Ebb and Flow* already fails to hold water, *Black* further examines the romanticization of rural subjects as the guardians of a local tradition against an outside industrial force.

Most relevant to this attempt is the film's presentation of the rice farmers, who are allotted the most screen time relative to other social actors such as factory employees, NGO workers, and governmental officials. In several interviews, the farmers express their frustration with the ongoing pollution in their respective areas. While it is safe to say that Ke himself strongly identifies with them, he does not shy away from showing some seemingly problematic aspects of their views. Indeed, the major discontent of many farmers targets not so much the industrial waste that has polluted the irrigation water as the local governments' "unfair" system of examination, which conducts survey sampling from a few selected fields in a potentially contaminated area instead of a comprehensive check-up of the entire place. As a result, some farmers are still able to grow and sell their contaminated rice simply because their fields have not been tested, which would lead to them being banned from future cultivation. Two parts of the film show Ke directly asking the farmers who have escaped testing whether they are conscious of having profited from polluted crops. Both frankly admit it and say that they would never eat their own harvests or use the irrigation water to prepare their food.

This is not to say that *Black* blames these farmers for jeopardizing public food safety. In fact, the film conveys a sympathetic attitude toward them when, during their responses, it cuts away from accusatory close-ups of their faces to illustrative shots, such as ones that record the compulsory destruction of some contaminated crops that other farmers have had to experience. That said, while these farmers are certainly not guilty of producing the pollution, the film touches upon their complicity in its further dissemination. We might think of Ke's decision to present their so-called confessions as a response to the strategic downplaying of the pro-development discourse at the local level in *Ebb and Flow*. Their confessions articulate a strong sense of struggle and contradiction in most of the locals' desires to improve their livelihood. These desires can easily supersede environmentalist and public health concerns when there is no greener, healthier alternative.

From *Black* onward, Ke's films have more consciously revealed such a conflicted situation for many rural subjects. Take, for instance, his study of polluted underground water in *Undercurrent* (2015). In one scene, the camera follows an executive of Citizen of the Earth (a Taiwanese environmentalist NGO) and several activists as they examine the underground water collected in a well next to a broccoli field. The pungent smell of the water, indexical of various organic solvents released from nearby factories' wastewater, disgusts everyone. According to the NGO executive, the broccoli farmers have been selling their products to cities like Taipei despite the obvious toxicity of their irrigation water. When one of the activists asks him if the farmers would eat their own vegetables, an awkward knowing laugh is all he can offer. Consider, too, a similar episode in *The Age of Awakening* in which Ke interviews a fisherman who lives close to Formosa's sixth naphtha cracker complex in Yunlin County (where it was eventually built after being vetoed by the Magistrate of Yilan County, as mentioned above). The fisherman complains that the complex has contaminated the area, which has resulted in declining yields from his fish farm. When asked about what could be done to improve Formosa's environmental impacts, he bluntly suggests that "it will be better for the complex to relocate to Vietnam . . . Taiwan is too small for all these factory smokestacks."

Dubious as the ethics of these rural subjects' actions and views might be, Ke's inclusion of them in his films issues not so much a critique of them as a rethinking of a specific kind of nativist exclusivity that favors local interests at the expense of others (such as Taipei residents or the Vietnamese), even if industrial pollution of air, water, and land ultimately defies any regional barrier. The fisherman's proposal decidedly reflects one of the logical outcomes when the nativist romanticization of locality is taken to the extreme: a Taiwan-centric, not-in-my-backyard worldview that achieves local conservation by outsourcing industrial pollution to developing or underdeveloped areas. One cannot ignore the involvement of Taiwanese enterprises in several recent high-profile cases of environmental injustice, such as a

Formosa's $500 million settlement for its steel plant's massive water pollution in Ha Tinh, Vietnam. Or the ongoing protests of African American communities in a strip of land between New Orleans and Baton Rouge, nicknamed "Cancer Alley," against a planned Formosa petrochemical facility, set to double the toxic emissions in the already gravely contaminated area. Not to mention Taiwan's current status as "a weak undeveloped green economy" according to several environment and health indexes, such as per capita carbon dioxide emissions (more than twice the global average), due to the general lack of governmental regulation, market-based and nonmarket alike.[16] If, in Max Liboiron's words, "pollution is not a manifestation or side effect of colonialism but is rather an enactment of ongoing colonial relations to Land," then Taiwan as a whole has transformed from a historically colonized region into an active colonizer of the Global South in the era of global capitalism and reactionary neoliberalism.[17] The next section examines how Ke's most recent films accentuate this grave issue, which environmentalism in Taiwan today must address.

Cypress Geopolitics

Taiwanese corporate offshoring of high-polluting industries to other rising economies has not gone unnoticed in Ke's work. As early as *Formosa vs. Formosa,* a sequence details a Formosa plant's destructive pollution in Cambodia to support the film's condemnation of the transnational corporation. Because of the film's nativist framework, however, such a critique targets the specific alliance of governmental and corporate powers, rather than the framework itself through which the condemnation is conducted. In *The Age of Awakening,* which revisits this ideological formulation a decade later, Ke's critique of major Taiwanese corporations instead highlights the liquidation of the opposing tension between the two Formosas—no longer Formosa versus Formosa but Formosa *and* Formosa. Here, the island, rather than being an exploited object of natural resources, has itself become the center of a hegemonic force, against which activists in other countries act through the very discourse of Taiwanese nativism itself.

Consider the film's follow-up tracing of the development of the Kuokuang petrochemical plant beyond Taiwan. Due to several unforeseen reasons, the original construction in Fangyuan did not materialize, and the company instead chose Pengerang in southern Malaysia as the new site. The decision triggered several local protests. During one of them, as the film shows, a Malaysian activist powerfully recites, in Mandarin, the following lines from the Taiwanese nativist writer Wu

16. Lin Mu-Xing, Lee Tsung-Yi, and Chou Kuei-Tien, "The Environmental Policy Stringency in Taiwan and Its Challenges on Green Economy Transition," *Development and Society* 47, no. 3 (2018): 479.
17. Max Liboiron, *Pollution Is Colonialism* (Durham, NC: Duke University Press, 2021), 6.

Sheng's poem "Can Only Write You a Poem," originally created for the campaign against Kuokuang's construction in Fangyuan: "How I wish my poems / Could be cast into bullets / To shoot through avaricious brains, / Or forged into swords / To penetrate chests that host proliferating greed. / But I cannot." When she reads these lines out loud in public, through split screen the film overlaps her voice with Wu's own reading of the same lines in a prior protest in Taipei. As the direct mirroring of the Malaysian activist on the left half of the frame and Wu on the right takes place through cinematic mediation (Figure 8.2), a transregional dialogue transpires across different times. While we might consider this juxtaposition as an alliance between various "local" agents against a shared transnational corporate target, the film's inclusion of the Yunlin fisherman's discourse of exclusivity forces us to rethink this conventional understanding of the local altogether. The Malaysian activist's recitation, in effect, destabilizes the kind of locality specified in Wu's poem as "the remaining mudflat wetland" in the coastal area of western Taiwan (namely Fangyuan).[18] If such a particular site can now refer to Pengerang or, by implication, any other area, then the target of the poem's criticism likewise becomes unstable, not inherently tied to its original configuration of Taiwanese state and corporate forces. Locality thus becomes a slippery concept, referring to and reacting against different entities depending on the specific context in which it is mobilized.

The Age of Awakening insists on rejecting an essentialist understanding of the local, its conceptual antithesis (the Sinocentric, the transregional, or the global), and the ecopolitical implications associated with them. In another scene that examines the ongoing movement against the construction of Taiwan's fourth nuclear power

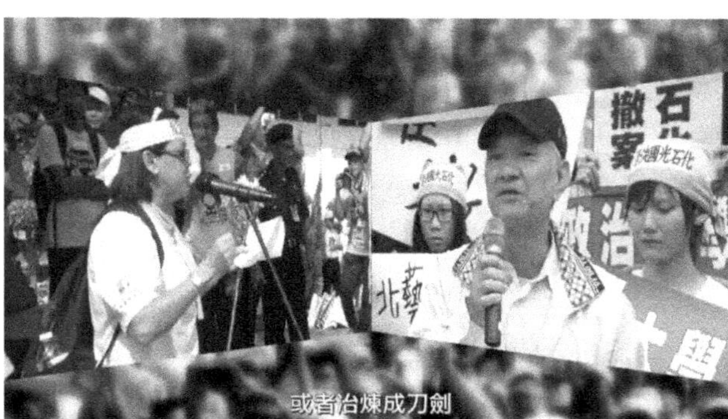

Figure 8.2: Overlapping recitations of the poem in Taiwan and Malaysia. Courtesy of Ke Chin-yuan.

18. Wu Sheng, "Zhineng weini xie yishou shi," Huanjing zixun zhongxin, June 27, 2010, https://e-info.org.tw/node/56856.

plant since the late 1980s, the film starts out by showing several black-and-white photographs of the street protests in the late 1980s, wherein the slogans on a few banners explicitly connect the anti-nuclear movement with the advancement of Taiwanese independent statehood. Yet this collaboration between ecopolitics and nationalism, the trace of which can still be seen in *Formosa vs. Formosa* (as previously explored), is now situated as a product of that very historical moment. Following this review of the 1980s, the film moves onto the early 2000s. With the election of Chen Shui-bian as president in 2000, the DPP, which had supported the anti-nuclear movement, ended the KMT's continuous rule for more than half a century. The new government, however, soon betrayed its electoral promise and announced the continuation of the plant's construction in 2001. Concluding with an interview with Lai Wei-jie, the director of Green Citizens' Action Alliance, this section of the film reflects on the reduction of pro- versus anti-development to the partisan conflict between the KMT and the DPP, namely, between Sinocentrism and nativism. The nativist discourse that used to work effectively on both nationalist and environmentalist fronts no longer serves as a proper activist strategy, insofar as all locales in Taiwan are now fully encompassed in the sphere of global capital, from which both political parties have benefited.

One way of thinking about the film's conscious self-distantiation from the nativist discourse is Jameson's widely cited concept of "cognitive mapping," a political act that "hold[s] to the truth of postmodernism, that is to say, to its fundamental object—the world space of multinational capital—at the same time at which it achieves a breakthrough to some yet unimaginable new mode of representing this last, in which we may again begin to grasp our positioning as individual and collective subjects and regain a capacity to act and struggle which is at present neutralized by our spatial as well as our social confusion."[19] To what extent might Ke's environmentalist documentary qualify as a piece of postmodern art is debatable, but undoubtedly it endeavors to outline for the viewer a new mode of representing Taiwan's position in the world so as to act, and be an activist, in it. While Jameson does not specify if cognitive mapping has a certain formal constitution, I would like to suggest that various aesthetic devices in the film could be seen as attempts to audiovisualize the intersection between Taiwanese geopolitics and ecopolitics. The distance that the film generates between the scenes of social movements now and then, between itself and past media, takes the form not only of Lai's verbal rejection of the 80s activism based on the model of nativism-cum-nationalism but also of a stylistic mediation by which old images are presented anew.

19. Fredric Jameson, *Postmodernism, or the Cultural Logic of Late Capitalism* (Durham, NC: Duke University Press, 1991), 54.

Consider the film's opening for an example of this mediation: against the light of a table lamp in an otherwise dark office, Ke alone examines numerous photographic negatives of the activist scenes that he has recorded throughout his career. The next few shots see the placement of these negatives into a scanner and their gradual transformations into digital files on a computer screen. Not merely an act of preservation, the virtualization of these analog images facilitates the defamiliarization of their original ideological claims. At various points when Ke incorporates past images (including archival news footage and sequences from his previous work) into the film, they are inserted onto TV screens in everyday spaces, such as a casual restaurant (Figure 8.3). Unlike the two bits of news footage in the opening of *Formosa vs. Formosa*, which serve as the building blocks on which the film constructs its conceptual oppositions, here their importance drastically decreases. Their size is reduced; their presence is relegated to just one audiovisual element among many in a random setting; and their command of spectatorial attention is diminished to something that people might or might not notice or care about during a lunch break. The sense of detachment that permeates these shots, created out of Ke's stylized treatment, carries the weight of an acknowledgement of the insufficiency of his past approach in addressing the strengths and weaknesses of a Taiwan-centric environmentalism today. If images used to carry any truth claim, today they are just images and nothing more.

Beyond either a local site of the oppressed or a hegemonic center of global capitalism, where should Taiwanese eco-media go from here in the collective imagination of the island's ecological present and future after the legacy of nativism? No

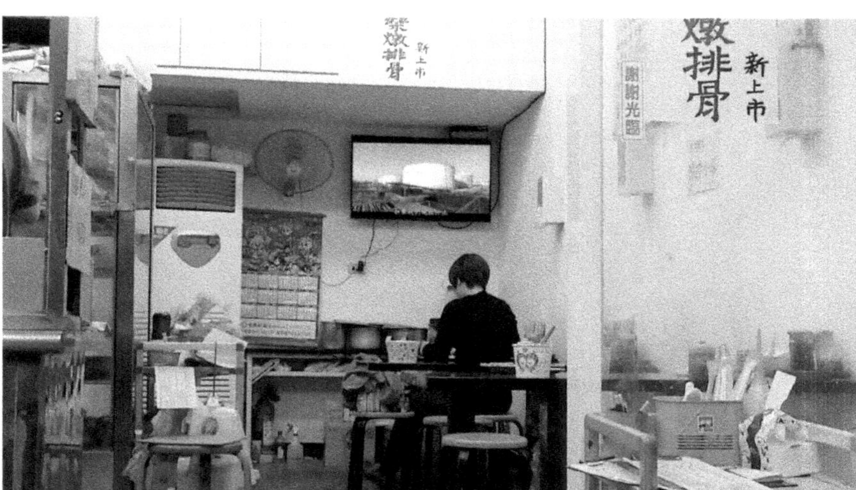

Figure 8.3: Old news footage on the TV screen. Courtesy of Ke Chin-yuan.

clear answer seems to be provided in *The Age of Awakening*, but some clues appear in Ke's subsequent film, *Sacred Forest* (*Shendian* 神殿, 2019), which explores Taiwan's astounding high-mountain forests. As the camera follows several groups of people—from hikers to scientists to patrol guards—into the island's oldest and tallest forests, reaching 4,000 meters above sea level, new ways of conceiving environmentalism beyond the nativist framework emerge out of the people's encounter with the species and ecosystems there. A memorable discussion by Chen Yu-feng, whose critique of the DPP is previously cited, dives into the deep time of ecology. As he recounts during a hike in a cypress forest:

> Sixty to seventy million years ago, when the continents of North America and Asia were still connected, the ancestors of these cypresses grew in the convergent boundaries. When the continents split about sixty-five to seventy million years ago, half of them traveled to what is now North America and evolved into three different species; the other half traveled to what is now Japan and evolved into another three species. The latter further traveled to Taiwan and evolved into a fourth species unique to the place, namely Taiwan red cypress . . . As you can see, the cypresses in Taiwan and North America were all originally related. With the knowledge we have today, perhaps we should not limit ourselves to twentieth-century notions of nationalism, regionalism, and other parochial concepts. We should instead think from a global perspective; conservation defies national borders.

While this cypress-inspired worldview might not be nuanced enough for contemporary ecocriticism, in which debates surrounding the tension between the planetary, the global, and the postcolonial have long reminded us of the entanglement of these theoretical conceptualizations, the centrality of Chen's perspective in one of Ke's latest films clarifies the trajectory of his evolving aesthetics and a new vision of Taiwanese geopolitics.

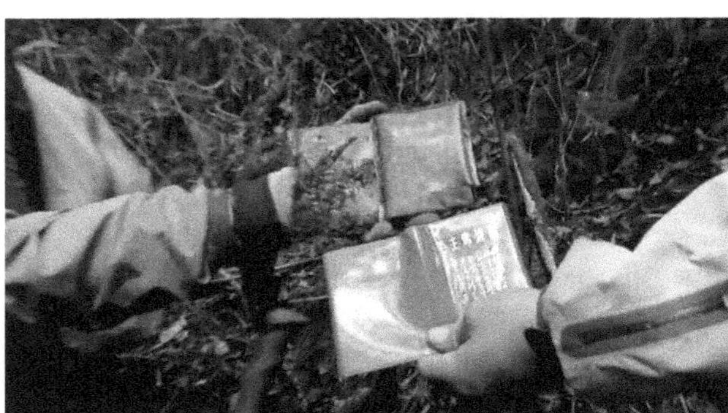

Figure 8.4: Mao in the forests. Courtesy of Ke Chin-yuan.

I shall conclude this chapter with one such moment when the film whimsically practices Chen's vegetal cognitive mapping. At one point, when the camera follows several members of the Bunun Mountaineering Team into the forest, someone finds an old copy of *Mao Zedong Poems*, published in 1972 (Figure 8.4)—the film never explains how this book, which would be either banned or viewed as politically sensitive in Taiwanese society over the past few decades, made it up to the mountains. As a team member flips through Mao's writings and shows a page to the camera, an unidentified off-screen voice asks: "Did he mention anything about cypress?" On hearing this question, everyone bursts out laughing. Perhaps likely a ghostly figure, the cross-strait tension between "free Taiwan" and "authoritarian China" as well as other Cold War ideologies still haunts all aspects of Taiwanese geopolitics, even in unexpected places high up in the mountains. But the fellow teammates' genuine laughter in response to the seemingly naive inquiry signals, however elusively, the presence of a much grander ecological reality, which just might hold the seed for a reconfiguration of the existing (eco)political structure.

Section IV

Digital Embodiment in Neoliberal Capitalism

9

Live Streaming and *Present.Perfect.*

Digital Able-Bodiedness, Liveness, and Disabilities

Chang-Min Yu

In the past decade, live streaming has become ubiquitous with the development and adoption of high-speed Internet.[1] With a digital device, a built-in camera, and a set of broadcasting programs such as OBS studio, one can easily generate content in the continuous present from the bedroom to showcase ludic talent and facial beauty—an audiovisual body image enhanced by interfacing with the screen. These streams present the body as malleable materials to be integrated. With gaming, it is the incredible nimbleness of the hand moving through screen configuration. With performance, it is the face that has become fully imbricated with transformative filters that seek to remake every countenance as a culturally determined ideal. This ability, furthermore, is inseparable from the liveness of the image. Situated in the temporality of "now," live streaming exudes an alluring liveliness that enacts enviable corporeal autonomy and full-bodied communication with the viewers. The interactions with streamers, as implied, are stereotypically gendered.

The majority of live streams, in terms of viewership, can be largely divided into two polarized categories: male video game live streams and female performance live streams. For example, Stuart Cunningham et al. have noted the intersection between industrial and social dimensions of online broadcasts in China.[2] On the one hand, the booming esports industry has taken advantage of the media exposure gained by live streaming from competitive players that are predominantly male.[3] On the other

1. T. L. Taylor, *Watch Me Play* (Cambridge, MA: MIT Press, 2018), 3.
2. In this article, I am focusing primarily on Chinese live streaming—instead of Chinese-language streaming—as representative of larger trends on the rise. The disinction, though crucial elsewhere, is not as productive here.
3. Recent news that the Chinese government calls for less "effeminate men" in gaming, though

hand, they surmise that the gender imbalance in the Chinese population has popularized the talk show format hosted by female live streamers, who can soothe the loneliness of male migrant workers disillusioned by the false hope of social mobility. Their popularity has demonstrated the "success of gendered livestreaming."[4] In their view, the social hierarchy of gendered economy is more problematically robust than ever.[5]

Cunningham et al. are not alone in considering live streaming as promisingly problematic in the Chinese context.[6] Much scholarship on Chinese live streaming focuses on online streaming's interactive mechanism,[7] the interfacial monetization,[8] the gift-giving socialization,[9] vicarious experiences,[10] as well as emotional labor and its impact on user stickiness.[11] These studies are interested in gauging and clarifying the social influence of livestreaming in a positivistic way. Yet no scholarship so far has attempted to investigate mainstream live streaming as a phenomenological experience; such sensual understanding should not be treated as a given fact in social constellation of add-ons or a self-evident pursuit slotted into the landscape of digital

---

representative of a broader trend in media, is itself equally symptomatic of this dichotomy. See Andy Chalk, "China Calls for Less 'Effeminate' Men in Videogames," *PC Gamer*. September 16, 2021.

4. Cunningham et al., "China's Livestreaming Industry," *International Journal of Cultural Studies* 22, no. 6 (2019): 727. Other researchers also focus on how the digital platform might be patriarchal. Xiaofei Han has analyzed the "platform-as-daddys" discourses, while Zhang and Hjorth argue that such hierarchical organization might be subvertible through gender performativity. See Xiaofei Han, "Platform as new 'Daddy': China's Gendered Wanghong Economy and Patriarchal Platforms Behind," *Internet Policy Review* 11, no. 1 (2022); Ge Zhang and Larrisa Hjorth, "Live-streaming, Games and Politics of Gender Performance: The Case of *Nüzhubo* in China," *Convergence* 25, no. 5–6 (2019): 807–25.
5. Live streaming is understood as online broadcasts, as the streamer can choose when to be "on air." This is the legacy from broadcasting industries, such as radio and television. See Taylor, *Watch Me Play*, 23–65.
6. Most of the media texts discussed in this essay will be Chinese. Some people might argue it is crucial to justify their "Chineseness." I think this is mistaken. One should be able to come to terms with fundamental debates about media operations with African, Asian or any other non-occidental texts. This is what Naoki Sakai is insistent on deconstructing. See Naoki Sakai, "Modernity and its Critique," in *Postmodernism and Japan*, ed. Masao Mitoshi and H. D. Harootunian (Durham, NC: Duke University Press), 93–122.
7. Xinru Chen and Zhuo Chen, "Between the Marked and the Unmarked," *Media, Culture, & Society* 42, no. 5 (2020): 727–44.
8. Zhen Ye, "Streamer-Interface-Viewer Entanglement in Popular Chinese Social Media Apps," *MedieKulture* 70 (2021): 131–50.
9. Yu et al., "Impact of Viewer Engagement on Gift-giving in Live Video Streaming," *Telematics and Informatics* 35 (2018): 1450–60.
10. Lu et al., "Vicariously Experiencing it all without Going Outside," *Proceedings of the ACM on Human-Computer Interaction* 3, No. CSCW (2019): 1–28.
11. Shi et al., "The Impact of Emotional Labor on User Stickiness in the Context of Livestreaming Service," *Frontiers in Psychology* 12 (2019): 698510.

culture. Can we provide a tentative description of the body image in live streaming? What is entailed in the act of putting oneself, through the hand and face, on the Internet? How does this body image relate to the viewer? How do we reflect on the perennial *liveness* and *presentness* of the broadcast? Finally, what is left after the broadcast? These are the questions that prompt my research.

This chapter does not intend to tackle live streaming in its entirety. I aim to provide a preliminary account of live streaming from the perspective of the body image and how the mainstream practice of live streaming can be *disabled* through the intervention of another, earlier, medium of cinema and its inflection on the body, as well as the ontology of media. In the first part of the chapter, I argue that live streaming depends on the digital presentation of an able body in liveness. Such living ability is what undergirds the dominant genres in live streaming—male gaming and female performance—their gendered division being more of a spectrum.[12] Both digital able-bodiedness and liveness are challenged in Shengze Zhu's 2019 *Present.Perfect.* (*Wanmei xianzaishi* 完美現在時). In the second part of the article, I will unpack the textual strategies deployed in Zhu's cinematic experiment to analyze its critical, cross-medial refraction of live streaming and its many perfect bodies. In particular, Zhu chooses to spotlight what is marginalized in live streaming platforms—quasi-surveillance sequences as well as bodies grounded in their actual existence, disabled and otherwise—through a compilation of past broadcasts. Her engagement with disabilities in the immense archive of bygone streams opens a new path to reflect on the cultural ideals of the body and a politics of remediation. Both digital able-bodiedness and its disablement will elucidate how live streaming technologies produce digital cyborgs and serve the function of plastic surgeries. Our understanding of the body and its wellness, normatively relegated to professional medicine, would have to accommodate media's capacity to redefine what an able body is.

Enabling Live Streams

Live streaming is enabled by digital able-bodiedness. It is not a relationship of determination, as testified by the diversity and variety of streaming communities celebrating and empowering disabilities, though not without some setbacks.[13] Instead, the able-bodiedness is a smoothly enhanced coordination between body and screen image, an idealized kinetic capacity. The facilitated able-bodiedness is most forcibly felt in video game live streams, one of the earliest and still-dominant

12. Other genres similarly intersect with this gender division, such as influencer marketing or *daihuo* in the Chinese context. I want to acknowledge that these are not strict categories. What the division showcases is a persistent patriarchal culture that regulates gender performances.
13. Ed Nightingale, "Twitch Streamers Campaign for Disability Pride Month," *Eurogamer*, January 19, 2022.

genres on broadcast platforms. In the image, we often—but not always—see a miniaturized close-up of the streamer positioned at one corner, so as not to block the ludic action. The main layer of the image is the game, including but not limited to *Dread Hunger, League of Legends, Honor of Kings, Counter Strike, Escape from Tarkov,* and many more. Within the frame, there can be a visually customizable champion moving in a simulated arena. Or, equally likely, we are seeing the battleground from the character's first-person perspective, with goggles, telescopic sights, and other tactical modules. In between the rounds, the streamer switches back to his desktop and browses through game-related web pages or others' streams to see how others have fared. The cursor, without the enframing game, helps to guide the viewers' attention. The movement of the mouse is, dependent on sensitivity and frame anchorage settings, transformed into the movement of the frame. One moves the mouse to shift focus to another part of the battlefield (*League of Legends*) or adjust and enhance the view in order to better eliminate the incoming threats (*Counter Strike*). In these scenarios, the hand is not simply substituted by another icon—the cute little white arrow—on the screen. The hand becomes the integral orientation of the frame. The live streaming image, with the superimposed face cam footage and the agile hand movement integrated, mutates into a weird body configuration.

Therefore, this able-bodiedness is first and foremost digital, that of the digits.[14] It is not, for instance, primarily defined by social accommodation that allows one kind of body to freely move in the living world while denying another kind such freedom, as defined by Elizabeth Barnes's *The Minority Body* (2016).[15] We can think of it in the literal sense, to evoke a feeling of one's fingers moving through keys and buttons as part of the input system. Haptics aside, manual porting is not enough; the streamer has to be quick and swift in entering commands. In that sense, digital integration needs a kind of dexterity that requires postural and visual coordination to produce suitable reactive responses. The gamer is seated at an appropriate height and cushioned in a gaming chair to support the neck and alleviate the pressure from the back. The eyes are looking straight ahead at the screen, which is shared on live streaming. The viewers can sense that their movement is tracking what change we should be paying attention to in the image. The streamer provides a voice commentary to explain what we should be looking for in the game: his cleverness in maneuvering the character, his comprehension of what the situation is, and his computation of what is about to happen. Live streaming provides a mutated body

14. Chang-Min Yu, "Cinema's Turing Test," *NECSUS: European Journal of Media Studies* 6 (2017): 189–207.

15. Barnes argues that "[b]eing disabled is simply something that makes you a minority—it is a way of having a minority body" (78). This view is meant to be value neutral; that is, having nothing to do with well-being. See Elizabeth Barnes, *The Minority Body: A Theory of Disability* (Oxford: Oxford University Press, 2018).

image with the face, voice, posture, hands, and eyes all reconstituted in the digital environment as an entertaining construct.

What are the characteristics of this mutation, then? We might say the sensorimotor schema is completely reformulated on screen. The sensorimotor, known as the body schema, is the body's existential feedback loop with the spatialized world, a concept popularized by Maurice Merleau-Ponty's phenomenology.[16] Later in film studies, Deleuze's *Cinema 1* (1980) and *Cinema 2* (1983) retooled the concept for a narratology of cinema, understood as the circuit of perception, affection, and then action. Both applications rely on an image of the moving body realizing its intentionality in the world. In contrast, the gaming or live streaming body is assimilated with the screen surface that shuttles between gaming environment and computer interface. Such amalgamation is graphically represented in the first-person shooters, where the two arms and one gun are awkwardly attached to the unobstructed, non-distorted field of vision. This gamic vision is enclosed within the desktop of an operating system, presenting a flattened canvas for image sources. In this dispositif of electronic vision, it is not merely that the body is liberated from its structural integrity of flesh, channeled through what Vivian Sobchack has named as "a simultaneous, dispersed, and insubstantial transmission,"[17] and reorganized as an avatar image that is pieced together by the streamer's sensory inputs and computer modding. It is imbued with manual nimbleness—as a token of mental acuity—that is showcased in gaming, as well as manifested in the multiplied windows on stream. Instead of tactility, the live streaming image of gaming is pointedly *the invisible hand*.

The invisible hand sustains live steaming's able-bodiedness. This is not to say that a successful live streamer cannot expose his own inadequacy, or that the hands cannot appear on camera. They are commonly seen in live streaming. The argument nevertheless stands for the fact that the interfacial image of live streaming has embodied the body's intentionality for completing tasks in the virtual world. The sensorimotor schema is in the trajectory of the actions performed on-screen. In the constantly moving image, the coordination of perception and action can now be simultaneously experienced, with or without the representation of the body on-screen. In spectatorship, the cohesiveness of this computational vision is acutely sensed, since the viewer is not the actual streaming gamer. We are watching how the imagined hand seems able to traverse through layers of the digital image and evinces a coherent intention. Digital able-bodiedness lies in its manifestation of technical

16. Mark Paterson has argued that the research about the sensorimotor body had gradually come into being in the nineteenth century and fully matured by the time Merleau-Ponty published *Phénoménologie de la perception* (1945). See Mark Paterson, *How We Became Sensorimotor* (Minneapolis: University of Minnesota Press, 2021).

17. Vivian Sobchack, "The Scene of the Screen," in *Post-Cinema: Theorizing 21st-Century Film*, ed. Shane Denson and Julia Leyda (Falmer: REFRAME Books, 2016), 111.

manipulation, a digital smoothness aided by the computer environment. The evanescence of digitality—the manual and electrical digits moving in sync—allows us to enjoy the automation of the image, free of our own control.

That said, live streaming has reformed the presentation of the body image on screen in another sense. The other dimension is the body's beautification—particularly the that of the face—with all the feature, proportion, and ratio adjusting filters freely available for the presentation of the self. This is a very different kind of digital able-bodiedness that is equally imbricated with the capacity of the screen. The assistance empowers as well as enhances the body image's boosted valuation in a given cultural environment. And on this other end of the live streaming spectrum, we have female performance, specifically the talk shows. In contrast to the freely roaming invisible hand on the virtual battleground, female performance is primarily defined by the face and the upper body that appear glaringly whitened and softened. But the filter is not simply *filtering,* as in the original sense of applying a layer of material to modulate color hue and saturation. It is more appropriately termed as a transformative lens that is powered by facial recognition technology that distinguishes the face from other aleatory elements in the frame.[18] In so doing, the contour of the face in the frame is turned malleable, its volume slimmed down and the texture scrubbed clean, while automatically adapting the area around the face according to the movement of the host's body. The modulating effect is prominent at the border of the face. The neighboring area would have a slight undulation that does not appear to come from the muscle. The outline can appear extra clean, smooth, and fluid. The chin, in the dramatization of ethereality, blends into the neck; the glasses, in the amplification of the soulful look, are robbed of the rims. This portrait is endowed with a machinic and even animistic capacity.

Interfacially virtualized, the etherealized face does not point to the Platonic idea of beauty, since all the parameters of adjustment are tailored to specific cultural expectations of the consuming viewers. The face needs to be whitewashed, the shape triangulated, the eyes blown up, and the lips blushed. Ticking one box would place the face higher on the ladder of fairness. Now, fairness is easily achieved by automated modulation. The automaticity of the beautifying camera exemplifies another kind of digital able-bodiedness—to use one's own face as raw material for the mold of an artificial ideal. At the visible threshold of the live streaming face is a digital liveliness that serves as a thin layer of the magical veil. It is this capability to reshape the matter of the face that the viewer might mistake as otherworldliness. The filtered face in live streaming is halfway between matter and spirit. This able body is a body without physical blemishes. It might be what postmodern philosophers like Jean

18. For an in-depth analysis of the technology, see Lila Lee-Morrison, *Portraits of Automated Facial Recognition* (Bielefeld: Transcript Verlag, 2019).

Baudrillad would call "simulation," since the real, biological body is nowhere to be found. All we have is an image of computational ideality that calls forth the perfection of facial femininity.[19] Baudrillard's damning term does not explain this image's specific attraction other than the Cartesian edict to escape the burden of the body. I would argue that it is more appropriate to see this face in the act of performance to effectuate digital able-bodiedness.

In these broadcasts, the medium shot is the privileged scale—a view that shows from the chest up to accentuate the "assets." The scale is rarely the extreme magnification of an eye that can be horrifying and confrontational, or the more distant view that allows more space to enter the frame. It is a tight portrait. Within this frame, the female host interpellates her viewer in flirtation with ad hoc responses, thanks, and pleas for more monetary appreciation. The undistracted view can sometimes create an effect of hypnotic immersion through the voice. Sometimes—for the media environment of live streaming is necessarily full of distractions—the viewer habitually watches live streaming along with many other channels of information. In the ideal circumstance, her face speaks to every viewer individually in digital intimacy. Her angelic close-up is juxtaposed with the anonymous digital multitude that can only individualize themselves by gifting announcements; the streaming *danmu* is largely anonymized to present the response from a collective point of view, the entirety of viewers who are watching the stream.[20] In order to match up with the magnitude of the face, an eager viewer's only noticeable form of individualized interaction is through gifting. In this situation—singular and yet widespread among all heterogenous possibilities of online broadcast—live streaming is returned to a female streamer with many lonely male viewers. These men, faced with the screened close-up in a monadic way, might imagine this is a one-to-one conversation in suspending their disbelief. The dream comes true, intermittently and repeatedly, with donation.

The female talk shows in live streaming disclose how the images are imbricated with the audiovisual disposition of the platform to produce an alluring digital able-bodiedness. It is the face, the proximity as well as how their combination is seen. Traditionally, the image of the face is where appearance and identity, expressive surface and psychological depth, all intersect—as expertly examined by Noa Steimatsky.[21] The face might not be straightforward in communication, but it figures an equivocal and yet possible path toward truth, as cinema has explored in films like *The Wrong Man* (1953, dir. Alfred Hitchcock) and *Persona* (1965, dir. Ingmar Bergman) through a narrative of psychological interrogation. No such path is given

19. Jean Baudrillard, *Simulacres et Simulation* (Paris: Éditions Galilée, 1981).
20. *Danmu* can be roughly translated as "bullet screen." It is usually a series of chat room transcripts following from right to left, as if there are bullets slowed down.
21. Noa Steimatsky, *The Face on Film* (Oxford: Oxford University Press, 2017).

in the live streaming genre of female talk shows. The face and its endowed power of hypnosis seem closer to that of Dr. Mabuse in *Dr. Mabuse, the Gambler* (1922, dir. Fritz Lang), a demonic figure aided by the cutting-edge technology at the time, such as broadcasting and the telephone.[22] The pleading and teasing face in the window is a digital construct that, on the basis of gendered interactions, allocates attention according to fiscal contribution. The digital countenance originates from its seamless and yet seamy—as the effect is quite observable and uncanny—integration with the filters, as well as from its infrastructure of communication on the streaming platform. The simulation as such is exactly why this face is powerful.

The invisible hand and malleable face are live streaming's two-faced Janus that actualizes digital able-bodiedness. This is no coincidence. The bipolar expressiveness of the body is articulated by paleontologist André Leroi-Gourhan. He argues that "a link therefore exists between the hand and the facial organs, and the twin poles of the anterior field attest their equal participation in the construction of communication symbols."[23] The digital environment remakes their communicational capacity. The invisible hand furnishes agile mobility and intentionality—inseparable from the computational media—in gaming and, more broadly, the digital environment. Manual input is translated as the shifting angle of perspective and orientation and the timely reaction to change on the virtual arena. A fantasy of flawless connection with the screen, so to speak. The interpellating face, on the other, is fashioned in geometric, undulating perfection that implies some sort of digital animism. The countenance is made less corporeal and more prone to shapeshifting, according to a system of values. In the semi-material state, faciality in live streaming both shrinks and broadens the gap between two parties in communication. The face appears to be so close and yet far away in its presencing against the anonymized crowd as digitally mandated. In other words, digital able-bodiedness is how the body is suffused with computational and platformic capabilities.

One particular trait of live streaming makes the hand and face even more alive on screen: the liveness of live streaming. When the viewer is consuming live streaming, the awareness of "this is happening now" is intensified, since the genre defines itself as "live" in its namesake. Such is an ideological construction, as Jane Feuer demonstrates in her analysis of the complicit relationship between live television and the feeling of real presence: "Live television is *not* recorded; live television is alive; television is living, real, no dead . . . television's meta-discourse generates a circuit of meanings from the single term 'live.'"[24] As a direct descendent of broadcast

22. Tom Gunning, *The Films of Fritz Lang* (London: BFI, 2001).
23. André Leroi-Gourhan, *Gesture and Speech* (Cambridge, MA: The MIT Press, 2018), 113.
24. Jane Feuer, "The Concept of Live Television," in *Regarding Television: Critical Approaches*, ed. E. A. Kaplan (Lanham: University Publications of America, 1983), 14.

TV, the discursive construction of liveness in live streaming is equally potent.[25] Many features on the interface accentuate the shared synchronicity between streamer and viewer. For example, on the video player of the stream, a right-pointing triangle play button, once clicked, is replaced by the double line of a pause button. The absence of a video timeline implies the video on-screen is uninterruptable. A red dot would occasionally appear at the bottom corner of the image to evoke past memories about live recording. More importantly, it is the chat room function that allows the virtual crowd to enjoy liveness as an instantaneous mechanism of feedback. The viewer sends out the message that is immediately visualized and shared with other viewers and the streamer. These messages might appear on live stream in a microcosm or as *danmu*. The loop provides, through real-time interaction, enhancement for the stream's liveness.

In live streaming spectatorship, digital able-bodiedness is consumed in the temporal flow of liveness as constructed by many graphic indications and interactive mechanisms. Its presumed real-time quality lessens the suspicion that the performance on-screen is prerecorded and hence less convincing or demanding.[26] It is because of liveness that the skillful invisible hand in gaming seems more awe-inspiring than ever in its timeliness. It is because of liveness that the alluring face in female talk shows seems more urgent in that there seems every chance to make direct contact with her. Liveness points to excellence as well as interpellation. Both of these qualities, as I have previously argued, are nothing less than a digital construction, the automatism of computational mechanisms. Yet liveness restores an affect of corporeal agency. The viewer can imagine there is a *living* body inside live streaming's special effects. The imaginary body anchors the male gamer and female performer in their virtual interactions. Aside from this fantasy of virtual corporeality, in the more general and diffuse interaction of live streaming, the assumed temporal simultaneity shared by streamer and viewer engenders a feeling of togetherness and communitarian bonding that is further strengthened by the emojis granted along with donation or subscription to the channel. This is why liveness is not simply a supplemental quality but an essential part of the live streaming experience in negotiating the line between private and public.

Watching live streams, in my personal experience, is to engage with a porous screen through which the subject's privacy is reformulated. This idea is inspired by Stanley Cavell's concept of film "as a moving image of skepticism."[27] In his judgment, the fascination with cinema originates from the condition of the modern subject, for

25. Taylor, *Watch Me Play*, chapter 1.
26. While some performance onstream is lip-synced and thus not exactly live, we can also consider the synchronization to be an enactment of liveness.
27. Stanley Cavell, *The World Viewed* (Cambridge, MA: Harvard University Press, 1979), 188.

whom the cinematic world is *screened*; that is, ontologically separate from the audience. The world on-screen exists and progresses without me. The state of alienation confirms the subject's skeptical attitude toward the world, while also alleviating its responsibility from doing anything to change the world. The privacy, paradoxically, is enjoyed with the other audience members in the darkened theater—this was cinema's "private-in-public" spectatorship, at least for the period of American cinema that Cavell was writing about.[28] In the era of live streaming, one's consumption of online broadcasts remains screened. It is not incumbent upon the viewer to be part of the crowd in the chat room. He can look at the number of viewers to summon the feeling of sharedness.[29] Moreover, in contrast to the pastness of the cinematic image, the live streaming image is perennially now. If Cavell thinks the world projected on the cinematic screen exists without the subject, the world presented in live streaming bolsters this effect with its liveness: it is going on, now, automatically without me. Perhaps the fascination with an imaginary unburdened state of spectatorship in live streaming, shrouded by the anonymity of Internet monikers, is our dreamed response to the demands of social media. This fantasy is distinguished by its porous possibility of interaction: I can be part of the world through the given digital protocols of interactivity. My interaction and agency in the world are visualized and witnessed in the chat room and on the stream. This is television's mode of transmission: to bring the public into the private.[30] Livestreaming comes with an added benefit of (limited) two-way communication.

With these reconstitutions of the body, one can see digital able-bodiedness as providing a negative definition of what the body is in medical media. It serves a centrifugal vision toward simulation, either in the ludic environment or for pure exteriority, rather than a centripetal excavation that burrows into carnal malfunction. The former sees the body as infinitely enhanceable and the latter sees it as in desperate need of examination and possibly treatment. Live streaming performs the liveness of the body, while medical media strive to see where the body isn't alive enough (necrotic tissue) or too much alive (cancerous malignancy). These experiences of temporality and aliveness can be further triangulated with the communication of privacy. While live streaming channels manufactured privacy in the titillating interaction with the viewer, medical media, even with explicit consent, necessarily violates a sense of corporeal confidentiality. Such a dynamic is shown, most experimentally, in Lucien Castaing-Taylor and Verena Paravel's *De Humani Corpororis*

28. Paul Young, *The Cinema Dreams of Its Rivals* (Minneapolis: University of Minnesota Press, 2006).
29. The male pronoun here pointing to Cavell's ideal spectator is very much supposed to be masculine—solitary and deliberate—in the canonic tradition of American literature that is at least traceable to Thoreau.
30. For the host, the opposite would be the case: many of them are live streaming directly from their bedrooms.

Fabrica (2022), in which microscoped bodily tissues are blown up to full screen to feel their pulsation and, on a second thought, an intimate proximity with a stranger's innermost depth. This juxtaposition is not the only way to think through live streaming's body image. In the second half of this essay, I will shift focus to *Present. Perfect.* to elucidate how the director, in reimagining what the archive is in the digital era through her found-footage practice, deconstructs digital able-bodiedness—the invisible hand, the alluring face—with human vulnerabilities in their suspended temporality.

The Disabled Archive of Live Streaming: *Present.Perfect.*

Present.Perfect. should be characterized as a compilation or found-footage film—I am using the term in a broadly institutional sense—in that its source materials are collected from past broadcasts on live streaming platforms. The practice itself, as Jay Leyda found out seventy years ago, defies naming. Its core components, such as selecting footage and editing them together, are essential for every kind of filmmaking, so the act of isolating the practice in a different nomological category feels awkward, if not outright counterintuitive. For the genre's nominal defiance, Leyda jokingly asks the reader: "Can you suggest a right term?"[31] As if the issue of naming is not sufficiently thorny, the footage in *Present.Perfect.* does not come from any particular archive, public or private, in the traditional sense; they are from the ever-expanding collection of automatic broadcast storage on the platforms themselves. The streamers can decide whether they want to save their past broadcasts in the video format for the viewer to easily access, mostly in the interest of advertisement revenues. Their genesis is thus, less than ever before, not an intentional act of documenting *actualités*, but rather the data-driven push to amass more and more information for machine-learning programs to profitably process the collection of infinitely multiplied self-presenting live streams in the pursuit of digital multitude. Appropriating these videos is a bold attempt to think through how individual artistic practices situated in the found-footage tradition can help expose how these image artifacts are digitally and ideologically constructed.

Shengze Zhu does this in several ways, ranging from the removal of the streams from their liveness to the film's narrativization of disabilities and bodies in their grounded environment. Two cinematic quirks stand out. First, the film is composed with long takes in monochrome. The long take, harking back to live streaming's continuous broadcast, can force the audience to ruminate on representation, drained of colors as if somewhat spiritualized. At the film's opening, three slates of intertitles explain the definition of live streaming and its meteoric rise in China. What follows

31. Jay Leyda, *Film Begets Film* (New York: Hill and Wang, 1964), 7.

is a series of shots about construction and work sites, views that resemble surveillance more than live streaming. The first shot, panning to the left with a heavy load hung in midair, is taken from the driver's seat of a crane positioned at the top of a high-rise. The banal image, in its 360-degree rotation, brings the multicolored title of the film in view, flowing as an unmissable line of *danmu*. The second shot shows the demolition of a building. The first ten minutes of the film are made with these views of human and machine labor. No one is talking; all the sounds would seem to originate from the actions represented on-screen. The sequence serves a twofold function. The first is live streaming's surveillant imbrication. Live streaming's self-presentation cannot be separated from a self-enforced public surveillance, either by the government or big-tech companies. The surveillant aspect of live streaming is neglected because it is seen as entertainment rather than as an archive of footage for future examination and prosecution. Second, the views remind the audience of their kindred spirits with traditional documentary. We are invited to reach into the unseen, banal, and yet fascinating aspects of modern life and how people can voluntarily, without much effort, make the sight available for a bigger audience—demonstrated by one bearer's adjustment of the camera.

The representation of static banality veers away from one's customary consumption of live streaming. In the network of digital archives, the videos are usually recorded in the same predictable manner: desktop and cam footage for male gamers, facial close-ups for female performers, accessible through their individual channel in a different tab or column. Zhu opts to piece together the streams mostly from the IRL—in real life—genre: to perform as oneself as "in real life" and interact with the viewer's comments and requests in real time. The streamers in this genre operate in the mode of "unexpected views." What I mean by unexpected is that they produce content that might be eye-opening for its supposed unfamiliarity, for it is removed from either the usual format of gaming or talk shows. IRL positions against the general background of live streaming's preference for the digital environment. The name indicates its aspiration to represent a snapshot of reality, similar to what documentary is believed to achieve. The film's first section features monotonous labor and then shifts toward a human-centered representation of the streamers in their lived environments. They showcase and comment on various pursuits, including public dancing, farm plowing, livestock raising, underwear sewing, and many others—a true expression of "variety" streaming.[32] The diversity of these representations would point to live streaming's unfulfilled promise to cultivate a media landscape in which everyone, in the ease of digital technology, can produce content directly from living and gain access to an interested audience. It is by returning to live streaming's

32. Variety streaming means a broadcaster is able to play a variety of games onstream, in contrast to the one for which he is famous. This is a very limited view of "variety."

archive that Zhu can recover this potential. One might consider live streaming's archived broadcasts as *disabling* in a technical sense. These materials are disabled in their temporality. They present diverse experiences that are able to escape from the limitation of digital able-bodiedness in its sole engagement with virtuality.

There is another form of disability featured in *Present.Perfect.*: the bodies with disabilities. As the film goes on, a few characters, though their names are left unstated, emerge from its storytelling. Some performers explicitly present their own disabilities to the viewers, such as self-castration, phocomelia (congenital malformation in limbs), and facial burn trauma. The castrated man, moving in a landscape of demolished ruins from land requisition and gentrification, has the appearance of a ten-year-old. The phocomelic man is seen lying on all fours in a busy street to solicit sympathetic donations. The burn survivor, facing the camera frontally to allow a clear view of the trauma, shares the carnal experiences of his twisted flesh. With a light touch, they interact with the people in the profilmic environment and in the virtual world. Their humor is so graciously deadpan that it can make the offline and online interactions cringey. They take the questions about their body and how they live in the world with an emotional levity. For example, the castrated man, carrying the camera with a selfie stick, tells his online audience that he needs to find a way out of the rubbles while convincing them that he is *really* castrated: "I cut it myself . . . it is useless!" Obviously, his way out of destruction is not physical but through the connection with a virtual crowd. His interaction with them leads the audience to believe that some have gathered to see a curious specimen as well as offer their support in finding a way out.

In another case, the phocomelic man directs his viewers' attention to the passing people who dressed as the pokemon *pikachu,* while no pedestrians feel the need to pay attention *to him*. Both the welcoming attitude and apparent need to engage the online viewers put the film's audience in an affective bind. We might feel embarrassed to have witnessed these awkward interactions, because they are the visible proof for the public's distrust and neglect toward people with disabilities. We might also be attracted to these self-exhibitions, with a possibility to connect with the streamers and provide heartfelt and monetary support in solidarity.[33] However, the exact quality of the affection seems ambivalent. The IRL footage provides a chance for the director to return to the bodies that are neither invisible nor alluring in the public eye. The film highlights, through contesting the mainstream practice of live

33. This is Zhang Ling's view: "By establishing online communities, these livestreamers seek emotional connections and mutual understanding, even though some of their followers' interest may be based in curiosity or even voyeurism." (70). See Zhang Ling, "Foreshadowing the Future of Capitalism: Surveillance Technology and Digital Realism in Xu Bing's *Dragfly Eyes* (2017)," *Comparative Cinema* 8, no. 14: 62–81.

streaming, what is refused to be noticed by the general public in an emotionally charged manner.

In the film's narrative, Zhu reveals, quite carefully, these people in an expanding as well as deepening series of their nameless portraits. The expansion is of a spatial kind, in comparison to how live streaming paradigmatically presents an identical environment through innumerous iterations. In the case of the burn survivor, the audience first sees him in a room, seated to talk to the viewer about his own injury in detail. He is not afraid of showing his disfiguration to the camera and presents himself as a defiant hero "who goes against the will of god." One viewer, whose message we do not get to see, says that "live streaming does not suit him." In response, the broadcaster retorts by saying "I chose live streaming . . . if you don't think this suits me, you can gift something and leave. I would not hold you responsible." The verbal abuse is deftly countered by taking advantage of the potential guilt. Our understanding of his rebellious personality is enriched the next time he is shown on-screen, singing in a karaoke bar all by himself. With stroboscopic flashes, the lights of a disco ball lamp float through the space. After signaling to the camera that he is about to begin, the audience hears a voice accompanying the song. A few lines in, the broadcaster puts the microphone down, his eyes cast toward the off-screen right with apparent frustration. He comes toward the foreground and says "they don't let me sing" before going back to follow a few more lines and yelling "let me do it!" During the song's acoustic interlude, the audience gets the context with more explanation: "one girl was driven out by me." The line implies that the karaoke bar's owner did not want him to sing and, by (over)taking his voice, the venue can get rid of this unwelcome guest. By insisting on projecting his voice, he persists in the profilmic space as well as his live streaming community. The men represented in the film defy their incorporation with the screen, as seen in the genre of male gaming, in their proud performance of othered, awkward bodies.

The women, in contrast, are not disembodied faces and voices beautified by the animism of the digital environment—it is as if, in choosing what footage to include, *Present.Perfect.* strips away the cosmetic magic of animating filtering. Every one of them resists the stereotype of an alluring face; they are seen and grounded with a corporeal existence in the mundane, everyday world. For instance, the first woman seen in the film gives the audience a tour of her family's pig farm, while casually parrying away the viewer's sexist insult ("The sow is more popular!") before showing and going to use the bathroom—a biological exposé unthinkable in a usual female live stream (Figure 9.1). She even mutes the sound as the excretory noises are considered a bannable offense by the platform. Another woman is seen hovering outside in an alleyway. The bumpiness of the frame suggests the camera is locked on some kind of vehicle moving sideways. After a while—along with the film's refusal to editorialize—the audience comes to realize that she is possibly paralyzed from the

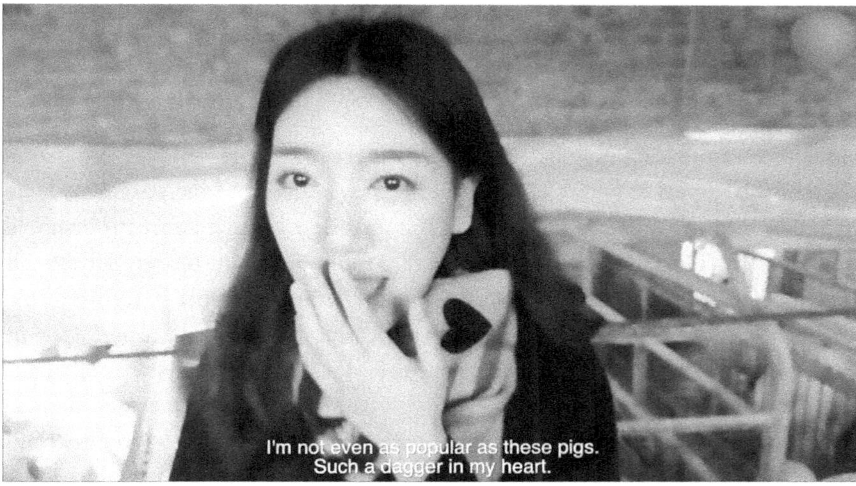
I'm not even as popular as these pigs.
Such a dagger in my heart.

Figure 9.1: Tactful deflection and exposure. Courtesy of Shengze Zhu.

waist down. Expressionless and hard to read, the woman says that she refuses to read the *danmu* because it is hard to read through the reflection outside, along with other morbid responses to the chat room. Toward the end of the shot, at the request of a viewer, she tilts the camera down to introduce her ride and expresses her gratitude for the virtual gifts. We cannot help but feel these live streams for their corporeality, the body's existential connection with the screened reality.

The idea of digital able-bodiedness in live streaming is contested through the presentation of disabled bodies as well as *laboring bodies*. The sense of the latter in the film is strategically developed with the female worker in an underwear factory. This time, it is about a woman's experience with labor and child-rearing in rural China. The audience's first encounter with her is on the sewing table in a factory. No obvious digital filter is visible. The chat room interface rarely appears to show incoming donations. In the shot, her hands never stop sewing together fabric pieces, while reading out loud and responding to the messages from the chat room. Within the frame, between the clothes on the left and the machine on the right, there seems to be an empty space opened by the live streaming camera and inhabited by her virtual community. The spatial caesura allows her to take a rest, in time, from the flanking mechanical repetition. Her hands are not symbolized by the graphic icons or indicated by the virtual agency in the gaming environment; their constant motion points to how her body is integrated into the industrial infrastructure of labor. Live streaming, instead of being a job, is her *pastime* and social escape from the constricting and exhausting female labor. Her reliance on live streaming as an emotional outlet appears increasingly obvious in the four different scenes. And the interaction with the chat room, like other clips included within the film, provides an evolving commentary on the woman's current situation.

In the first clip, one viewer promises that "he has arranged for the rest of their lives . . . how much do you need for the bride token?" The broadcaster gives a number and goes on to discuss how her live streams present a "more real life." No matter whether this appeal to reality is verifiable, we can understand the statement as an invitation into the scene of lived labor. The inclusion of such affirmation should be read as the film's intention to encourage a more profound recognition of this human being. The second time around, while mentioning that her sixteen-year-old coworker has dropped out of school, the broadcaster makes a grimace and declares that "I was once married and am now single . . . does my marriage status influence whether you tune in?" It is reasonable to guess, without seeing the message, that the live streaming viewers keep harassing her over her marriage status—an important question for female live streamers, whose presumed celibacy can enable a more potent spectatorial fantasy. Toward the end of the scene, she casually brings up a daughter who would become the focus in the streamer's next sequence. We then see her at home reprimanding the crying daughter. She temporarily loses the nonchalant look before putting on a smile to welcome a new viewer. The audience, and the viewer, witnesses how the broadcaster responds to her child's weeping, heard off-screen, with negative reinforcement: "Nobody likes you!" In slight exasperation, we come to a gradual realization, through her matter-of-fact explanation, that the woman is under immense stress from wage labor as well as domestic labor, including nannying her brother's child and cooking. In the kitchen, the mother and daughter make up eventually. In the last time, the woman brings her daughter to the factory and promises to buy a new toy with the money these male undies would make. In the film's serialized construction, the mother and daughter can be happy, in a complicated way as always, with each other; no digital able-bodiedness can accomplish such a feat.

Zhu juxtaposes these streamers, progressively threading their stories in a living tapestry. The animated quality of such imagery originates not from the liveness of the broadcast. Live streaming constructs itself as perennially now, with no sense of living progression; there is always another round of battle in gaming as well as another song to hear in performance. In narrativizing the grounded existence of these streamers, the film returns a kind of temporality for the image, to allow an existence in time, for the streamers, while highlighting their temporal distance from the audience. In that operation, even without the photographic index, we can say as Roland Barthes does, "that has been."[34] *Present.Perfect.* eponymously suggests that it is an experiment on the temporality of the live stream image—"present perfect"

34. Roland Barthes, *Camera Lucida* (New York: Hill and Wang, 1987), 76.

as in starting in the past and continuing indefinitely into the future—and the "presentation" of "perfected" human bodies in manual dexterity and facial ideality. The alliance of liveness and digital able-bodiedness is reformulated through human vulnerabilities. The vulnerabilities are not merely altered human figures with the so-called defects, but people that expose themselves in the banality of insufficiencies—occupational hazards, infrastructural inadequacies, and existential loneliness. These minority bodies, while calling for more accommodation in the digital community, are not lacking. We might interpret "present perfect" in another way: the film's presentation of these bodies is, at present, *perfect* instead of *perfected*.

The terminological distinction can assist us in contextualizing live streaming and *Present.Perfect.* in the larger field of medical and health humanities. In contrast to mainstream narratives about disabled bodies, Zhu's film does not provide an uplifting narrative of advocacy for eventual triumph over bodily limitations—such as breast cancer memoirs critiqued by Anne Boyer's incisive biography *The Undying* (2019). The medial operations in the film are more interested in parsing out how bodily representation is never simply representational; media's corporeality concerns with its own ontology. That entanglement comes with a mandate to demand a certain ability from the body, both in performing for the screen and in soliciting the body's interaction. These mandates, once enforced, enable us to forget how such ability is defined against disabilities whose critical character has been thoroughly dissected by Jonathan Sterne.[35] *Present.Perfect* might be similarly characterized as providing, to borrow Sterne's words, a *disabling* political phenomenology for live streaming.

Cinema as a Disabled Medium

When live streaming is remediated through cinema, the interruption of real-time communication—and the loss of a community—is acutely felt. Here the disabled liveness and the subject's disability are superimposed. Recycling live stream broadcasts, the film calls attention to the seeming paradox of *liveness in the past* through the representation of unfulfilled interaction. The apparent liveness amplifies the on-screen presence of the broadcaster that, in the polar case of showcasing disabilities to elicit sympathy, becomes almost piercing. The phocomelic man, at one point, brings up how people are mostly "fair-weather friends." He continues to differentiate between acquaintances online and friends in real life. The one viewer who has been interacting with the streamer voices the intention to leave and play a game. The man begs the viewer to stay and says video games are predictable and addictive, before

35. Jonathan Sterne, *Diminished Faculties: A Political Phenomenology of Impairment* (Durham, NC: Duke University Press, 2022), 193–208.

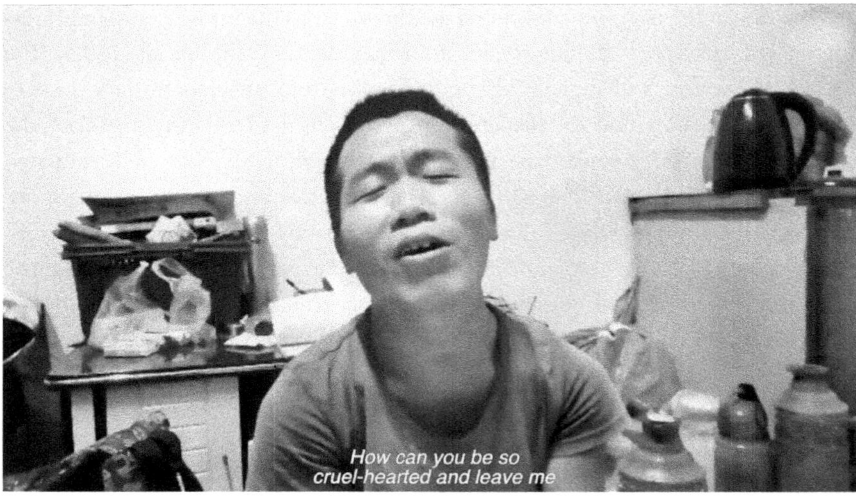

Figure 9.2: Arrested communication. Courtesy of Shengze Zhu.

singing a song to elegize the viewer's departure with his hand raising in the air to bid farewell (Figure 9.2). A long silent look into the screen ensues. Here, the arrest of the moving image from live streaming allows us to experience the liveness of his look while cogitating its situatedness in the past. His loss of connection with the viewer cannot be, in any usual broadcast, mitigated by one's entrance into the chat room as timely replacement. The screen is no longer porous. The audience might feel, more keenly than ever, the impossible responsibility to interact—our digital integration, evoked in watching that interaction, is dissected.

In this case, cinema keeps its distance from the immediate pulse of capitalism that trembles through the propagation of beguiling images on the Internet and in live streaming. Live streaming is sustained by digital able-bodiedness. Its practice continues and strengthens the constriction of our patriarchal culture. The narrative strategies in *Present.Perfect.* help us reconsider the digital and cultural parameters undergirding live streaming's mainstream genres, an incorporation of manual ableism and facial attraction in their interfacial enhancement. Disability in the film is a representational as well as ontological engagement that can refract liveness through the lens of screened cinema. The past liveness of human bodies expedites a disenchantment of digital embodiment.

10

"The Most Calming Thing You Have Done on the Internet"

Healing Vlogs and the Aesthetics of Li Ziqi

Lilian Kong

"Healing" has become a powerful commodity label and popular culture niche. Holistic wellness practices have been passed down for centuries across multiple cultures, but widespread commercial consumption of media for healing purposes holds a shorter history, traceable to late twentieth-century Japan. Especially in the 1990s, products ranging from relaxation toys to sound therapy took off, reflecting the impact of an economic bubble burst, subway gas attacks, and the 1995 Kobe earthquake. Whether self-promoted as "healing" or not, these products soothed consumers so effectively that marketers declared a nationwide "healing boom" in the early 2000s.[1]

The 2008 financial recession helped catapult this boom into global circulation, resonating with Euro-American self-care, slow living, and psychotherapeutic movements, as well as Mainland China's own "healing culture" (*zhiyuxi wenhua* 治癒系文化) movement. In China, this movement is tied to three factors. First, psychology became an institutionally established field in the 1980s, incorporating mental health awareness into both Chinese traditional medicine and Western medicine practices.[2] Second, from the twenty-first century onward, popular discourses that express anxieties and desires—all inseparable from China's reentry into the global market and subsequent privatization—skyrocketed. In the past decade, for example, the term "happiness fever" (*xingfu re* 幸福熱) became popular, signaling middle-class aspirations toward a meaningful life in the face of collective moral ambiguity

1. Paul Roquet provides an overall account of twentieth-century Japanese healing booms, which culminated in this most pronounced, explicitly articulated "healing boom" of the 1990s. Paul Roquet, *Ambient Media: Japanese Atmospheres of Self* (Minneapolis, MN: University of Minnesota Press, 2016), 151–52.
2. Li Zhang, *Anxious China: Inner Revolution and the Politics of Psychotherapy* (Oakland, CA: University of California Press 2020), 41–43.

and financial instability.[3] Other viral terms such as "involution" (*neijuan* 内卷) or "inner depletion" (*neihao* 内耗) also articulate anxieties around overly competitive environments and lack of work-life balance.

Third and often overlooked in English-language research, China's commercialized multimedia environment has provided its own conditions for healing. It is no coincidence that the term "healing" appeared early on through the publicity campaign of a romantic comedy film: Teng Hua-Tao's *Love Is Not Blind* (*shilian sanshisan tian* 失戀33天, 2011) was advertised as "China's first healing romance film."[4] Chinese "healing culture" has since repurposed canonical literature, traditional art, cartoons, and other aesthetic media forms in a way that provides comfort to everyday lives, inspired by but rarely strictly adhering to medical or counseling practices.[5]

The mid-2010s witnessed the emergence of online healing media. Content creators on user-generated content platforms, at first mainly East Asian video bloggers (vloggers), began to brand themselves as "healing." The label's reach expanded with the increase of anxiety and depression during the COVID-19 pandemic, "public feelings" embroiled in the varied politics of crisis-ridden capitalist systems.[6] The pandemic has led to a mushrooming of more comforting online spaces: therapists on TikTok offer mental health tips, live streamers endorse "wholesome" or "cozy" video games, and YouTubers romanticize cottage living as a cure for burnout.[7] "Healing" has become an ever-lucrative, exponentially growing label in the global online platform economy.

---

3. Zhang, *Anxious China*, 134–35.
4. Wu Kang, "Qingnian qunti zhiyuxi wenhua liuxing xianxiang touxi," *Qingnian tansuo*, no. 5 (2017): 95–96.
5. Wu, "Qingnian qunti zhiyuxi wenhua liuxing xianxiang touxi."
6. The term "public feelings" is borrowed from Ann Cvetkovich, *Depression: A Public Feeling* (Durham, NC: Duke University Press, 2002). Cvetkovich was part of the early 2000s Public Feelings group that conceptualized negative emotions as public and political within American capitalist contexts, rather than as personally confined mental illnesses. Amid the also very political, public reactions to the pandemic, I expand this term beyond an immediate American context.
7. #therapytok is a TikTok video niche where licensed therapists and less professional content creators alike post mental health tips. Dani Blum, "Therapists Are on TikTok. And How Does That Make You Feel?" *New York Times*, May 7, 2021, https://www.nytimes.com/2021/01/12/well/mind/tiktok-therapists.html. "Wholesome" or "cozy" video games separate themselves from more action-focused video games, instead often described and promoted as cute, casual, and uplifting. They skyrocketed in popularity during and after 2020, in part due to the 2020 founding of a live stream that curates wholesome games, Wholesome Direct. For more on the Cottagecore trend, see Ambar Pardilla, "What Is Cottagecore? Meet The Biggest Trend During Quarantine," *Huffington Post*, September 11, 2020, https://www.huffpost.com/entry/cottagecore-trend-quarantine-diy_l_5ecd875ec5b6e3f6739dbdfc, and Isabel Slone, "Escape into Cottagecore, Calming Ethos for Our Febrile Moment," *New York Times*, March 10, 2020, https://www.nytimes.com/2020/03/10/style/cottagecore.html.

As a flourishing label, however, online healing media encompass an overwhelming array of approaches to holistic well-being, which attract varied users and consumption habits. How do we theorize the way such a heterogenous category heals? One productive method is virtual ethnography, which assesses viewer demographics, experiences, and opinions. While I take online comments of healing affects into account, my chapter focuses on how much these affects are themselves stylistic constructions, part of an online media aesthetic. Be it through layered ocean sounds or earth-toned cottage-living videos, online healing media engage primarily through its use of media-specific formats, as well as intermedial formal elements, which are not without their own effects or connotations. They generate sensorial fields for viewers to experience.

More concretely, I explore the aesthetics of healing vlogs, with a focus on Internet star Li Ziqi. Li is a vlogger who uploads videos of her making handicrafts, cooking from scratch, and performing other routines in rural Mianyang, Sichuan. Her signature style has catapulted her to global fame. Especially in 2020, the subscriber count on Li's YouTube channel doubled, earning her the Guinness World Record for most subscribers on a Chinese account. The reasons for Li's unprecedented popularity are many, but I analyze how "[this] quiet, resourceful farmer in China's southwestern countryside seemed to heal all wounds."[8] Considering such responses from critics toward her content, what formal techniques ground Li's capacity to "heal all wounds?" How do they engage specific vlogging formats and modes of online platform consumption to create their own functional media aesthetics, which reshape our understanding of online healing media's role?

I address these questions by teasing out three intertwined aspects of Li's videos: soft ambience, escapist impulse, and processual slowness. Each aspect is capable of capturing attention, the core currency of the platform economy, through therapeutic registers. They come together to immerse viewers in digital atmospheres of calm. Indeed, this chapter approaches Li's healing aesthetics through the framework of atmosphere. Indebted to Paul Roquet's theory of ambient media as well as Friedlind Riedel's emphasis on atmosphere as kinetic force field, my conceptualization of atmosphere places equal pressure on its simultaneously homogenizing and differential modalities. It is able to capture the immersive quality of Li's aesthetics without reducing their healing affects to a singular function. My chapter ultimately argues that Li's vlogs configure healing as an internally distributed atmospheric field. Rather than a "quick fix" cure for (mental) health issues,[9] then, healing becomes a

---

8. Caio Yurgel, "Li Ziqi: A Romantic in the Year of the Plague," *Sixth Tone*, December 9, 2021, https://www.sixthtone.com/news/1009177/li-ziqi-a-romantic-in-the-year-of-the-plague.
9. This definition of "healing" is inspired by Jie Yang's critical analysis of psychotherapeutic practices in post-Mao China. Jie Yang, *Unknotting the Heart: Unemployment and Therapeutic Governance in China* (Ithaca, NY: Cornell University Press, 2015), xix.

process of perpetual calibration to the polarized tensions, desires, and affects that make up life under capitalist conditions. This process structures the affective framework of Li's aesthetics and is furthermore embodied in online healing media's own twin impulses of turning away from and profiting off of digital economies.

Rural Vlogs, Healing Vlogs: The Rise of Li Ziqi

Li (legal birth name Li Jiajia) began making videos during difficult times.[10] Abandoned by divorced parents, Li lived with her grandparents in Mianyang, found a city job at fourteen, and returned to care for her grandmother in 2016. That year, she began uploading food-centered videos on the Chinese streaming platform Youku, quickly becoming a domestic online star (*wanghong* 網紅). Followers could not get enough of her graceful farming and cooking skills, as well as the splendor of her rural abode. By 2017, Li had turned this internet fame into a cross-platform brand. She developed Sichuan Ziqi Culture Limited Co. and commenced her now-terminated collaboration with multichannel network company Hangzhou Weinian. This collaboration led to "a rare leap for Chinese influencers" because both parties decided to upload Li's videos to YouTube, hoping she could be "just as popular with a global audience."[11] Two years later, this hope was realized.[12] She profited immensely as viewership from both Chinese and American servers skyrocketed,[13] eliciting commentary from a wide array of sources, including *The New York Times*, *The New Yorker*, and the *Los Angeles Review of Books*.[14]

10. See Zhang Zijun, "Shidaorujin, cai zhenzheng kandongle Li Ziqi de shipin," *Elle China*, February 19, 2020, https://www.ellechina.com/celeb/gossip/a30991715/liziqi-20220219/, "Behind the scenes with Li Ziqi, the mysterious Chinese internet celebrity with 58 million fans," *South China Morning Post*, September 17, 2019, https://www.scmp.com/lifestyle/entertainment/article/3027602/behind-scenes-li-ziqi-mysterious-chinese-internet-celebrity, and "Exclusive Interview with Li Ziqi, China's Most Mysterious Internet Celebrity," Goldthread, Youtube, September 12, 2019, https://www.youtube.com/watch?v=J9CfVcXoYh4.
11. Oscar Schwarz, "Li Ziqi's Online Pastoral Poetics," *New Yorker*, August 4, 2023, https://www.newyorker.com/culture/rabbit-holes/li-ziqis-online-pastoral-poetics.
12. By the end of 2019, Li had a quarter million Weibo subscribers and 9 million YouTube subscribers.
13. There have been educated estimates that Li earns around US$24 million per year. Even if Li's revenue is half of or a quarter of $24 million, however, that is still a substantial income. "Chinese YouTube star Li Ziqi dismisses claim she makes US $24 million a year," *South China Morning Post*, January 10, 2020. For Li's viewer demographics, see "YouTube Stats and Analytics for Li Ziqi," *Hypeauditor*, accessed February 2022, https://hypeauditor.com/youtube/li_zi_qi_liziqi-UCoC47do520os_4DBMEFGg4A/.
14. See Stephanie Wong, "The Life of Nostalgic Content: On Li Ziqi," *Los Angeles Review of Books*, February 12, 2022, https://lareviewofbooks.org/article/the-life-of-nostalgic-content-on-li-ziqi/; Tejal Ral, "The Reclusive Food Celebrity Li Ziqi is my Quarantine Queen," *New York Times*, April 22, 2020, https://www.nytimes.com/2020/04/22/dining/li-ziqi-chinese-food.html; Schwarz, "Li Ziqi's Online Pastoral Poetics," *New Yorker*, April 22, 2020.

Li's international success was lauded by official Chinese organizations,[15] a move that has made her relationship with the state a center of both scholarly and popular speculation.[16] My chapter, however, extends the significance of Li's fame beyond her speculated connections with the Chinese state. This section first outlines the state-market forces at play in the broader vlogging phenomena that contributed to Li's rise. I then both situate her vlogs within domestic and global capitalist platform economies and place her signature aesthetics in dialogue with national, regional, and transregional vlogging trends.

Chinese streaming platforms such as Youku and Tudou launched in 2005, spurring modest interest in vlog creation. But it was not until 2018, after vlogging's commercial potential became evident and domestic user-generated content became pervasively monetizable, that China experienced its own "vlogging boom." Vlog trends from the mid-2010s paved the way for this boom: just two years prior, a cluster of rural "microcelebrities"[17] had gained traction as they documented themselves performing tasks, such as catching fish or harvesting fruit. They take advantage of vlogging's autoethnographic format to position themselves as both "active bearers" and "witnesses" of rural culture.[18] Rural vloggers and local officials even worked together to transform villages into "*wanghong* villages," exporting specialty products and boosting tourism.[19] Witnessing this phenomenon in 2017, Xi Jinping

15. To name two accolades, Li received an award from a state-sponsored newspaper and accepted an offer to serve as ambassador of the Communist Youth League. "Behind the scenes with Li Ziqi, the mysterious Chinese internet celebrity with 58 million fans," *South China Morning Post*, September 17, 2019.
16. For English-language scholarship focused on Li's role as a cultural export, see Limin Liang, "Consuming the Pastoral Desire: Li Ziqi, Food Vlogging and the Structure of Feeling in the Era of Microcelebrity," *Global Storytelling: Journal of Digital and Moving Images* 1, no. 2 (2022): 7–39 and Fangfei Wang, "Narrating China: Reading Li Ziqi and Fangfang from a Nationalist Perspective," Masters thesis (Duke University, 2021). For popular debates, see Lei Silin, "Li Ziqi zenme jiu bushi wenhua shuchu le," *WeChat Blog*, December 5, 2019, https://mp.weixin.qq.com/s/NWEEIW2ntGbjUpKUJmHf3Q; and "Liziqi yu Kongzixueyuan: wuyi jiangshu de 'Zhongguo gushi' yu lingren yanwu de 'wenhua shuchu'," BBC, January 21, 2020, https://www.bbc.com/zhongwen/trad/chinese-news-51191109?fbclid=IwAR1C1zLciB9RwlNGbAjZJLBDQX_rCB4fC6mEW9M6E0vpmtjvPZiWWEH6TJc.
17. This term is oft used in scholarship on the rural influencer phenomenon. See Limin Liang, "Consuming the Pastoral Desire: Li Ziqi, Food Vlogging and the Structure of Feeling in the Era of Microcelebrity," and Han Li, "From Disenchantment to Re-enchantment: Rural Microcelebrities, Short Video, and the Spectacle-ization of the Rural Lifescape on Chinese Social Media," *International Journal of Communication* 14 (2020): 3769–87.
18. For an overview on autoethnographic creative practices, see Lisa Ortiz-Vilarelle, "Autoethnography and Beyond: Genealogy, Memory, Media, Witness," *Life Writing* 18, no. 4 (2021): 475–82.
19. Li Xiangjuan, "'Wanghong cun' de zhifujing," *Fujian Daily*, May 20, 2020, http://fjrb.fjsen.com/fjrb/html/2020-05/20/content_1259041.htm?div=-1.

called for rural youth to implement new media to lift their communities out of poverty.[20]

The popularity of these rural microcelebrities partially enabled Li's rise, but their vlogs are stylistically at odds with Li's. The formal techniques employed in rural vlogs are worth unpacking, so as to better situate Li's vlogs within broader online self-documentation conventions. In Fisherman Ah Feng's 2019 YouTube vlog, for example, rural vlogger Ah Feng sticks with a consistent mode of address. He stands in front of the camera and shouts from the seashore:[21] "Hi everyone, I'm Ah Feng! I'm going to look at the wine jars I buried yesterday and see if there are goods in store today!" He talks to and looks at us, using direct address to invite engagement and feedback. A 2019 tutorial video on Chinese platform Bilibili explicitly instructs vloggers to focus on direct address. The video outlines two building blocks of a successful vlog: the A-roll, where you narrate events while facing your camera, and B-roll, comprised of supplementary footage that mellow out gaps within your main narration.[22]

These expectations are not exclusive to Chinese vlogs. Instead, they reflect how widespread vlogging conventions have been across user-generated content (UGC) platforms.[23] At the turn of the century, online participatory networks had been lauded for fostering spaces of nonhierarchical communication. Scholarship since the mid-2000s has problematized such optimism,[24] but on UGC platforms, expectations for direct participation persist, for economic reasons. It is assumed that online influencers must rely on amicable, relatable self-branding and "quantifiable 'assess[ments] of social values'" to maintain a fan base.[25] Thus, the expectation of

20. Zhang Jinfeng. "Zimeiti shiyuxia xiangcun qingnian 'zouhong' xianxiang de chuanboxue tanjiu," *Shiting*, no. 5 (2020): 210–12. His statement was followed by Three Rurals (*sannong* 三農) conferences that offered funding for rural content creators, see "Jinri toutiao jindaohui jihua: 5 yi butie sannong chuangzuozhe," *EBRun*, July 8, 2018, http://www.ebrun.com/20180703/284595.shtml.

21. "Afeng zhanshi shichuan yijiu de ganhai fangfa," Yumin afeng, April 10, 2019, https://www.youtube.com/watch?v=3CJkOzTVP_M&t=4s.

22. "Ruguo wo de shenghuo pingpingwuqi you zhiyou shouji name gai ruhe pai vlog ne?" Bushifuposhu. January 27, 2019, https://www.bilibili.com/video/BV1Ht411t7QG/?spm_id_from=333.788.recommend_more_video.-1.

23. Both Chinese and English scholarship on vlogs also reinforce the centrality of direct address for vloggers, as well as live streamers and other content creators. See Bin Zhenyu, "Vlog Zhongguo fazhan xianzhuang yu qianjing qianxi," *Shiting*, no. 3 (2019) and Jean Burgess and Joshua Green, *YouTube: Online Video and Participatory Culture* (Hoboken, NJ: John Wiley & Sons, 2018).

24. See José van Dijck, *The Culture of Connectivity: A Critical History of Social Media* (Oxford: Oxford University Press, 2013), Tiziana Terranova, "Free Labor: Producing Culture for the Digital Economy," *Social Text* 18, no. 2 (2000): 33–58 and Robyn Caplan and Tarleton Gillespie, "Tiered Governance and Demonetization: The Shifting Terms of Labor and Compensation in the Platform Economy," *Social Media + Society* 6, no. 2 (2020): 1–13.

25. Brooke Erin Duffy, Annika Pinch, Shruti Sannon, and Megan Sawey, "The Nested Precarities of Creative Labor on Social Media," *Social Media+ Society* 7, no. 2 (2021): 3.

direct address in vlogs shapes a media aesthetics, one that makes sensible a dominant—but narrow—understanding of digital sociality and economy.

To uphold such an aesthetics as *the* standard means of maintaining user interest makes alternative vlog techniques seem trivial. This also implies that the media aesthetics these alternative techniques point to can reshape our conceptualization of online participatory culture. But first, what might these alternative techniques refer to? In her most popular video,[26] Li roasts chestnuts and makes the delectable Chinese sweet *tanghulu*. She is alone and silent, feigning unawareness of the camera. Viewers are drawn to the sound of foliage crunching on the forest floor and to Li's serene profile. Her voice is only present when she speaks to her grandmother, but even then, background music subdues their chats. Such an aesthetics untethers the vlogger from any direct interaction with the vlog camera, but still manages to generate sustained pleasure for viewers. "When I'm stressed or worried," Tien Trung comments under Li's video, "I watch her videos and feel *instantly* better."[27]

The aesthetics that propelled Li to international stardom, since then emulated by rural vloggers such as Dianxi Xiaoge and Ermichuiyan, resonate with a broader East Asian healing vlog niche. Vloggers, many of which are urban-dwelling women, have aestheticized self-documentation for soothing purposes since the mid-2010s. Such healing vlogs are pervasive on Chinese short video platforms. Examples include Linzimu's "Healing Vlog. A girl Living Alone" (*Zhiyu* vlog. *duju nuhai* 自癒 vlog 獨居女孩), where our vlogger whisks eggs in a glass bowl and lights candles. Living alone, she does not talk or even show her face. South Korean YouTuber Sueddu also records days in her apartment. Background music and tingly ASMR emanate out of daily tasks and mundanities, lulling viewers.[28] Both channels aestheticize slow living, a "slow culture" pedagogy that advocates measured, intentional consumption of food, information, commodities, and everyday processes.[29] In particular, Sueddu

26. "Peanut and Melon Seeds, Dried Meat, Dried Fruit, Snowflake Cake," Li Ziqi, January 31, 2019, https://www.youtube.com/watch?v=FWMIPukvdsQ&t=30s.

27. Tien Trung, comment on "Peanut and Melon Seeds," 2019. Emphasis mine.

28. "Autonomous Sensory Meridian Response" refers to a tingly sensation triggered by certain sensory cues. ASMR has become a genre of online healing videos. Rob Gallagher, "Eliciting Euphoria Online: The Aesthetics of 'ASMR' Video Culture," *Film Criticism* 40, no.2 (2016), https://quod.lib.umich.edu/f/fc/13761232.0040.202/--eliciting-euphoria-online-the-aesthetics-of-asmr-video?rgn=main;view=fulltext.

29. The term "slow culture," which encompasses the slow food and slow living movements, grew popular in late 1980s Europe and the United States. The slow living movement emerged as an extension of an Italian slow food movement and is generally associated with minimalist and essentialist lifestyles. Suzanne Zuppello, "Slow Food's Elitism Only Fueled My Cravings for McDonald's," *Eater*, October 18, 2018, https://www.eater.com/2018/10/18/17943358/slow-food-manifesto-elitist-fast-food, and Wendy Parkins and Geoffrey Craig, *Slow Living* (Oxford: Berg Publishing, 2006).

labels her videos as "silent vlogs." This term refers to the muting of direct address and has since been intertwined with "healing vlogs" in general.[30]

Li's videos are influenced by both domestic rural vlog and regional healing vlog trends. Moreover, her deliberate choice to eschew direct address has the potential to reconfigure affects, subjectivities, and socialities typically associated with platform networks. In other words, indirect virtual communication gives rise to its own media aesthetics, introducing complexity to the dominant role that direct participatory aesthetics still play in analyses of user-generated content.

Li Ziqi's Healing Atmospheres

What, then, exactly comprises Li's aesthetics? What kind of Internet sociality and subjectivity do they condition, as videos that not only completely lack "A-roll" but also aim to give everyday self-documentation therapeutic function? This section explores how Li's formal techniques generate atmospheres of ambience, escapism, and slowness. Her ambient and escapist aesthetics form polar impulses, simultaneously inviting viewers to melt into their environments and cultivating a strong urge to get away. These impulses begin to pluralize the therapeutic functions of Li's videos, and how these functions become commodifiable. Lastly, these impulses are held together through her videos' implementation of the serial vlog format, which I argue reconceptualizes "healing" as itself a mode of ceaseless navigation through internally complex sensorial, temporal fields.

Ambient Tableau

Ambience expresses its own healing atmosphere in Li's videos. Her 2018 video on hang-dried persimmons,[31] for example, commences with an extreme long shot as the camera lingers on tree-laden mountain peaks. The ridges of the mountains are softened by dense blue fog. In a slightly closer long shot, Li appears. Her faraway body, encircled by persimmon fruit branches, occupies center frame but remains out of focus. The indigo color of her clothes blurs into the overall tableau as she pauses in her steps. After an interweaving of close-ups and long shots, we see Li harvest the persimmons by snipping the fruit and dropping them into her basket, snipping and dropping. Throughout the video, Li is at times no more than a speck of indigo floating across green fields, flitting amid blue mountains and orange persimmon clusters.

30. Makato Meoka, "What's All the Noise about Silent Vlogs?" *YouTube Official Blog*, July 26, 2021, https://blog.youtube/culture-and-trends/whats-all-the-noise-about-silent-vlogs/.
31. "It's a Red Mountain, and in the Fall, it's Natural to Make Some Sweet Persimmons," October 8, 2018, https://www.youtube.com/watch?v=QHTnuI9IKBA&t=39s.

Other times, she occupies the blurred background, blending again into the overall flora and fauna. Even after she returns home with her bountiful harvest, green, blue, and orange infuse the shots where Li peels the persimmons with her grandmother. This tricolor palette and blur focus gives the video a painterly feel and encourages a dispersed gaze that dissolves the boundaries between natural landscapes and human bodies.

It is not in passing that I emphasize the prominence of pictorial landscapes in these videos. Much scholarship on atmosphere arises from analyses of landscape paintings and design.[32] Riedel, mapping out the Western theoretical genealogy of "atmosphere," initially defines atmosphere as the rendering of "diverse elements" into "seamless hue, just as a sunset tinges the entire 'world' in shades of red."[33] Atmosphere theorist Gernot Böhme directly grounds his theory in C. C. L. Hirschfeld's work on garden art. For Böhme, atmosphere radiates out from matter, diffusing viewers within a mood, a "spatially extended common reality."[34] In turn, atmosphere pushes for a "new aesthetics," which extends beyond any frame or border to envelop viewers in their "everyday life."[35]

The presence of this kind of atmosphere on online platforms changes how online vlogs engage viewers. Indeed, this atmosphere attunes us to how Internet sociality can exist as indirect, scattered "common reality," rather than direct verbal and visual communication. In Li's vlogs, this sensorial engagement with viewers materializes as healing affects, best conceptualized via Roquet's analytical lens. In *Ambient Media*, Roquet connects ambient atmospherics to Japanese healing media, defining ambience as a formal means of "dissolv[ing] the self into a stream of sense impressions."[36] For example, ambient novels melt readers into descriptions of plush couches or warm lighting, enveloping us in the haptic comforts of colors, temperatures, and textures,[37] while ambient films emanate calm through a minimalist style. Roquet states of the film *Toni Takitani* (Ichikawa Jun, 2004) that most objects are "*gray, black, white, indigo* . . . [and] *out-of-focus walls* slide by close to the camera."[38] This attention to color and camera blur echoes the techniques within Li's persimmons video, as well as Riedel and Böhme's theorizations.

32. In the late eighteenth century, German landscape artists and art critics such as Carl Ludwig Fernow and Carl Gustav Carus drew inspiration from Friedrich Schiller's notion of "world soul" and Immanuel Kant's conceptualizations of *Stimmung*.
33. Friedlind Riedel, "Atmosphere," in *Affective Societies: Key Concepts*, ed. Jan Slaby and Christian von Scheve (London: Routledge, 2019), 90.
34. Gernot Böhme, "Atmosphere as the Fundamental Concept of a New Aesthetics," *Thesis Eleven* 36, no. 1 (1993): 122.
35. Böhme, "Atmosphere as the Fundamental Concept of a New Aesthetics," 125.
36. Roquet, *Ambient Media*, 15.
37. Roquet, *Ambient Media*, 159.
38. Roquet, *Ambient Media*, 127. Emphasis mine.

Beyond highlighting the connection between ambient atmosphere and healing media, Roquet provides insight on its sociopolitical implications. Namely, he emphasizes that ambience is "low-affect." Be it through background music or still landscapes on TV, ambient media in urban spaces (hotel lobbies, restaurants, etc.) relax the environment without drawing attention to themselves. Informed by Foucault, Roquet then argues that ambient media heal through subtle mood regulation, allowing consumers to tune our emotions at our own pace.[39] Chinese scholarship echoes this more optimistically, lauding Chinese healing culture as a lubricant (*runhuaji* 潤滑劑) that can ease youth back into "harmoniously engag[ing] with society."[40] Ambience foregrounds "healing" as a mechanism for biopolitical attunement.

Li's videos undeniably harbor the healing ambience conceptualized by Roquet. As her persimmons video draws to a close, it is already wintertime. We hear the soft howl of winter wind as Li pours tea into a cup, its steam rising slowly next to the now fully dried persimmons, their once-vibrant hue dusted with white marks of dehydration. It is no wonder that her viewers often experience a sense of soft, sleepy comfort, even developing "a habit of watching her videos before going to bed . . . like a relaxation therapy."[41] However, closer analyses of where and when her videos are set—spatiotemporal locations that differentiate her from most urban-set East Asian healing vlogs—will lead us to question if the entirety of Li's atmosphere can be categorized as low-affect ambience, or whether alternative aesthetic tendencies and sociopolitical implications can also arise.

Eremitic Mise-en-Scène

In another video on magnolia blossoms, Li rides a horse through the forest, wearing traditional Han-style garments, or *hanfu* 漢服.[42] Craggy tree trunks cocoon her from screen-left as pink magnolia clusters frame her from screen-right. Behind her is a hut, its contours made hazy by the fog. Ambient elements pervade this video as much as her other videos. Yet, the way branches, flowers, and bushes frame Li's body evokes a different kind of atmosphere. Such long shots echo paintings where, perhaps, a lone figure walks along a path, his silhouette framed on multiple sides. Willow trees

39. Roquet, *Ambient Media*, 14.
40. Wang Xiajing, "'Wei' shidaixia zhiyuxi wenhua liuxing xianxiang jiedu," *Qingnianjizhe*, no. 32 (2018): 30. It is also noteworthy that Wang's emphasis on harmonious (*hexie*) engagement has particular resonance with more official projects of building a harmonious society (*hexie shehui* 和諧社會). Thus, as Zhang Li states succinctly, this subjectivity modulation process incorporates not only "the usual neoliberalism story of self-advancement but [also] a more complicated picture of [state-market] assemblages." Zhang, *Anxious China: Inner Revolution and the Politics of Psychotherapy*, 114.
41. Seema Alim, comment on "It's a Red Mountain," 2018.
42. "Riding a Horse to Find Magnolia Liliflora Blossoms for my Lovely Fans," April 6, 2019, https://www.youtube.com/watch?v=F8O3fRC4tSk&t=52s.

droop from the right and flat rocks ground him from below as his straw hut peeks through from behind the trees. What I have just described mirrors the "atmosphere of isolation"[43] that permeates *Mr. Five Willows* (*Wuliu* 五柳), Ming dynasty artist Chen Hongshou's painting of Daoist hermit and literati poet Tao Yuanming (AD 365–427). In many hermit paintings, natural elements partially conceal the hermit to accentuate the distance between his world and the viewers, in effect drawing viewers further into his withdrawn recluse.

Similar shots in Li's videos thus create an eremitic mise-en-scène. For urban viewers, this mise-en-scène conjures an atmosphere that cannot be adequately described as ambient. Exacerbated by the natural framing that places partial barriers between us and Li, long shots emphasize a spatiotemporal discrepancy between Li's world and ours. One YouTube commenter shows how this discrepancy generates intense affects, claiming that Li's videos are "so hypnotic and soothing that I can't finish what I'm eating while watching."[44] Another commenter expresses an escapist desire sparked by the compositions of Li's shots: "this channel makes me want to forsake civilization and go live in the forest."[45]

Here, Li's vlog style strays from other East Asian healing vlogs, revealing the influence of Chinese healing culture specifically. Eremitic seclusion in nature is an important element of Li's vlog style, but it by no means entails that Li seriously promotes eremitism, traditionally a practice of retreating from government duties, court positions, and social interaction more generally.[46] Instead, Li's eremitic mise-en-scène indexes how musings on nature by premodern literati have regained popularity as a healing culture subtrend.[47] Chinese journalists and critics thus repeatedly tie Li's aesthetics to Tao Yuanming's poems, in turn circulating snippets of premodern poetry widely online as little doses of therapy. Dai Wangyun evokes *Peach Blossom Spring*, "Tao's classic story of a secluded utopian paradise,"[48] to describe Li's "idyllic

---

43. Dianne Lorell Morton, "Paintings as Social Rhetoric: Wei-Jin Themes in Ming dynasty Illustrations and Inscriptions," PhD diss. (University of Kansas, 2001): 141.
44. Asteria, comment on "A pot of wine among watermelon fields," September 14, 2020, https://www.youtube.com/watch?v=kgEgOi32CE0&t=1073s.
45. Asia Amazing, comment on "It's a Red Mountain," 2018.
46. Eremitism was officially acknowledged through writing in China during the Han (206 BC–AD 220) and Six Dynasties (AD 220–589) periods, and paintings of hermits proliferated in the Ming dynasty. For an overview of Ming dynasty hermit painting and poetry, see *The Artful Recluse: Painting, Poetry, and Politics in Seventeenth-Century China*, ed. Peter Charles Sturman and Susan Tai (Santa Barbara, CA: Santa Barbara Museum of Art, 2012).
47. Wu, "Qingnian qunti zhiyuxi wenhua liuxing xianxiang touxi," 98.
48. Dai Wangyun, "How Li Ziqi Repackages Rural China for Urban Fantasies," *Sixth Tone*, December 27, 2019, https://www.sixthtone.com/news/1005007/how-li-ziqi-repackages-rural-china-for-urban-fantasies.

repose," and *Elle China*[49] introduces her by citing from a couplet in Tao's *Drinking Wine* series:

> I built my cottage in a peopled place
> Yet hear no sounds of passing carts and horses . . .
> Gathering chrysanthemums by the Eastern fence
> I catch sight of South Mountain in the distance;
> The mountain air is lovely as the sun sets
> And flocks of flying birds return together.[50]

Tapping into eremitic aesthetics, Li Ziqi's atmosphere cultivates an urge to move across thresholds. This urge is articulated in Riedel's chapter, which initially introduces ambient theories of atmosphere, but then moves toward alternative theorizations that draw on early eighteenth-century European etymological associations between atmosphere and a magnetic force field or human effluvia. She articulates atmosphere as a mereological arena made up of movements, rather than an emanating but otherwise preexisting air. Movement is often generated through "affective thresholds": atmosphere "produce[s] meaning in their difference from" our reality.[51]

"Affective thresholds" generate a satisfyingly intense movement toward fantasy worlds, exacerbating dissatisfactions with our everyday lives. This healing function thus acquires complicated implications as it thrives on online platforms. On the one hand, it uniquely romanticizes the fact that being online is always both a public and private act: even as we acquire thousands of Facebook friends or comment on and like countless TikTok videos, there is often a component of isolation that accompanies the act of going online. Rather than feeding the fantasy of constant social connection, Li's escapist atmosphere creatively plays with the inherent asocial sociality of our digital experience, to feed a more critical eremitic fantasy, a haven that seems to exist outside of society as such. On the other, the foregrounding of a virtually unpopulated, distinctly Asian rural haven exploits both gentrifying and Orientalizing thresholds for commercial profit. Domestically, Li tames the countryside for the urban viewer. Dai highlights how, "after sanding off the rough edges of rural life," Li turns "what's left into . . . audio-visual treats for urbanites to consume."[52] Internationally, another layer is added to this urban-rural threshold. Though Li's on-screen costumes reflect a broader domestic *hanfu* trend circulating among Chinese

49. Zhang, "Shidaorujin, cai zhenzheng kandongle Liziqi de shipin," https://www.ellechina.com/celeb/gossip/a30991715/liziqi-20220219/.
50. This translation, featuring all but four lines in Tao's couplet, is from Susan E. Nelson, "Catching Sight of South Mountain: Tao Yuanming, Mount Lu, and the Iconographies of Escape," *Archives of Asian Art* 52 (2000/2001): 11–43.
51. Riedel, "Atmosphere," 92.
52. Dai, "How Li Ziqi Repackages Rural China."

youth,[53] when she strategically circulates these videos to non-Chinese audiences on YouTube, these costumes combine with unpopulated landscapes to reduce China to a forever preindustrial refuge.[54] This "China" echoes a provocative dialogue in Benjamin Hoff's *The Tao of Pooh*, a bestseller that Disney-fies Daoism:

> "the easiest way to [understand Taoism] would be for us to go to China . . ."
> "What?" said Pooh, his eyes wide open in amazement. "Right now?"
> "Of course. All we need to do is lean back, relax, and there we are."[55]

Li projects China as the embodiment of calm itself. One goes there just by "leaning back" into a healing state of mind. Her escapist atmosphere in many ways tailors the ongoing commodification of mystical Asian philosophies to the online platform attention economy.

So far, this chapter has argued that Li's vlogs aesthetically produce polarized atmospheres that correspond to distinct healing affects and configurations of Internet sociality. Her ambient atmosphere extends low-affect calm, scattering viewers' subjective orientations into dispersed, regulatable mood. Eremitic shot compositions create thresholds that draw urban viewers into an "atmosphere of isolation" that exists on the edge of sociality as such. Two questions linger. First, if the healing functions of Li's ambient and eremitic atmospheres cannot simply be merged together, how do they engage each other, and what theorizations of healing does their intertwinement express? Second, my chapter's current focus on long-shot compositions almost exclusively prioritizes intermedial, spatial expressions of atmosphere. Are there significant temporal aesthetics at play? The next section shows how Li's videos form a durational atmosphere that holds together the twin impulses of ambient diffusion and escapist urge, fundamentally redefining what "healing" entails within the vlog format's medium-specific rhythms.

---

53. For a general overview of *hanfu* culture, one of China's most popular Gen-Z trends, see Xinyi Wang, François Colbert, and Renaud Legoux, "From Niche Interest to Fashion Trend: *Hanfu* Clothing as a Rising Industry in China," *International Journal of Arts Management* 23, no. 1 (2020): 79–89.
54. Chinese literature professor Michel Hockx cautions that Li Ziqi's vlogs index the proliferation of "views of Chinese culture and Chinese tradition as 'exotic and different.'" Jill Li, "As China's Vloggers Draw International Fans, Beijing Sees Soft Power Opportunity," *VOA*, August 12, 2020, https://www.voanews.com/a/east-asia-pacific_voa-news-china_chinas-vloggers-draw-international-fans-beijing-sees-soft-power/6194341.html. See also Zhen Troy Chen and Thomas William Whyke, "Manufacturing and Commodifying 'Chineseness': Micro-Celebrity Li Ziqi's Construction of an Idyllic Rural China and her Media Representation on YouTube," in *China's International Communication and Relationship Building*, ed. Xiaoling Zhang and Corey Schultz (London: Routledge, 2022), 150–64.
55. Benjamin Hoff, *The Tao of Pooh* (New York: Dutton Books, 1982): 1.

Slow Atmospheres

Vlogs chronicle daily life, and so are structured around processes. We have seen that processes occupy center stage in Li's vlogs, be it harvesting and peeling persimmons, or plucking magnolias to make into jam. During an episode of the WBUR *Endless Thread* podcast,[56] host Amory Sivertson narrates the start of Li's video on the process of planting cucumbers.[57] Li first bundles together bamboo to make a fence. She then wets soil and breaks off chunks. In real time, she forms two little soil spheres in her hands, then shows via time-lapse how she molds the others. Li presses seeds onto these spheres before watering them and covering them with dry soil. Reacting to the same video, *Endless Thread* cohost Ben Johnson describes Li's "extremely slow-moving, long set of videos" as "the most calming thing you have done on the internet in weeks."

Li's processes indeed feel slow. In one minute, she exhibits her seed-planting process, repeating some steps to further decelerate the task's progression. This processual aesthetics affects one differently than, say, aggressive, short video cooking tutorials that teach viewers an entire recipe within some fifteen seconds. However, Li's processes also are still bite-size, inundated with quick cuts and time-lapses. In addition, the start of Li's cucumber video weaves together the two unrelated processes of seed planting and fence building. So, if Roquet highlights *Toni Takitani*'s singular long takes and "slow cinema" aesthetics as formative to its healing atmosphere,[58] Li's "extremely slow-moving" duration holds a different valence, toggling multiple temporalities at once. To grasp this valence is to tap into the broader atmospheric field opened by Li's healing aesthetics.

In film and media studies, healing affects have already been linked to depictions of process. In *The Process Genre: Cinema and the Aesthetic of Labor*, Salomé Aguilera Skvirsky theorizes process as its own transmedial genre, the "ordered representation of someone making or doing something."[59] Accordingly, she analyzes affects generated by this genre,[60] centering on how processes draw viewers in. Absorption, as defined by Skvirsky, is a state of productive fixation where viewers become engrossed in "causally linked" steps that lead to a final product.[61] However, some

56. Ben Brock Johnson and Amory Sivertson, "Li Ziqi, China's Quarantine Queen," *Endless Thread*, podcast audio, February 11, 2022, https://www.wbur.org/endlessthread/2022/02/11/li-ziqi-chinas-quarantine-queen.
57. "The Life of Cucumbers," July 20, 2020, https://www.youtube.com/watch?v=oi38cQMORQY.
58. Roquet, *Ambient Media*, 128, 143.
59. Salomé Aguilera Skvirsky, *The Process Genre: Cinema and the Aesthetic of Labor* (Durham, NC: Duke University Press, 2020), 2.
60. Skvirsky, *The Process Genre*, 4.
61. Skvirsky, *The Process Genre*, 80.

of her examples complicate this definition, revealing how the genre can create less goal-oriented healing affects.

At the start of her chapter dedicated to absorption, Skvirsky elaborates on a now-viral six-minute segment from *Mister Rogers' Neighborhood*. We are shown how crayons are produced in a factory. Guided by Fred Rogers's mellow, slightly monotone voice—by now a popular ASMR treat[62]—this processual depiction could make one's gaze glaze over. Skvirsky acknowledges the "dull," lulling quality of the video but also cites comments on how the episode is "hypnotic," making the viewer "forget about" stress "and just get lost in the relaxing mundanity of watching crayons get made."[63] Processes, then, can dissolve viewers into a "Zen-like" mood, while also pushing us to flee from "times of panic and desperation."[64] They bring together ambient and escapist healing atmospherics.

This polarized absorption, which does not necessitate productive progress, quasi-participation, or the satisfaction of closure, is present in Li's processes.[65] The start of her video on making ice cream both disperses and transfixes attention through two acts: snipping and plucking.[66] She reaches up to a tree weighed down by juicy berries and snips the berries off three times in succession. She places them in a basket before plucking other fruit. Back at home, she plucks tea leaves from a bush fourteen times. These movements offer a repetitive lull as well as an intense immersion into Li's momentum. In addition, just like in her cucumber video, most of Li's processes are nonlinear, mingling with other incomplete processes and adhering to a serial pattern of vlog uploads. The main process in Li's ice cream video, for example, is intercut with segments of her cooking fresh tea leaves and making a miniature garden.

A process is no longer a step-by-step path; it is a site of possibility. Look at all the things Li does with a persimmon, or harvests through the gesture of plucking. Likewise, the slowness associated with processual depiction becomes a site that viewers can "just get lost in." Decelerated affective experiences do not just lead to time slowing down but also open viewers up to different temporal threads. To paraphrase Riedel, atmosphere becomes force field, assembling the shifts and tensions

62. See retox44 Relaxing Voices ASMR, "Unintentional ASMR Relaxing Voice Fred Rogers 1969 Senate Testimony," *YouTube*, May 28, 2023, https://www.youtube.com/watch?v=zdLDKwuTqA0, and White Noise Television, "1 Hour of Mister Rogers ASMR Clips Relax and Sleep," *YouTube*, August 1, 2022, https://www.youtube.com/watch?v=ddA9n_ofQ1M.
63. Skvirsky, *The Process Genre*, 77.
64. Dayna Evans, quoted in Skvirsky, *The Process Genre*, 30.
65. In contrast, for Skvirsky, the process genre upholds efficiently, modern techniques and ideological aspirations toward progress even in depictions of so-called "primitive" processes. See Skvirsky, *The Process Genre*, 146–92.
66. "Cool and Sweet Berry Ice Cream, the Taste of Summer," July 1, 2019, https://www.youtube.com/watch?v=vaf3Z-tNXqM&t=250s.

among distinct entities and suggested movements.[67] The healing power of Li's slowness thus neither pulls viewers away from nor quickly dissolves their current situations but rather allows them to make sense of the present as inherently dynamic, subject to multiplication, tension, and change.[68]

This atmospheric conceptualization of slowness reconfigures attitudes toward global capitalism. Along with many other healing vlogs, Li's vlogs crucially do not position "slowness" as external to a monolithic capitalist "speed," aiming to rescue viewers from such an exploitative temporality.[69] Straying from more attention-grabbing participatory aesthetics, Li still manages to break records within the digital attention economy. More than anything, the profitability of her slow aesthetics exhibits that capitalism is not reducible to a singular rate-of-speed. Slowness, then, operates as a strategic mediator within our inherently plural experience of capitalism. As Lutz Koepniz conceptualizes, it "*sharpens our senses for the coexistence of different and often incompatible vectors of time* . . . [opening us] up to the opulence and manifoldness of the present."[70]

Conclusion

Li Ziqi's vlogs assemble contrasting and cohering aesthetic techniques. Taken separately, these techniques have their own healing effects, each creating its own conditions for Internet sociality and profitability. Ambience comforts the viewer via regulatory, low-affect tone. Eremitic escapism inspires the intense urge to move across affective thresholds, to imagine what life might be like at the edges of sociality. These impulses intertwine through Li's processual configuration of the vlog format. Together, they redefine healing, a label shaped by online platform distribution and dependent on aesthetic appeal. To heal is to open the present into an atmospheric force field, to explore soothing means of exploring the affects, temporalities, and social relations within this field.

Since the summer of 2021, Li stopped uploading videos, primarily due to conflicts with Hangzhou Weinian. Her pastoral fantasy world has become, for now, a relic of the recent past. Healing vlogs, however, continue to enchant, transforming

67. Riedel, "Atmosphere," 93.

68. Caetlin Benson-Allott coined the term "temporal escapism" as the reconfiguration and expansion of present durations for us to find reassurance and potential in. Benson-Allott describes how she has been relying on American films that employ temporal escapism to get through the COVID-19 pandemic blues. Caetlin Benson-Allott, "In Praise of Escapism," *Film Quarterly* 74, no. 1 (2020): 79.

69. See, for example, the overlapping and mutual interruption of various processes in Japanese vlogger Choki's "A Warm Holiday in the Life of a Japanese Living Alone," November 10, 2020, https://www.youtube.com/watch?v=taGPCVtdgKA.

70. Lutz Koepnick, *On Slowness: Toward an Aesthetic of the Contemporary* (New York: Columbia University Press, 2014), 4. Emphasis mine.

the social and economic potentials of online self-documentation. Transregional curiosity about the East Asian healing vlog phenomenon has intensified since 2020, as expressed by online articles.[71] In these articles, poetic descriptions of the vlogs often bleed into reflections on the author's own life. Novelist Crystal Kim writes that she cried often during the COVID-19 quarantine, overwhelmed by her pregnancy, her doctor husband being on the front lines, and endless Zoom meetings. As she was accompanied regularly by anonymous women performing tasks in their earth-hued abodes, she began to get playfully lost in her own everyday routines. As she noticed slanted rays of light flooding her house and the sounds of her cooking, "my perspective shifted."[72] It remains to be seen to what extent healing vlogs will transform the dynamics of online sociality, both within social media platforms and in engagement with other audiovisual media.

71. For examples of English-language coverage of East Asian healing vlogs (also known as silent vlogs), see Crystal Kim, "Slow Living with Korea's Silent Vloggers," *Elle*, May 21, 2021, https://www.elle.com/culture/a36451963/korea-silent-vloggers/; Meoka, "What's All the Noise about Silent Vlogs?"; and Emily Lehmann, "Serenity Now: The Immersive World of Silent Vlogs," *Verily Magazine*, May 27, 2022, https://verilymag.com/2022/05/serenity-now-the-immersive-world-of-silent-youtube-video-vlogs-2022.
72. Kim, "Slow Living with Korea's Silent Vloggers."

Bibliography

Akashi, Kaijin 明石海人. *Hakubyō* 白描 [Ink sketches]. Tokyo: Kaizō-sha, 1938.

Alpert, Robert, Merle Eisenberg, and Lee Mordechai. *Diseased Cinema: Plagues, Pandemics and Zombies in American Movies*. Edinburgh: Edinburgh University Press, 2023.

Alschuler, Sari. "Humanities." In *Keywords for Health Humanities*, edited by Sari Alschuler, Jonathan M. Metzl, and Priscilla Wald, 109–12. New York: New York University Press, 2023.

An, Rui 安瑞. "Shijunti zhiliao de qianshi, jinsheng, yu weilai" 噬菌體治療的前世、今生與未來 [Past, present, and future of phage therapy]. *Kexue tongbao* 科學通報, no. 23 (2017): 2577–80.

Anderson, Joseph L., and Donald Richie, *The Japanese Film: Art and Industry*. Princeton, NJ: Princeton University Press, 1982.

Andrews, Bridie. *The Making of Modern Chinese Medicine, 1850–1960*. Vancouver: UBC Press, 2014.

Aoki, Bunzō 青木文象. "*Kojima no Haru* to tanka no sekai" 『小島の春』と短歌の世界 [*Spring on the Small Island* and the world of Poetry]. *Eiga hyōron* 映画評論 [Film criticism] 22, no. 9 (1940): 59–63.

"Apeun 100nyeonui yeoksa donghaenghaneun Sorokdo" [Sorok island with its painful 100-year-long history], National Sorokdo Hosptial Museum of Hansen's Disease. http://www.sorokdo.go.kr/museum/html/content.do?menu_cd=05_04&depth=mi.

Arai, Eiko 新井英子. *Hansen-byō to kirisuto-kyō* ハンセン病とキリスト教 [Hansen's disease and Christianity]. Tokyo: Iwanami Shoten, 1996.

Arai, Yuki 荒井 裕樹. *Kakuri no bungaku: Hansen-byō ryōyōsho no jiko hyōgen-shi* 隔離の文学ーンセン病療養所の自己表現史 [Literature of quarantine: A history of self-expression in Hansen's disease sanatoria]. Tokyo: Shoshi arusu, 2011.

Ba, Jin 巴金. "Yichang wanjiu shengming de zhandou" 一場挽救生命的戰鬥 [A battle for life]. *Renmin wenxue* 人民文學 no. 8 (1958): 107–12.

Badiou, Alain. *Théorie du sujet*. Paris: Éditions du seul, 1982.

Baek, Seon Lye. "1919–20nyeon singminji Joseonui kollera yuhaenggwa bangyeokwaldong" [Choleraepidemics in colonial Korea and the activities of preventive epidemics in 1919–20]. MA thesis, Hanyang University, 2011.

Baker, Rodney. *The Hiroshima Maidens: A Story of Courage, Compassion, and Survival.* New York: Penguin Books, 1986.

Bakhtin, M. M. *The Dialogic Imagination.* Edited by Michael Holquist. Translated by Caryl Emerson and Michael Holquist. Austin, TX: University of Texas, 1981.

"Bandoui mulsangwa munhwa, sipsamdo gakdoreul jeonmanghamyeo" [Industry and culture of peninsula, overlooking thirteen provinces respectively]. *Samcheolli,* May 1940.

Barnes, Elizabeth. *The Minority Body: A Theory of Disability*. Oxford: Oxford University Press, 2018.

Barnes, Nicole Elizabeth. *Intimate Communities: Wartime Healthcare and the Birth of Modern China, 1937–1945*. Oakland, CA: University of California Press, 2018.

Barthes, Roland. *Camera Lucida.* Translated by Richard Howard. New York: Hill and Wang, 1981.

Baudrillard, Jean. *Simulacres et Simulation.* Paris: Éditions Galilée, 1981.

"Behind the scenes with Li Ziqi, the mysterious Chinese internet celebrity with 58 million fans." *South China Morning Post,* September 17, 2019. https://www.scmp.com/lifestyle/entertainment/article/3027602/behind-scenes-li-ziqi-mysterious-chinese-internet-celebrity.

Belmonte, Laura A. *Selling the American Way: U.S. Propaganda and the Cold War*. Philadelphia, PA: University of Pennsylvania Press, 2008.

Benson-Allott, Caetlin. "In Praise of Escapism." *Film Quarterly* 74, no. 1 (2020): 75–79.

Bethune, Norman. *The Wounds*. Ontario: Alive Press, 1939.

Bin, Zhenyu 賓振宇. "Vlog Zhongguo fazhan xianzhuang yu qianjing qianxi" Vlog中國發展現狀與景淺析 [Vlog's developmental trajectory and prospects in China vlog]. *Shiting 視聽*, no. 3 (2019): 147–49.

Blum, Dani. "Therapists Are on TikTok. And How Does That Make You Feel?" *The New York Times,* May 7, 2021. https://www.nytimes.com/2021/01/12/well/mind/tiktok-therapists.html.

Boddice, Rob. "Introduction." In *Pain and Emotion in Modern History,* edited by Rob Boddice, 1–15. New York: Palgrave Macmillan, 2014.

Böhme, Gernot. "Atmosphere as the Fundamental Concept of a New Aesthetics." *Thesis Eleven* 36, no. 1 (1993): 113–26.

Bok, Hyesook. "Naui gyoyurok wolloyeoryu-ga yeongneun hoego (83) yeonghwa debwi (13)" [My memoir, a veteran actress's retrospect (83) film debut [13]]. *Donga ilbo,* May 6, 1981.

Boyer, Anne. *The Undying*. New York: Macmillan Publishers, 2019.

Brazelton, Mary Augusta. *Mass Vaccination: Citizen's Bodies and State Power in Modern China.* Ithaca, NY: Cornell University Press, 2019.

Bray, Francesca. "Introduction." In *Gender, Health, and History in Modern East Asia,* edited by Angela Ki Che Leung and Izumi Nakayama, 1–34. Hong Kong: Hong Kong University Press, 2017.

Brives, Charlotte, and Jessica Pourraz. "Phage Therapy as a Potential Solution in the Fight Against AMR: Obstacles and Possible Futures." *Palgrave Communication* 100, no. 6 (2020): 1–11.

Buckingham, Jane. *Leprosy in Colonial South India: Medicine and Confinement*. New York: Palgrave Macmillan, 2002.

Burgess, Jean, and Joshua Green. *YouTube: Online Video and Participatory Culture*. 2nd edition. Hoboken, NJ: John Wiley & Sons, 2018.

Burns, Susan L. "Constructing the National Body: Public Health and Nation in Meiji Japan." In *Nation Work: Asian Elites and National Identities*, edited by Timothy Brooks and Andre Schmid, 17–50. Ann Arbor, MI: University of Michigan Press, 2000.

Burns, Susan L. *Kingdom of the Sick: A History of Leprosy and Japan*. Honolulu, HI: University of Hawai'i Press, 2019.

Byŏn, Chae-ran. "Taehan nyusŭ, munhwa yŏnghwa, kŭndaejŏk kihoek ŭrosŏŭi 'kajok kyehoek'" [Daehan news, cultural film, and family planning programs as "modern project"]. *Yŏnghea yŏngu* 52 (2012): 207–35.

Caplan, Robyn, and Tarleton Gillespie. "Tiered Governance and Demonetization: The Shifting Terms of Labor and Compensation in the Platform Economy." *Social Media + Society* 6, no. 2 (2020): 1–13.

Cavell, Stanley. *The World Viewed: Reflections on the Ontology of Film*. Cambridge, MA: Harvard University Press, 1979.

Chalk, Andy. "China Calls for Less 'Effeminate' Men in Videogames." *PC Gamer*. September 16, 2021. https://www.pcgamer.com/china-slows-new-game-approvals-calls-for-less-effeminate-men-in-videogames/.

Chang, Chia-ju. "Frankenstein's Migratory Subject: *Under the Dome* and *Formosa vs. Formosa*." *Journal of Modern Literature in Chinese* 15, no. 2 (2018): 209–32.

Chee, Liz P. Y. *Mao's Bestiary: Medical Animals and Modern China*. Durham, NC: Duke University Press, 2021.

Chee, Liz P. Y. "'To Cure a Hundred Diseases': Animal Blood Therapies in Mao's China." *Science, Technology and Society* 23, no. 2 (2018): 195–213.

Cheek, Timothy. *Mao Zedong and China's Revolution: A Brief History with Documents*. Boston: Bedford/St. Martin's, 2002.

Chen, C. C. *Medicine in Rural China: A Personal Account*. Berkeley, CA: University of California Press, 1989.

Chen, Gongmin 陳恭敏, and Wang Lian 王煉. Gongchan zhuyi de kaige 共產主義的凱歌 [A victorious song of communism]. Shanghai: Shanghai wenyi chubanshe, 1958.

Chen, Lincoln C., Michael R. Reich, and Jennifer Ryan, eds. *Medical Education in East Asia Past and Future*. Bloomington, IA: Indiana University Press, 2017.

Chen, Pin-juin 陳品君. "Jilupian zuowei guozu yuyan: women de lingyitang dilike" 紀錄片作為國族寓言：我們的另一堂地理課 [Documentary as a national allegory: learning another geography lesson]. *Xinwenxue yanjiu* 新聞學研究 12 (2016): 1–32.

Chen, Shaochang 陳紹昌. "Wo yu renyi de yidian yuanyuan" 我與人藝的一點淵源 [My connection with the Beijing People's Art Theater]. *Xinmin wanbao* 新民晚報, June 23, 2012.

Chen, Shu 陳述, ed. *Sulian chuanranbing yufang zhidao* 蘇聯傳染病預防指導 [Guidance for epidemic prevention in the Soviet Union]. Shanghai: Huadong yiwu shenghuo chubanshe, 1952.

Chen, Tina Mai. "The Human-Machine Continuum in Maoism: The Intersection of Soviet Socialist Realism, Japanese Theoretical Physics, and Chinese Revolutionary Theory." *Cultural Critique*, no. 80 (2012): 151–81.

Chen, Xinru, and Zhuo Chen. "Between the Marked and the Unmarked: Twin Semiotic Paradoxes of the Barrage in China's Livestreaming Fandom." *Media, Culture, & Society* 42, no. 5 (2020): 727–44.

Chen, Yu-feng 陳玉峯. "Qianjin yu Aige: ke chin-yuan daoyan jilupian shouying yinyan" 《前進》與〈哀歌〉——柯金源導演紀錄片首映引言 [*The Age of Awakening* and Lamentations: Introduction at the premier of director Ke Chin-yuan's documentary]. *Shanlin shuyuan* 山林書院, May 12, 2018. http://slyfchen.blogspot.com/2018/05/blog-post_12.html.

Chen, Zhen Troy, and Thomas William Whyke. "Manufacturing and Commodifying 'Chineseness': Micro-Celebrity Li Ziqi's Construction of an Idyllic Rural China and her Media Representation on YouTube." In *China's International Communication and Relationship Building*, edited by Xiaoling Zhang and Corey Schultz, 150–64. London: Routledge, 2022.

Cheng, Dan'an 承澹庵. "Zhenci zhixiao zhi yanjiu" 針刺治效之研究 [A study of the treatment effect of acupuncture needling]. *Xingtan yixue yuebao* 杏壇醫學月報, no. 47 (1933): 12–15.

"Chinese YouTube Star Li Ziqi Dismisses Claim She Makes US $24 Million a Year." *South China Morning Post*, January 10, 2020. https://www.scmp.com/news/china/society/article/3045620/chinese-youtube-star-li-ziqi-dismisses-claim-she-makes-us24m.

Chiou, Yen-bin 邱彥斌. "Hengchang yu wuchang: lun Zhutianxin 'Gudou' zhong de kongjian, shenti, yu zhengzhi jingjixue" 恆常與無常：論朱天心〈古都〉中的空間、身體與政治經濟學 [Mutability and immutability: Space, body, and political economy in Chu Tien-Hsin's "Ancient Capital"]. *Zhongwai wenxue* 中外文學 35, no. 4 (2006): 57–94.

Chivers, Sally. *The Silvering Screen: Old Age and Disability in Cinema*. Toronto: University of Toronto Press, 2011.

Cho, Chun-hyŏng. "Kukka ka shijangŭl chibae haessŭl ttae: 1970-nyŏndae chunghuban usu yŏnghwa-oehwa suip k'wŏt'ŏ k'ŏneksyŏn kwa han'guk yŏnghwa" [When the state ruled the market: The connection between superior film selection program and foreign film import quota system and Korean cinema in the mid-to-late 1970s]. *Yŏnghwa yŏn'gu* 96 (2023): 5–53.

Cho, Yeong Hee. "Geundae Hanguk sigakgyoyuk midieoroseoui hwandeunghoe yeongu" [A study of magic lantern shows as the media of visual education in modern Korea]. PhD diss., Seoul National University, 2018.

Choe, Jae-Seong. "Ilje gyeongchalgiguui wisaeng seonjeon" [Propaganda of sanitation by Japanese police organizations]. *Hanilminjongmunjeyeongu* 40 (2021): 5–53.

Ch'oe, U-yŏng. "1970-nyŏndae chubu tam'ron ŭi hwaksan kwa kŭ yŏnghyang: Chubu tŭlŭi chilbyŏng kwa 'talson' ŭl chungsim ŭro" [The spread of housewife discourse in the 1970s and its impact: Focusing on housewives' illnesses and "deviation"]. Master's Thesis. Kookmin University, 2021.

Chŏng, Yŏng-hong. *Chayŏn ŭi haebang kwa minjung ŭi soyo han'guk ŭi hwan'gyŏng munje e taehan kwan'gyeronjŏk chŏpkŭn* [The liberation of nature and the wandering of *minjung*]. P'aju: Hanul ak'ademi, 2008.

Cole, Thomas R., Nathan S. Carlin, and Roald A. Carson. *Medical Humanities: An Introduction*. Cambridge: Cambridge University Press, 2015.

Chōsensōtokufu 朝鮮總督府, ed. *Chōsensōtokufu oyobi shozokukansho shokuinroku* 朝鮮總督府所屬官署職員錄 [Red book of the government-general of Korea]. Keijō: Chōsensōtokufu, 1941.

Chōsensōtokufu 朝鮮總督府, ed. *Taishō hachinen korerabyō bōekishi* 大正八年コレラ病防疫誌 [Record of cholera control in Taisho 8th year]. Seoul: Chōsensōtokufu, 1920.

Chōsensōtokufu 朝鮮總督府, ed. *Taishō kyūnen korerabyō bōekishi* 大正九年コレラ病防疫誌 [Record of cholera control in Taisho 9th year]. Seoul: Chōsensōtokufu, 1921.

Chujo, Kazuo 中条一雄. *Genbaku otome* 原爆乙女 [Atomic maidens]. Tokyo: Asahi Shinbunsha, 1984.

Chung, Yuehtsen Juliette. "Sovereignty and Imperial Hygiene: Japan and the 1919 Cholera Epidemic in East Asia." In *The Decade of the Great War: Japan and the Wider World in the 1910s*, edited by Tosh Minohara, Tze-ki Hon, and Evan Dawley, 439–60. Leiden: Brill, 2014.

Cousins, Norman. "The Maidens Are Coming." *The Saturday Review*, April 9, 1955. www.unz.org/Pub/SaturdayRev-1955apr09-00024.

Cunningham, Stuart, David Craig, and Junyi Lv. "China's Livestreaming Industry: Platforms, Politics, and Precarity." *International Journal of Cultural Studies* 22, no. 6 (2019): 719–36.

Cvetkovich, Ann. *Depression: A Public Feeling*. Durham, NC: Duke University Press, 2012.

Dai, Wangyun. "How Li Ziqi Repackages Rural China for Urban Fantasies." *Sixth Tone*, December 27, 2019. https://www.sixthtone.com/news/1005007/how-li-ziqi-repackages-rural-china-for urban-fantasies.

Dan, Shao. "Red Star over Medicine: Redefining Doctor-Patient Relationship in Early CPC History (1930s–1960s)." *East Asian Science, Technology and Society: An International Journal* 14 (2022): 1–31.

Dauncey, Sarah. "Screening Disability in the PRC: The Politics of Looking Good." *China Information* 21, no. 3 (2007): 481–506.

Dauncey, Sarah. *Disability in Contemporary China: Citizenship, Identity and Culture*. Cambridge: Cambridge University Press, 2020.

Davis, Darrell William, and Emilie Yueh-yu Yeh. *Taiwan Film Directors: A Treasure Island*. New York: Columbia University Press, 2005.

Deleuze, Gilles. *Cinema 1: The Movement-Image*. Translated by Hugh Tomlinson. London: The Athlone Press, 2002 [1983].

Deleuze, Gilles. *Cinema 2: The Time-Image*. Translated by Hugh Tomlinson. London: The Athlone Press, 2005 [1985].

Deng, Xinmin 鄧新民. "Zimeiti: xinmeiti fazhan de zuixin jieduan ji tedian" 自媒體：新媒體發展的最新階段及其特點 [Self-media: The evolution and special aspects of new media development]. *Tansuo* 探索, no. 2 (2006): 134–38.

Deng, Yuancheng 鄧元誠, et al. "Longya zheng" 聾啞症 [Deaf-mutism]. *Zhongji yikan* 中級醫刊, no. 9 (1956): 28–31.

DeTora, Lisa M., and Stephanie M. Hilger. "Foreword." In *Bodies in Transition in The Health Humanities: Representation of Corporeality*, edited by Lisa M. DeTora and Stephanie M. Hilger, xiv–xxii. London: Routledge, 2020.

DeTora, Lisa M., and Stephanie M. Hilger. "Introduction: Bodies and Transitions in the Health Humanities." In *Bodies in Transition in The Health Humanities: Representation of Corporeality*, edited by Lisa M. DeTora and Stephanie M. Hilger, 1–8. London: Routledge, 2020.

Dikötter, Frank. *Mao's Great Famine: The History of China's Most Devastating Catastrophe, 1958–1962*. London: Bloomsbury, 2010.

Donga Entertainment. "Kŭngnyŏnghwa '*Yŏngnyŏ*' chejak shin'go chajin ch'wiha" [Voluntary withdrawal of production declaration for feature fiction film *Zero Woman*]. November 2, 1977. Reference number RK03318004. Held at Korean Film Archive, Seoul, South Korea.

Donga Entertainment. "Yŏnghwa chejak shin'gosŏ" [Declaration of film production form]. May 30, 1978. Reference number RK03318006. Held at Korean Film Archive, Seoul, South Korea.

Dower, John. *War Without Mercy: Race and Power in the Pacific War*. New York: Pantheon Books, 1986.

Dubal, Samuel. "Humanity." In *Keywords for Health Humanities*, edited by Sari Alschuler, Jonathan M. Metzl, and Priscilla Wald, 113–16. New York: New York University Press, 2023.

Duffy, Brooke Erin, Annika Pinch, Shruti Sannon, and Megan Sawey. "The Nested Precarities of Creative Labor on Social Media." *Social Media + Society* 7, no. 2 (2021): 1–12.

Edelmann, Robert J. *The Psychology of Embarrassment*. New York: John Wiley & Sons, 1987.

Edmond, Rod. *Leprosy and Empire: A Medical and Cultural History*. Cambridge: Cambridge University Press, 2006.

"Eiga hihyō—*Kojima no Haru* kansō tokushū" 映画批評小島の春感想特集 [Film criticism: Special issue of reflections on *Spring on the Small Island*]. *Aisei* 愛生 11, no. 3 (1941): 7–17.

"Eiga *Kojima no Haru*" 映画小島の春. *Chiryō Kusurihō* 治療薬報 [Medicine and treatment newsletter] 485. September 1940.

Eisenstein, Sergei. *Eisenstein on Disney*. Edited by Jay Leyda. Translated by Alan Upchurch. Calcutta: Seagull Books, 1986.

Egan, Michael, and Robert Gottlieb. *Barry Commoner and the Science of Survival: The Remaking of American Environmentalism*. Cambridge, MA: The MIT Press, 2007.

Ehrlich, Paul. *The Population Bomb*. New York: Ballantine Books, 1968.

Family Planning Research Institute. "Chemyŏng '*Manwŏn*' yŏnghwa chejak e taehan t'ongbo" [Notification regarding the production of film titled *Crowded*]. June 8, 1977. Reference number RK03154004. Held at Korean Film Archive, Seoul, South Korea.

Fang, Xiaoping. *Barefoot Doctors and Western Medicine in China*. Rochester, NY: University of Rochester Press, 2012.

Fang, Xiaoping. "Changing Narratives and Persisting Tensions: Conflicts between Chinese and Western Medicine and Professional Profiles in Chinese Films and Literature, 1949–2009." *Medical History* 63, no. 4 (2019): 454–74.

Feuer, Jane. "The Concept of Live Television: Ontology as Ideology." In *Regarding Television: Critical Approaches*, edited by E. Ann Kaplan, 12–21. Lanham, MD: University Publications of America, 1983.

Forster, Hailey. "Hiroshima Victim Was Won by U.S." *New York Times*, November 7, 1956. https://www.nytimes.com/1956/11/07/archives/hiroshima-victim-was-won-by-us-back-in-japan-girl-tells-tearfully.html.

Foucault, Michel. *Society Must Be Defended*. New York: Picador, 2003.

Fraser, Benjamin, ed. *Cultures of Representation: Disability in World Cinema Contexts*. New York: Columbia University Press, 2016.

Fu, Lianzhang 傅連暲. "Yiwu gongzuozhe he bingren zhijian" 醫務工作者與病人之間 [Between medical workers and patients]. *Huli zazhi* 護理雜誌, no. 5 (1959): 137–39.

Fujii, Jinshi 藤井仁子. "'Joshi domo' no hanran—*Kojima no Haru* ni okeru sōryokusenka no shintai to sei" 「女子ども」の反乱ー『小島の春』における総力戦下の身体と性 ["Women and children" revolt: The body and sex under total war in *Spring on the Small Island*]. In *Eiga to shintai/sei* 映画と身体/性 [Film and the body/sex], edited by Saitō Ayako, 171–95. Tokyo: Shinwa-sha, 2006.

Fujii, Junji 藤井仁子. "*Kashi to fukashi no poritikusu—eiga Kojima no Haru to sōryoku taisei-ka ni okeru kattai no hyōshō (4) Metsubo no yūtopia*" 「可視と不可視のポリティクスー映画『小島の春』と総力戦体制下における〈癩〉の表象(4)」[Visible and invisible politics: representations of "leprosy" in the film *Kojima no Haru* and total mobilization (4) the destruction of utopia]. *UP* 364 (2003): 25–29.

Fujino, Yutaka 藤野豊. "'Inochi' no gendai shi" いのち"の現代史 [A modern history of "life"]. Tokyo: Shoshi arusu, 2011.

Furth, Charlotte. "Introduction: Hygienic Modernity in Chinese East Asia." In *Health and Hygiene in Chinese East Asia: Policies and Publics in the Long Twentieth Century*, edited by Angela Ki Che Leung and Charlotte Furth, 1–22. Durham, NC: Duke University Press, 2010.

Gallagher, Rob. "Eliciting Euphoria Online: The Aesthetics of 'ASMR' Video Culture." *Film Criticism* 40, no. 2 (2016). https://quod.lib.umich.edu/f/fc/13761232.0040.202/--eliciting-euphoria-online-the-aesthetics-of-asmr-video?rgn=main;view=fulltext.

Garner, D. L., and G. E. Sidel Jr. "History of Commercializing Sexed Semen for Cattle." *Theriogenology* 69, no. 7 (2008): 886–95.

Gilman, Sander L. *Illness and Image: Case Studies in the Medical Humanities*. London: Routledge, 2015.

Glasser, Brian. *Medicinema: Doctors in Films*. Oxon: Radcliffe, 2010.

"Gongchanzhuyi jingshen zhansheng sishen" 共產主義精神戰勝死神 [Communist spirit conquered the demon of death]. *Renmin ribao* 人民日報, June 29, 1958.

Goyal, Rishi, and Arden Hegele. "Introduction." In *Culture and Medicine: Critical Readings in the Health and Medical Humanities*, edited by Rishi Goyal and Arden Hegele, 1–19. London: Bloomsbury Academic, 2023.

Graham, Amanda J. "Re-Covering the Hiroshima Maidens." In *Medicine, Healing and Performance*, edited by Effie Gemi-Iordanou et al., 120–35. Oxford, PA: Oxbow Books, 2014.

Gross, Miriam. "Between Party, People, and Profession: The Many Faces of the 'Doctor' during the Cultural Revolution." *Medical History* 62, no. 3 (2018): 333–59.

Gross, Miriam. *Farewell to the God of Plague: Chairman Mao's Campaign to Deworm China*. Oakland, CA: University of California Press, 2016.

"Guangci yiyuan qiangjiu Qiu Caikang bingshi dang'an xuanzai" 廣慈醫院搶救邱財康病史檔案選載 [Selected archives of rescuing Qiu Caikang in Guangci Hospital]. *Dang'an zhencang* 檔案珍藏, no. 4 (1998): 52–58.

Gunning, Tom. *The Films of Fritz Lang: Allegories of Vision and Modernity*. London: BFI, 2001.

Hacking, Ian. "Making Up People." In *Reconstructing Individualism: Autonomy, Individuality, and the Self in Western Thought*, edited by Thomas Heller et al., 222–36. Stanford, CA: Stanford University Press, 1986.

"Hakjayeongusilsullye (1), baengman mundung gujecha segyunyeongu jungui ouihakbaksa" [Visit to researcher's office (1), Dr. Oh working on bacterial studies to save a million lepers]. *Samcheolli*, July 1930.

Han, Sang Eon. "1920nyeondae choban Joseonui yeonghwasaneopgwa Joseonyeonghwaui tansaeng" [The birth of film and its industry in Joseon during the early 1920s]. *Yeonghwa yeongu*, no. 55 (2013): 649–89.

Han, Sangeon. "1892–1925: Yeonghwa yuipgwa yeonghwasaneobui hyeongseong" [1892–1925: introduction of film and its industry]. In *Hangukgeundaeyeonghwasa: 1892nyeoneseo 1945nyeonkkaji* [History of modern Korean film: 1892–1945], edited by Yi Hyoin, Chung Chonghwa, and Han Sangeon, 15–99. Paju: Dolbaegae, 2019.

Han, Xiaofei. "Platform as New 'Daddy': China's Gendered Wanghong Economy and Patriarchal Platforms Behind." *Internet Policy Review* 11, no. 1 (2022). https://doi.org/10.14763/2022.1.1631.

Han'guk konghae munje yŏn'guso. *Han'guk ŭi konghae chido* [Pollution map of Korea]. Seoul: Irwŏlsŏgak, 1985.

"Hangungnabyeongyeonguwon jungongsik" [Dedication ceremony of Korean leprosy hospital]. *Donga ilbo*, September 25, 1976.

Hardt, Michael, and Antonio Negri, *Commonwealth*. Cambridge, MA: Harvard University Press, 2009.

Hardt, Michael, and Antonio Negri. *Multitude: War and Democracy in the Age of Empire*. New York: The Penguin Press, 2004.

Harper, Graeme, and Andrew Moor, eds. *Signs of life: Cinema and Medicine*. New York: Wallflower Press, 2005.

Harvey, David. *A Brief History of Neoliberalism*. Oxford: Oxford University Press, 2005.

Hayashi, Yukiko 林由貴子. "Tanka." In *Hagi no shimazato* 萩の島里 [Island home of the bush clover], edited by Uchida Morito 内田守人, 61–78. Tokyo: Fujokai-sha, 1939.

Hayashi, Yukiko 林由貴子. "Zakuro no nageki" 柘榴の嘆き [The sorrow of the pomegranate]. In *Seto no Akebono* 瀬戸の曙 [Daybreak over the inland sea], edited by Uchida Morito 内田守人, 139–73. Tokyo: Fujokai-sha, 1939.

Heise, Ursula K. "Plasmatic Nature: Environmentalism and Animated Film." *Public Culture* 26, no. 2 (2014): 301–18.

Henry, Todd A. *Assimilating Seoul: Japanese Rule and the Politics of Public Space in Colonial Korea, 1910–1945*. Oakland, CA: University of California Press, 2016.

High, Peter B. *The Imperial Screen: Japanese Film Culture in the Fifteen Years' War, 1931–1945*. Madison, WI: The University of Wisconson Press, 1995.

Hirano, Kyoko. "A Case Study of Japanese Film Exhibition in North America: The Japan Society, New York." In *Routledge Handbook of Japanese Cinema*, edited by Joanne Bernardi and Shota T. Ogawa, 314–30. London: Routledge, 2019.

Hirokawa, Waka 廣川和歌. *Kindai Nihon no Hansen-byō mondai to chiiki shakai* 近代日本のハンセン病問題と地域社会 [Modern Japan's Hansen's disease problem and local communities]. Osaka: Osaka daigaku shuppankai, 2011.

Hirokawa, Waka. "A Colony or a Sanatorium? A Comparative History of Segregation Politics of Hansen's Disease in Modern Japan." In *Science, Technology, and Medicine in the Modern Japanese Empire*, edited by David G. Wittner and Philip C. Brown, 117–29. London: Routledge, 2016.

"Hiroshima Maidens Coming to Capital," *Washington Post*, April 9, 1956. Archived in RG2/NY/M633 2.19, Montclair Monthly Meeting, Friends Historical Library, Swarthmore College.

Hoff, Benjamin. *The Tao of Pooh*. New York: Dutton Books, 1982.

Holdsworth, Amy, Karen Lury, and Hannah Tweed. Introduction to *Discourses of Care: Media Practices and Cultures*, edited by Amy Holdsworth, Karen Lury, and Hannah Tweed, 1–20. London: Bloomsbury Academic, 2020.

"Honkai shusai katsudoshashinkai" 本會主催活動寫眞會 [Film screening hosted by police bureau). *Keimu iho* 警務彙報, October 1922.

Horn, Joshua. *Away with All Pests: An English Surgeon in People's China, 1954–1969*. New York: Monthly Review Press, 1969.

Horn, Joshua. "The Mass Line." In *Health Care in China*, 1–14. London: Anglo-Chinese Educational Institute, 1976.

Houseworth, Lenora. "The Radical History of Self-Care." *Teen Vogue*. January 14, 2021. https://www.teenvogue.com/story/the-radical-history-of-self-care.

Hu, Jun 胡俊, and Zhen Cheng 甄橙. "Dayuejin qijian qiangjiu gangtie gongren Qiu Caikang: Zhang Disheng fangtan" 大躍進期間搶救鋼鐵工人邱財康：張滌生訪談 [Rescuing Qiu Caikang in the Great Leap Forward: Interviewing Zhang Disheng]. *Zhongguo kejishi zazhi* 中國科技史雜誌 32, no. 2 (2011): 222–30.

Hung, Chang-tai. "Reeducating a Blind Storyteller: Han Qixiang and the Chinese Communist Storytelling Campaign." *Modern China* 19, no. 4 (1993): 395–426.

Hwang, Kyung Moon. *Rationalizing Korea: The Rise of the Modern State, 1894–1945*. Oakland, CA: University of California Press, 2015.

Illich, Ivan. *Limits to Medicine: Medical Nemesis*. London: Marion Boyars Publishers, 2010.

Illich, Ivan. *Tools for Conviviality*. New York: Harper & Row, 1973.

Im, Chi-yŏn. "1960–70-nyŏndae Han'guk chŏngsin ŭihak tam'ron yŏngu: Chŏngsin wisaeng-hak eso hyŏndae chŏngsin ŭihak ŭro" [A study of the discussions on psychiatry of Korea in the 1960s and 1970s: From mental hygiene to modern psychiatry]. *Ŭisahak* 26, no. 2 (2017): 181–214.

Ishii, Hitonari 石居人也. "Hansen-byō byōzō to shite no eiga "Kojima no Haru"—1940 nen ni okeru kakuri no egakarekata to sono mirareru kata ハンセン表象としての映画「小島の春」1940年における隔離の描かれ方とその観られ方 [The film *Kojima no Haru* and the representation of Hansen: How isolation is depicted and viewed in 1940]. In *Kindai Nihon no "tasha" to mukiau* 近代日本の「他者」と向き合う [Facing The other in modern Japan], edited by Kurokawa Midori 黒川みどり, 148–73. Tokyo: Kaihō shuppan sha, 2010.

Izawa, Jun 井沢淳. "Yagi Yasutarō ron" 八木保太郎論 [Theories of Yagi Yasutarō]. *Shinario* シナリオ 14, no. 3 (1958): 26–28.

Jameson, Fredric. *Postmodernism, or, The Cultural Logic of Late Capitalism*. Durham, NC: Duke University Press, 1990.

Jannetta, Ann. *The Vaccinators: Smallpox, Medical Knowledge, and the Opening of Japan*. Stanford, CA: Stanford University Press, 2012.

Jefferys, W. Hamilton, and James Maxwell. *The Diseases of China, Including Formosa and Korea*. London: Bale & Danielsson, 1910.

"Jeong-jaegyeui sillyeokja . . . 'burussiseojulsu itgireul'" [Strong men of political and financial sectors . . . "Hoping to get rid of misfortune"]. *Chosun ilbo*, September 25, 1976.

"Jinri toutiao jindaohui jihua: 5 yi butie sannong chuangzuozhe" 今日頭條金稻穗計畫：5億補貼三農創作者 [Today's headline—golden rice grain plan: 5 billion to fund three-agricultures creators]. *ebrun*, July 8, 2018. http://www.ebrun.com/20180703/284595.shtml.

Johnson, Ben Brock, and Amory Sivertson. "Li Ziqi, China's Quarantine Queen." *Endless Thread*. Podcast audio. February 11, 2022. https://www.wbur.org/endlessthread/2022/02/11/li-ziqi-chinas-quarantine-queen.

Jones, Therese, Delese Wear, and Lester D. Friedman. "Introduction: The Why, the What, and the How of the Medical/Health Humanities." In *Health Humanities Reader*, edited by Therese Jones, Delese Wear, and Lester D. Friedman, 1–9. New Brunswick, NJ: Rutgers University Press, 2014.

Jŏng, Sae-kwŏn. "Shihŏmgwan agi esŏ ch'eoe sujŏng ŭro? 1970–80-nyŏndae saeroun kwahak kisul e taehan ŏllon podo pyŏnhwa" [From "test-tube baby" to "in vitro fertilization"? The changes of media report on new science and technology in the 1970–1980 Korea]. *Yŏksa pip'yŏng* 136 (2021): 462–96.

Jung, Keun-Sik. "Ilje malgiui Sorokdogaengsaengwongwa Ichunsang sageon" [Sorok island sanatorium in the late colonial period and Yi Choon-Sang accident]. *Yeoksabipyeong*, no. 72 (2005): 330–59.

Jung, Keunsik. "Singminji wisaenggyeongcharui hyeongseonggwa byeonhwa, geurigo yusan: singminji tongchiseongui sigageseo" [Formation, change, and legacy of the colonial sanitary police in modern Korea). *Sahoewa yeoksa* 90 (2011): 221–70.

Kaji, Hajime 一梶. "Suō Masasue enchō wo kataru" 周防正季園長を語る [Talking on director Suwa Masasue]. *Bunka chōsen* 文化朝鮮, May 1942.

Kang, Tae-Woong. "Jeonjeon ilbonui Hansenbyeong hwanja gyeongnijeongchaekgwa gukchaegyeonghwa jageun seomui bom" [Leprosy isolation policy and a propaganda film named *Spring on the Small Island* in prewar Japan]. *Ilbonyeoksayeongu* 54 (2021): 181–210.

Keiichi, Tsuneishi. "Unit 731 and the Japanese Imperial Army's Biological Warfare Program." In *Japan's Wartime Medical Atrocities: Comparative Inquiries in Science, History, and Ethics*, edited by Jing-Bao Nie, Nanyan Guo, Mark Selden, and Arthur Kleinman, 23–31. London: Routledge, 2010.

Keimukyoku eiseika. "Kyakuhon *Nama no hokori* (ge)" 脚本生之誇り（下）[*The Pride of Life* script [second]]. *Keimu iho* 警務彙報, July 1922.

Keimukyoku eiseika. "Kyakuhon *Nama no hokori* (jō)" 脚本生之誇り（上）[*The Pride of Life* script [first]]. *Keimu iho* 警務彙報, June 1922.

Kim, Crystal. "Slow Living with Korea's Silent Vloggers." *Elle*, May 21, 2021. https://www.elle.com/culture/a36451963/korea-silent-vloggers/.

Kim, Dong Hoon. *Eclipsed Cinema: The Film Culture of Colonial Korea*. Edinburgh: Edinburgh University Press, 2017.

Kim, Eunjung. *Curative Violence: Rehabilitating Disability, Gender, and Sexuality in Modern Korea*. Durham, NC: Duke University Press, 2017.

Kim, Gyewon. "Faces that Change: Physiognomy, Portraiture, and Photography in Colonial Korea." In *The Affect of Difference: Representations of Race in East Asian Empire*, edited by Christopher P. Hanscom and Dennis C. Washburn, 133–58. Honolulu, HI: University of Hawai'i Press, 2016.

Kim, Hoi-eun. *Doctors of Empire: Medical and Cultural Encounters in Between Imperial Germany and Meiji Japan*. Toronto: University of Toronto Press, 2014.

Kim, Hye-kyŏng. "Park Chung-hee ch'eje ha 'haekkajok' tamron ŭi byŏnhwa kwajŏng kwai wŏn kujo yŏngu: 'Chosŏn ilbo' rŭl chungsim ŭro" [The "nuclear" family discourse during the Park Chung Hee regime period: The discursive change and its dualism]. *Sahak wa yŏksa* 82 (2009): 169–212.

Kim Jae-Hyung. "Singminjigi Hansenbyeong Hwanjareul Dulleossan Jugeumgwa Saengjon" [A modern history of 'Imperial Medicine' surrounding Hansen's disease]. *Uisahak* 28, no. 2 (2019): 469–508.

Kim, Keum Dong. "Dogil wisaengyeonghwaeui suyongwa suneunghaneun shikminji juche hyeongseong" [Japan's acceptance of German's sanitary enlightenment film and the establishment of dutiful colonial subject]. *Yeonghwa Yeongu*, no. 51 (2012): 7–37.

Kim, Keum Dong. "Dogil wisaengyeonghwareul tonghae bon Joseon kollerawisaengyeonghwa(1920)wa cheonyeonduwisaengyeonghwa(1922)ui teukjinggwa hangye" [Characteristic and limitation of Joseon's cholera and smallpox sanitary film from the viewpoint of the Weimar republic]. *Yeonghwa Yeongu*, no. 55 (2013): 35–82.

Kim, Ryeo-Sil. *Tusahaneun jeguk tuyeonghaneun Singminji: 1901–1945nyeonui Hanguk yeonghwasarul doejibda* [Projecting empire and reflecting colony: Tracing the history of Korean film in 1901–1945]. Seoul: Samin, 2006.

Kim, Sang-hyun. "Science, Technology, and the Imaginaries of Development in South Korea." *Development and Society* 46, no. 2 (2017): 317–47.

Kim, Sangyong. "Nabyeongui yeongu geup chiryobeop" [A study on leprosy and its treatment]. *Gaebyeok*, June 1923.

Kim, Sonja M. *Imperatives of Care: Women and Medicine in Colonial Korea*. Honolulu, HI: University of Hawai'i Press, 2019.

Kim, Sun-yang. *Health Politics in Korea: The Political Dynamics of Healthcare Reform*. Seoul: Seoul National University Press, 2016.

Kim, Taek-joong. "1918nyeon dokgamgwa Joseonchongdokbu bangyeokjeongchaek" [The 1918 influenza pandemic and Japanese government-general of Korea's preventive measures against epidemics] *Inmun Nonchong* 74, no. 1 (2017): 163–214.

Kingston, Jeff. "Compensating Colonial Lepers, Slave Laborers and Hibakusha: Troubling Legacies and Evolving Standards of Postcolonial Justice in Japan." *The Asia-Pacific Journal: Japan Focus* 3, no. 11 (2005). https://apjjf.org/-Jeff-Kingston/1579/article.html.

Klein, Christina. *Cold War Orientalism: Asia in the Middlebrow Imagination, 1945–1961*. Berkeley, CA: University of California Press, 2003.

Kleinman, Arthur. *Patients and Healers in the Context of Culture: An Exploration of the Borderland between Anthropology, Medicine, and Psychiatry*. Berkeley, CA: University of California Press, 1980.

Klugman, Craig, and Erin Gentry Lamb, eds. *Research Methods in Health Humanities*. Oxford: Oxford University Press, 2019.

Ko, T'ae-u. "1970-nyŏndae Han'guk ŭi konghae sanghwang kwa chaenan insik" [Pollution problems and disaster awareness in 1970s South Korea]. *Kaenyŏm kwa sot'ong* 28 (2021): 7–52.

Koepnick, Lutz. *On Slowness: Toward an Aesthetic of the Contemporary*. New York: Columbia University Press, 2014.

Korean Performing Arts Ethics Committee. "Kŭngnyŏnghwa shinario shimŭi kyŏlgwa pogo" [Report on results of review of script for feature fiction film]. September 13, 1977. Reference number RK03318001. Held at Korean Film Archive, Seoul, South Korea.

"Kōtaigōhēka gokinei gokashi kaku kokuryū rairyōyōjohe" 皇太后御近影御下賜各國立癩療養所 へ [Empress dowager bestowing her portrait photographs to each national leprosy sanatorium]. *Chōsen shinbun* 朝鮮新聞, July 17, 1941.

Kovner, Sarah. "Allied POWs in Korea: Life and Death during the Pacific War." In *The Dismantling of Japan's Empire in East Asia: Deimperialization, Postwar Legitimation and Imperial Afterlife*, edited by Barak Kushner and Sherzod Muminov, 107–24. London: Routledge, 2018.

Kristeva, Julia, Marie Rose Moro, John Ødemark, and Eivind Engebretsen. "Cultural Crossings of Care: An Appeal to the Medical Humanities." *Medical Humanities* 44, no. 1 (2018): 55–58.

Lampton, David. "Development and Health Care: Is China's Medical Program Exportable?" *World Development* 6 (1978): 621–30.

Lampton, David M. *The Politics of Medicine in China: The Policy Process, 1949–1977*. London: Routledge, 1977.

Lee, Sun-jin. "Taean yŏnghwa eso sŏnjŏn yŏnghwa kkaji: Han'guk munhwa yŏnghwa ŭi yŏksa wa chaengjŏm" [From alternative films to propaganda films: The history and contested points of Korean culture films]. In *Chiwŏjin Han'guk yŏnghwasa: Munhwa yŏnghwa ŭi an kwa pakk* [The erased history of Korean film: Culture films inside and out], edited by Lee Byŏng-hun, 9–42. Seoul: Han'guk yŏngsang charyowŏn, 2014.

Lee, Taewoo. "Joseonyeonghwaui baljeon" [Development of film in Joseon]. *Kyunghyang Sinmun*, January 6, 1949.

Lee-Morrison, Lila. *Portraits of Automated Facial Recognition: On Machinic Ways of Seeing the Face*. Bielefeld: Transcript Verlag, 2019.

Lehmann, Emily. "Serenity Now: The Immersive World of Silent Vlogs." *Verily Magazine*, May 27, 2022. https://verilymag.com/2022/05/serenity-now-the-immersive-world-of-silent-youtube-video-vlogs-2022.

Lei, Hsiang-lin 雷祥麟. "Fuzeren de yisheng yu you xinyang de bingren: Zhongxiyi lunzheng yu yibing guanxi zai minguo shiqi de zhuanbian" 負責任的醫生與有信仰的病人：中西醫論爭與醫病關係在民國時期的轉變 [Responsible doctors and believing patients: Debates between Chinese and Western medicines and the transformation of the doctor-patient relationship in the Republican era]. *Xinshixue* 新史學 14, no. 1 (2003): 45–96.

Lei, Sean Hsiang-Lin. "Sovereignty and the Microscope: Constituting Notifiable Infectious Disease and Containing the Manchurian Plague (1910–11)." In *Health and Hygiene in Chinese East Asia: Policies and Publics in the Long Twentieth Century*, edited by Angela Ki-Che Leung and Charlotte Furth, 73–108. Durham, NC: Duke University Press, 2010.

Lei, Sean Hsiang-lin. *Neither Donkey nor Horse: Medicine in the Struggle Over China's Modernity*. Chicago: University of Chicago Press, 2014.

Lei, Silin 雷斯林. "Li Ziqi zenme jiu bushi wenhua shuchu le" 李子柒怎麼就不是文化輸出了 [Why isn't Li Ziqi a cultural export?]. *WeChat Blog*, December 5, 2019. https://mp.weixin.qq.com/s/NWEEIW2ntGbjUpKUJmHf3Q.

Lenig, Stuart. *The Bizarre World of Reality Television*. Santa Barbara, CA: ABC-Clio, 2017.

Leroi-Gourhan, André. *Gesture and Speech*. Translated by Anna Bostock Berger. Cambridge, MA: The MIT Press, 2018 [1964].

Lewis, Diane Wei. *Powers of the Real: Cinema, Gender, and Emotion in Interwar Japan*. Cambridge, MA: Harvard University Asia Center, 2019.

Leyda, Jay. *Films Begets Films: Compilation Films from Propaganda to Drama*. New York: Hill & Wang, 1964.

Li, Han. "From Disenchantment to Re-enchantment: Rural Microcelebrities, Short Video, and the Spectacle-ization of the Rural Lifescape on Chinese Social Media." *International Journal of Communication* 14 (2020): 3769–87.

Li, Jill. "As China's Vloggers Draw International Fans, Beijing Sees Soft Power Opportunity." *VOA*, August 12, 2020. https://www.voanews.com/a/east-asia-pacific_voa-news-china_chinas-vloggers-draw-international-fans-beijing-sees-soft-power/6194341.html.

Li, Victor H. "Politics and Health Care in China: The Barefoot Doctors." *Stanford Law Review* 27, no. 3 (1975): 827–40.

Li, Xiangjuan 李向娟. "'Wanghong cun' de zhifujing" '網紅村'的致富經 [A *wanghong* village's means of getting rich]. *Fujian Daily* 福建日報, May 20, 2020. http://fjrb.fjsen.com/fjrb/html/2020-05/20/content_1259041.htm?div=-1.

Liang, Limin. "Consuming the Pastoral Desire: Li Ziqi, Food Vlogging and the Structure of Feeling in the Era of Microcelebrity." *Global Storytelling: Journal of Digital and Moving Images* 1, no. 2 (2022): 7–39.

Liboiron, Max. *Pollution Is Colonialism*. Durham, NC: Duke University Press, 2021.

Lin, Mu-xing, Tsung-yi Lee, and Kuei-tien Chou. "The Environmental Policy Stringency in Taiwan and Its Challenges on Green Economy Transition." *Development and Society* 47, no. 3 (2018): 477–502.

Liu, Ruihua, Liu Qian, Li Lin, Deng Yuancheng, and Tan Huizhen. "A Statistical Study of 560 Cases of the Deaf in Peking." *Chinese Medical Journal* 75, no. 9 (1957): 753–63.

Liu, Sizhi 劉思職. "Shengming de qiyuan wenti" 生命的起源問題 [On the origin of life]. *Ziran bianzhengfa tongxun* 自然辯證法通訊, no. 1 (1956): 60–61.

"Liziqi yu Kongzixueyuan: wuyi jiangshu de 'zhongguo gushi' yu lingren yanwu de 'wenhua shuchu'" 李子柒與孔子學院：無意講述的'中國故事'與令人厭惡的'文化輸出' [Li Ziqi and the Confucius Institute: An unintentionally articulated "China's story" and the "cultural outreach" that disgusts people]. *BBC News*, January 21, 2020. https://www.bbc.com/zhongwen/trad/chinese-news-51191109?fbclid=IwAR1C1zLciB9RwlNGbAjZJLBDQX_rCB4fC6mEW9M6E0vpmtjvPZiWWEH6TJc.

Lo, Vivienne, Chris Berry, and Guo Liping, eds. *Film and the Chinese Medical Humanities*. London: Routledge, 2020.

Lu, Zhicong, Michelle Annett, and Daniel Wigdor. "Vicariously Experiencing it all without Going Outside: A Study of Outdoor Livestreaming in China." *Proceedings of the ACM on Human-Computer Interaction* 3, no. CSCW (2019), Article 25, 1–28.

Lucas, AnElissa. "Changing Medical Models in China: Organizational Options or Obstacles?" *The China Quarterly* 83 (1980): 461–89.

Lupke, Christopher. "Nativism and Localism in Taiwanese Literature." In *The Columbia Companion to Modern Chinese Literature*, edited by Kirk A. Denton, 258–66. New York: Columbia University Press, 2016.

Lynteris, Christos. "Photography, Zoonosis and Epistemic Suspension After the End of Epidemics." In *The Anthropology of Epidemics*, edited by Ann H. Kelly, Frédéric Keck, and Christos Lynteris, 84–101. London: Routledge, 2019.

Lynteris, Christos. *The Spirit of Selflessness in Maoist China: Socialist Medicine and the New Man*. London: Palgrave Macmillan, 2012.

Ma, Wen-yee. *Snow Glistens on the Great Wall: A New Translation of the Complete Collection of Mao Tse-tung's Poetry*. Santa Barbara, CA: Santa Barbara Press, 1986.

Ma, Xinde 馬信德 and Gu, Meizhong 顧美忠. *Dang jiuhuo le ta* 黨救活了他 [The Party saved his life]. Beijing: Zhongguo shaonian ertong chubanshe, 1958.

Mao, Tse-tung. "On Contradiction." In *Selected Works of Mao Tse-tung* 1, 311–47. Beijing: Foreign Languages Press, 1965.

Mao, Tse-tung. "On the Correct Handling of Contradictions among the People." In *Selected Works of Mao Tse-tung* 5, 384–421. Beijing: Foreign Languages Press, 1965.

Mao, Tse-tung. "Rectify the Party's Style of Work." In *Selected Works of Mao Tse-tung* 3, 35–51. Beijing: Foreign Languages Press, 1965.

Mao, Tse-tung. "Talks at the Yenan Forum on Literature and Art." In *Selected Works of Mao Tse-tung* 3, 69–98. Beijing: Foreign Languages Press, 1965.

Mao, Tse-tung. "The Foolish Old Man Who Removes the Mountains." In *Selected Works of Mao Tse-tung* 3, 312–24. Beijing: Foreign Languages Press, 1965.

Mao, Tse-tung. "The United Front in Cultural Work." In *Selected Works of Mao Tse-tung* 3, 235–37. Beijing: Foreign Languages Press, 1965.

"Mao Zedong sixiang shi zhenjiu liaofa huode xinde shengming: Shenyang budui kaizhan xin zhenjiu liaofa de diaocha baogao" 毛澤東思想使針灸療法獲得新的生命：瀋陽部隊開展新針灸療法的調查報告 [Mao Zedong thought gives new life to acupunctural therapy: survey report on the development of new acupunctural therapy by the Shenyang Army Unit]. *Remin ribao* 人民日報, September 16, 1969, 2.

"Mao Zhuxi geile wo zuida xingfu: ji longya xuesheng Zeng Jinguang canjun" 毛主席給了我最大幸福：記聾啞學生宗金廣參軍 [Chairman Mao has given me the greatest happiness: Deaf-mute student Zeng Junguang joins the army]. *Xinhua she xinwen gao* 新華社新聞稿, no. 811 (1971): 7–8.

"Mao zhuxi wuchan jieji luxian de shengli kage: Ji renmin jiefangjun 3125 budui Mao Zedong sixiang weisheng gongzuodui kaichuang zhiliao longyabing de xinluzi" 毛主席無產階級路線的勝利凱歌：記人民解放軍3125部隊毛澤東思想衛生工作隊開創治療聾啞病的新路子 [The triumph of Chairman Mao's proletarian line: The new way of treating deaf-mutism pioneered by the Maoist thought medical team of the 3125th Army]. *Remin ribao* 人民日報, December 16, 1968, 3.

Matsuoka, Hideaki 松岡秀明. "Hansen-byō to tanka: Eiga *Kojima no Haru* wo megutte" ハンセン病と短歌：映画〈小島の春〉をめぐって [Hansen's disease and tanka: A study of the film *Spring on the Small Island*]. *Communication Design* コミュニケーションデザイン 12 (2015): 39–52.

Matsuoka, Hiroyuki 松岡弘之. *Hansen-byō ryōyōjo to jichi no rekishi* ハンセン病療養所と自治の歴史 [The history of Hansen's disease sanatoria and patient autonomy]. Tokyo: Misuzu shobō, 2020.

Mbembe, Achille. "Necropolitics." Translated by Libby Meintjes. *Public Culture* 15, no. 1 (2003): 11–40.

McCurry, Justin. "South Korea Doctors' Strike: Government Moves to Suspend Thousands of Medical Licences." *The Guardian*, March 12, 2024. https://www.theguardian.com/world/2024/mar/12/south-korea-doctor-strike-government-suspends-medical-licenses.

McGettigan, Joan. "'The Whole World Shares Your Heartache': 'This Is Your Life' and 1950s Stardom." *Studies in Popular Culture* 35, no. 1 (2012): 109–20.

Meisner, Maurice. *Mao's China and After*. 3rd edition. New York: Free Press, 1999.

Meisner, Maurice. *Marxism, Maoism, and Utopianism*. Madison, WI: University of Wisconsin Press, 1982.

Meng, Qingyu 孟慶玉 and Wang Guizhen 王桂珍. "Qiannian tieshu kai le hua: zan caise jilu dianying *Kao Mao Zedong sixiang dakai longya jinqu*" 千年的鐵樹開了花：贊彩色紀

錄電影《靠毛澤東思想打開聾啞禁區》[A thousand-year iron tree blooms: in praise of color documentary *Opening the Forbidden Zone of Deaf-Mutism through Mao Zedong Thoughts*]. *Renmin ribao* 人民日報, November 12, 1971, 4.

Meoka, Makato. "What's All the Noise about Silent Vlogs?" *YouTube Official Blog*, July 26, 2021. https://blog.youtube/culture-and-trends/whats-all-the-noise-about-silent-vlogs/.

Merleau-Ponty, Maurice. *Phénoménologie de la perception*. Paris: Gallimard, 1945.

Ministry of Health and Social Affairs. "Kajok kyehoek yŏnghwa chejak hyŏpcho" [Cooperation on production of family planning film]. June 27, 1977. Refence number RK03154005. Held at Korean Film Archive, Seoul, South Korea.

Mitsuda, Kensuke 光田健輔. "*Kojima no haru* no kansō" 小島の春の可能 [Thoughts on *Spring on the Small Island*]. *Nihon iji shinpō* 日本医事新報 935 (1940): 58–59.

Miyao, Daisuke. "What's the Use of Culture? Cinematographers and the Culture Film in Japan in the Early 1940s." *Arts* 8, no. 42 (2019): 4–5.

Mizuguchi, Yasutoshi 水口安俊. *Sugamo senpan kōshukei: Aru senpan no gokuchū shuki* 巣鴨・戦犯絞首刑：ある戦犯の獄中手記 [Sugamo war criminals' death by hanging: A memoir of a convicted war criminal], edited by Fuyuko Kamisaka. Kyoto: Mineruva Shobō, 1981.

Modan, Nihonsha. *Ilbonjapji modeonilbongwa Joseon* 1940 [The Japanese modern Japan and Joseon 1940]. Translated by Hong Seunyoung, Park Mikyoung, Chae Youngnim, and Yoon Soyoung. Seoul: Eomunhaksa, 2009.

Montclair Monthly Meeting. Friends Historical Library, Swarthmore College, Swarthmore, PA.

Moran, Michelle T. *Colonizing Leprosy Imperialism and the Politics of Public Health in the United States*. Chapel Hill, NC: The University of North Carolina Press, 2012.

Morton, Diane Lorell. "Paintings as Social Rhetoric: Wei-Jin Themes in Ming dynasty Illustrations and Inscriptions." PhD diss., University of Kansas, 2001.

Mun, Man-yon. "Ijung ŭi noksaek hyŏkmyŏng Park Chung-hee sidae sikryang chŭngsan kwa sallim nok'wa" [The dual green revolution in South Korea: Reforestation and agricultural revolution under the authoritarian regime]. *Chŏnbuk sahak* 36 (2010): 155–84.

"Mundungbyeongeyakdoendago eorinaeganeulppaeeo" [Taking a child's liver to cure leprosy]. *Chosun ilbo*, July 5, 1927.

Myelnikov, Dmitriy. "An Alternative Cure: The Adoption and Survival of Bacteriophage Therapy in the USSR, 1922–1955." *Journal of the History of Medicine and Allied Sciences* 73, no. 4 (2018): 385–411.

Myelnikov, Dmitriy. "Creature Features: The Lively Narratives of Bacteriophages in Soviet Biology and Medicine." *Notes and Records* 74 (2020): 579–97.

"Nabyeonghwanjareul daepanseo songhwan" [Repatriation of lepers from Osaka]. *Maeil sinbo*, June 28, 1938.

Nam, Illan. *Democratizing Health Care: Welfare State in Korea and Thailand*. New York: Palgrave Macmillan, 2015.

[Name Redacted]. "Letter to Dr. Mitsuda." Nagashima Aisei-en Archives, May 6, 1943.

Nanda zhongwenxi yingpingzu [The film critics group of the Chinese department at Nanjing University] 南大中文系影評組. "Renlei lishi de xinchun: xikan *Chunman renjian*" 人類歷史的新春：喜看《春滿人間》[New spring in the human history: watching *Spring Reigns Everywhere*]. *Baihua* 百花, no. 11 (1960): 9–10.

Narita, Ryūichi 成田龍一. "*Kojima no Haru* no manazashi" 『小島の春』のまなざし [A look at *Kojima no Haru*]. In *Nihon kindai shisō taikei 22: sabetsu no shosō furoku "Geppō 15"* 日本近代思想体系22——差別の諸相付録月報 [Compendium of modern Japanese thought 22: Aspects of discrimination supplement monthly report 15], edited by Katō Shūichi et al., 4–7. Tokyo: Iwanami Shoten, 1990.

Narita, Ryūichi 成田龍一. *Rekishi" wa ika ni katarareruka: 1930 nendai "kokumin no monogatari hihan* 〈歴史〉はいかに語られるか1930年代「国民の物語」批判 [How can we talk about history? A critical look at the 1930s "story of citizens"]. Tokyo: Nihon hōsō shuppan kyokai, 2001.

"Night-shift Nurse Bonus Unhelpful: Survey." *Taipei Times*, October 21, 2023. https://www.taipeitimes.com/News/taiwan/archives/2023/10/21/2003808010.

Nightingale, Ed. "Twitch Streamers Campaign for Disability Pride Month." *Eurogamer*. January 19, 2022. https://www.eurogamer.net/articles/2022-01-19-twitch-streamers-campaign-for-disability-pride-month.

Nelson, Susan E. "Catching Sight of South Mountain: Tao Yuanming, Mount Lu, and the Iconographies of Escape." *Archives of Asian Art* 52 (2000/2001): 11–43.

New, Peter Kong-ming. "Barefoot Doctors and Health Care in the People's Republic and China." *Ekistics* 38, no. 226 (1974): 220–24.

New York Friends Center Records. Friends Historical Library, Swarthmore College, Swarthmore, PA.

"Nyuengan ni kan suru ken" 入園願ニ関スル件 [On a request for admittance]. Letter. Nagashima Aisei Archives, undated.

"Nyuengan ni kan suru ken" 入園願ニ関スル件 [On a request for admittance]. Letter. Nagashima Aisei Archives, September 4, 1940.

Office of the Director (Martin Steinberg) Records, 1939–1969. The Arthur H. Aufses Jr. MD Archives, Icahn School of Medicine at Mount Sinai, New York.

Ogawa, Masako 小川正子. *Kojima no Haru—Hansen-byō chiryō ni, shōgai wo sasageta aru joi no shuki* 小島の春ーハンセン病治療に生涯をささげたある女医の手記 [Spring on the small island: The notes of the woman doctor who gave her life to the treatment of Hansen's disease]. Tokyo: Nagasaki shuppan, 2009.

Ogawa, Masako 小川正子. "Tanka" 短歌 [Tanka poetry]. *Aisei Tokugo Kokumin Seishin Sōdōin* 愛生特号国民精神総動員 10, no. 4 (1940): cover.

Ogawa, Naohiro, Iqbal H. Shah, and Gayl D. Ness. "Introduction." In *Low Fertility and Reproductive Health in East Asia*, edited by Naohiro Ogawa and Iqbal H. Shah, 1–9. Dordrecht: Springer, 2015.

Oh, Chin-gon. "1970-nyŏndae Han'guk 'usu yŏnghwa' ŭi sidaejŏk t'ŭksusŏng koch'al: Yusin chŏngkwŏn sigi chedo, naeyong, sanŏp, hŭrŭm chungsim ŭro" [A study on the characteristics of the time of the Korean excellent film in the 1970s: Focused on the institution, contents, industry, and trend]. *Inmunhak yŏngu* 47 (2014): 621–50.

Oliver, Michael. *The Politics of Disablement*. London: Macmillan Education, 1990.

Ortiz-Vilarelle, Lisa. "Autoethnography and Beyond: Genealogy, Memory, Media, Witness." *Life Writing* 18, no. 4 (2021): 475–82.

Pai, Hyung Il. "Capturing Visions of Japan's Prehistoric Past: Torii Ryūzō's Field Photographs of 'Primitive' Races and Lost Civilizations (1896–1915)." In *Looking Modern: East Asian Visual Culture from Treaty Ports to World War II*, edited by Jennifer Purtle and Hans Bjarne Thomsen, 265–93. Chicago: Center for the Art of East Asia, University of Chicago; Art Media Resources, 2009.

Pang, Laikwan. *The Art of Cloning: Creative Production During China's Cultural Revolution*. London: Verso, 2017.

Pardilla, Ambar. "What Is Cottagecore? Meet The Biggest Trend During Quarantine." *Huffington Post*, September 11, 2020. https://www.huffpost.com/entry/cottagecore-trend-quarantine-diy_l_5ecd875ec5b6e3f6739dbdfc.

Park, Hyun Hee. "Tears in the Imperial Screen: Wartime Colonial Korean Cinema, 1936–1945." PhD diss., University of Chicago, 2017.

Park, Yun-Jae. "Hanmal, ilje Cho Hanseongwisaenghoeui hwaldonggwa singmin jibae" [The operation of Seoul sanitary organization and colonial rule from 1907 to 1914]. *Seoulhagyeongu* 22 (2004): 67–89.

Park, YunJae. "Sanitizing Korea: Anti-Cholera Activities of the Police in Early Colonial Korea." *Seoul Journal of Korean Studies* 23, no. 2 (2010): 151–71.

Parkins, Wendy, and Geoffrey Craig. *Slow Living*. Oxford: Berg Publishing, 2006.

Paterson, Mark. *How We Became Sensorimotor: Movement, Measurement, Sensation*. Minneapolis, MN: University of Minnesota Press, 2021.

Pendle Hill Records. Friends Historical Library, Swarthmore College, Swarthmore, PA.

Qian, Xinzhong. "Zhongxiyi qinmi hezuo renzhen de zhengli yanjiu zuguo yixue" 中西醫親密合作，認真地整理研究祖國醫學 [Chinese and Western medicine practitioners work closely together to seriously organize and study Chinese medicine]. In *Quanguo zhongyi jingluo zhenjiu xueshu zuotanhui ziliao xuanbian* 全國中醫經絡針灸學術座談會資料彙編 [Compendium of National Symposium on Chinese Meridian and Acupuncture], edited by Quanguo zhongyi jingluo zhenjiu xueshu zuotanhui mishuchu 全國中醫經絡針灸學術座談會秘書處, 3. Beijing: Renmin weisheng chubanshe, 1959.

Qin, Yi. "Yichang gonggong shijian de kuameiti chuangzuo: dui xianlipian *Chunman renjian* de kaocha" 一場公共事件的跨媒體創作：對獻禮片春滿人間的考察 [A cross-media creation of a public event: An examination of the tribute film *Spring Reigns Everywhere*]. *Zhongwai yingshi* 中外影史 2 (2020): 82–89.

"Rai yōgisha mishindan ni kan suru ken." 癩容疑者未診断に関する件 [On an undiagnosed suspected leprosy sufferer]. Letter. Nagashima Aisei Archives, August 16, 1940.

Reagan, Leslie J, Nancy Tomes, and Paula A. Treichler, ed. *Medicine's Moving Pictures: Medicine, Health, and Bodies in American Film and Television*. Rochester, NY: University of Rochester Press, 2007.

Riedel, Friedlind. "Atmosphere." In *Affective Societies: Key Concepts*, edited by Jan Slaby and Christian von Scheve, 85–95. London: Routledge, 2019.

Riskin, Carl. *China's Political Economy: The Quest for Development since 1949*. New York: Oxford University Press, 1988.

Rogaski, Ruth. *Hygienic Modernity: Meanings of Health and Disease in Treaty Port China*. Berkeley, CA: University of California Press, 2004.

Rogaski, Ruth. "The Manchurian Plague and COVID-19: China, the United States, and the 'Sick Man', Then and Now." *American Journal of Public Health* 111, no. 3 (2021): 423–29.

Rogaski, Ruth. "Vampires in Plagueland: The Multiple Meanings of *Weisheng* in Manchuria." In *Health and Hygiene in Chinese East Asia: Policies and Publics in the Long Twentieth Century*, edited by Angela Ki Che Leung and Charlotte Furth, 132–59. Durham, NC: Duke University Press, 2010.

Rojas, Carlos. "Contradiction." In *Afterlives of Chinese Communism: Political Concepts from Mao to Xi*, edited by Christian Sorace, Ivan Franceschini, and Nicholas Loubere, 43–48. Canberra: ANU Press, 2019.

Rojas, Carlos. *Homesickness: Culture, Contagion, and National Transformation in Modern China*. Cambridge, MA: Harvard University Press, 2015.

Roquet, Paul. *Ambient Media: Japanese Atmospheres of Self*. Minneapolis, MN: University of Minnesota Press, 2016.

Rothe, Anne. *Popular Trauma Culture: Selling the Pain of Others in the Mass Media*. New Brunswick, NJ: Rutgers University Press, 2011.

Rothman, Barbara Katz. *The Biomedical Empire: Lessons Learned from the COVID-19 Pandemic*. Stanford, CA: Stanford University Press, 2021.

Rui, Kunnze and Marc Matten. *Knowledge Production in Mao-Era China: Learning from the Masses*. Lanham, MD: Lexington Books, 2021.

"Saengganmeogeunnabyeongnyeo sahyeongeulguhyeong" [A female leper sentenced to death for eating a raw liver]. *Donga Ilbo*, September 7, 1928.

Sakai, Naoki. "Modernity and Its Critique: The Problem of Universalism and Particularism." In *Postmodernism and Japan*, edited by Masao Mitoshi and H. D. Harootunian, 93–122. Durham, NC: Duke University Press, 1989.

Sanders, Vicki. "Dancing and the Dark Soul of Japan: An Aesthetic Analysis of 'Butō'." *Asian Theatre Journal* 5, no. 2 (1988): 148–63.

Scheid, Volker. *Chinese Medicine in Contemporary China*. Durham, NC: Duke University Press, 2007.

Schmalzer, Sigrid. "Red and Expert." In *Afterlives of Chinese Communism: Political Concepts from Mao to Xi*, edited by Christian Sorace, Ivan Franceschini, and Nicholas Loubere, 215–20. Canberra: ANU Press, 2019.

Schmalzer, Sigrid. *Red Revolution, Green Revolution: Scientific Farming in Socialist China*. Chicago: University of Chicago Press, 2016.

Schneider, Lawrence. *Biology and Revolution in Twentieth-Century China*. Lanham, MD: Rowman & Littlefield, 2003.

Scholl, Lesa. "Introduction: Medicine and Modernity." In *Medicine, Health and Being Human*, edited by Lesa Scholl, 1–12. London: Routledge, 2018.

Schwarz, Wendy. *Reading Tao Yuanming: Shifting Paradigms of Historical Reception (427–1900)*. Cambridge: Cambridge University Press, 2008.

Selden, Mark. *The Yenan Way in Revolutionary China*. Cambridge, MA: Harvard University Press, 1974.

Seo, Gijae. "Hansenbyeongeul dulleossan jeguguihagui geundaesa: Ilboneo midieoreul tonghae bon daejunggwanri jeollyak" [A modern history of imperial medicine surrounding Hansen's disease: Strategies to manage public opinion in modern Japanese media]. *Uisahak* 26, no. 3 (2017): 417–54.

Seo, Gijae. *Joseon Yeohaenge Tteodoneun Jeguk* [Empire wandering by travels to Joseon]. Seoul: Somyeong chulpan, 2011.

Seraphim, Franziska. "Spaces of Punishment." In *The Tokyo Tribunal: Perspectives on Law, History and Memory*, edited by Viviane E. Dittrich, Kerstin von Lingen, Philipp Osten, and Jolana Makraiová, 369–98. Brussels: Torkel Opsahl Academic EPublisher, 2020.

Shaanxi sheng zhongyi jinxiu xuexiao fushe menzhenbu 陝西省中醫進修學校附設門診部 [Shaanxi Province Chinese Medicine School Clinic]. "Zhenjiu shizhi longya 42 li de baogao" 針灸施治聾啞42例的報告 [Report on 42 deaf-mute cases treated by acupuncture]. *Zhongyi zazhi* 中醫雜誌, no. 1 (1956): 31.

Shanghai zhongyi xueyuan fushu dishiyi renmin yiyuan 上海中醫學院附屬第十一人民醫院 [11th Affiliated Hospital of Shanghai Chinese Medicine School]. "Zhenci chuangzao qiji: longzi ting daole zongluxian xuanchuan; yaba kaikou huijiang shehui zhuyi hao" 針刺創造奇跡 [Acupuncture creates miracles]. In *Quanguo yiliao weisheng jishu geminig jingyan jiaoliu dahui huikan* 全國醫療衛生技術革命經驗交流大會彙刊 [Compendium of the National Healthcare Technology Revolution Experience Exchange Conference], edited by *Quanguo yiliiao weisheng jishu geminig jingyan jiaoliu dahui mishuchu* 全國醫療衛生技術革命經驗交流大會秘書處, 246–47. Beijing: Renmin weisheng chubanshe, 1958.

Shaw, Claire L. *Deaf in USSR: Marginality, Community, and Soviet Identity, 1917–1991*. Ithaca, NY: Cornell University Press, 2017.

Shenyang zhongyi xuehui 瀋陽中醫學會 [Shenyang Chinese Medicine Association]. "Guanyu zhenjiu liaofa duiyu zhiliao longya zheng de jiaoliu jingyan zuotanhui zongjie" 關於針灸療法對於治療聾啞症的交流經驗座談會總結 [Symposium on treating deaf-mutism through acupuncture]. *Beijing zhongyi* 北京中醫3, no. 2 (1954): 31–32.

Shepherd, Sophia. "The Enemy is the Knife: Native Americans, Medical Genocide, and the Prohibition of Nonconsensual Sterilizations." *Michigan Journal of Race and Law* 27 (2021): 89–106.

Shi, Liu 石流, and Si Qi 思齊. "Kao Mao Zedong sixiang dakai le longya 'jinqu': 3016 budui weishengke Mao Zedong sixiang yiliao xuanchuangdui zai Liaoyuan Longya Xuexiao zhiliao longyabing de shiji" 靠毛澤東思想打開了聾啞"禁區": 3016部隊衛生科毛澤東思想醫療宣傳隊在遼源聾啞學校治療聾啞病的事蹟 [Relying on Mao Zedong thought to open the forbidden zone of deaf-mutism: The 3016th army health department's Mao Zedong thought medical team's treatment of deaf-mutism at Liaoyuan Deaf-Mute School]. *Renmin ribao* 人民日報, October 30, 1968, 4.

Shi, Yunxia, Chuhao Ma, and Yuxin Zhu. "The Impact of Emotional Labor on User Stickiness in the Context of Livestreaming Service—Evidence from China." *Frontiers in Psychology* 12 (2021): 698510.

Shibusawa, Naoko. *America's Geisha Ally: Reimagining the Japanese Enemy*. Cambridge, MA: Harvard University Press, 2006.

Shikiba, Ryūzaburō 式場隆三郎. "Igakuteki ni mita *Kojima no Haru*" 医学的にみた「小島の春」 [Watching Kojima no Haru medically]. *Nihon Eiga* 日本映画 5, no. 9 (1940): 36–38.

Shin, Dong Won. *Hoyeolja, Joseoneul Seupgyeokhada* [Cholera raids Joseon]. Seoul: Yuksabipyungsa, 2004.

Si, Chengdong 司程東, and Yu Zhili 於智籬. "Liji shanghan ji fushanghanyi shijunti fenli fangfa de yanjiu" 痢疾傷寒及副傷寒乙噬菌體分離方法的研究 [A study of methods for the detection of dysentery, typhoid, and paratyphoid B phages]. *Weishengwu xuebao* 微生物學報, no. 2 (1955): 145–50.

Shin, Hye-ju. "1900nyeondae gisaeng hwandeunghoe yeongu" [A study on lantern slide of *gisaeng* during the 1900s]. *Hangugeumaksahakbo* 58 (2017): 99–136.

Sidel, Victor W. "The Barefoot Doctors of the People's Republic of China." *New England Journal of Medicine* 286, no. 24 (1972): 1292–300.

Skvirsky, Salomé Aguilera. *The Process Genre: Cinema and the Aesthetic of Labor*. Durham, NC: Duke University Press, 2020.

Slone, Isabel. "Escape Into Cottagecore, Calming Ethos for Our Febrile Moment." *New York Times*, March 10, 2020. https://www.nytimes.com/2020/03/10/style/cottagecore.html.

Slovic, Scott, Swarnalatha Rangarajan, and Vidya Sarveswaran. "Introduction: Toward a Medical-Environmental Humanities. Why Now?" In *The Bloomsbury Handbook to The Medical-Environmental Humanities*, edited by Scott Slovic, Swarnalatha Rangarajan, and Vidya Sarveswaran, 1–10. London: Bloomsbury Academic, 2022.

Snelders, Stephen. *Leprosy and Colonialism: Suriname under Dutch Rule, 1750–1950*. Manchester: Manchester University Press, 2017.

So, Hyŏn-suk. "1956-nyŏn kajŏng pŏpryul sangdamso sŏlrip kwa hojujae p'yeji rŭl hyanghan kinagin yŏjŏng" [The long journey toward the abolition of "hojuje" in South Korea]. *Yŏksa pip'yŏng* 113 (2015): 72–94.

Sobchack, Vivian. "The Scene of the Screen: Envisioning Photographic, Cinematic, and Electronic 'Presence.'" In *Post-Cinema: Theorizing 21st-Century Film*, edited by Shane Denson and Julia Leyda, 88–128. Falmer: REFRAME Books, 2016.

Solomon-Godeau, Abigail. *Photography at the Dock*. Minneapolis, MN: University of Minnesota Press, 1991.

Song, Xiaobin 宋小濵. *Jiali jiawai hua xiejin* 家裡家外話謝晉 [Anecdotes about Xie Jin]. Beijing: Zhongguo shehui chubanshe, 2013.

Soon, Wayne. "Blood, Soy Milk, and Vitality: The Wartime Origins of Blood Banking in China, 1943–45." *Bulletin of the History of Medicine* 90, no. 3 (2016): 424–54.

Soon, Wayne. *Global Medicine in China: A Diasporic History*. Stanford, CA: Stanford University Press, 2020.

Sorace, Christian. "Saint Mao." *Telos*, no. 151 (2010): 173–91.

"Sorokdo yeonghwahwae chongdokbu wonjo" [Sorok island film screening supported by the government-general]. *Maeil sinbo*, January 10, 1941.

"Sorokutō no haru "小鹿島の春 [Spring on Sorok Island]. *Kankō Chōsen* 觀光朝鮮, March 1940.

"Sorokutō tanbōki: Chōsen'no *Kojima No Haru*" 小鹿島探訪記：朝鮮の小島の春 [Travel journal of Sorok island: Joseon's *Spring on the Small Island*]. *Modan Nippon Chōsenhan* モダン日本 朝鮮板, 1940.

Sorokutōkōseien 小鹿島更生院, ed. *Sorokutōkōseien nenpō* 小鹿島更生院年表 [A chronology of Sorok sanitarium]. Sorokutō: Sorokutōkōseien, 1937.

"Sotsugyōsei: Keijōteikokudaigaku" 卒業生：京城帝國大學 [Graduates: Keijō imperial university]. *Chōsensōtokufu kanpō* 朝鮮總督府官報, April 5, 1941.

Stam, Robert. *Subversive Pleasures: Bakhtin, Cultural Criticism, and Film*. Baltimore, MD: Johns Hopkins University Press, 1989.

Steimatsky, Noa. *The Face on Film*. Oxford: Oxford University Press, 2017.

Sterne, Jonathan. *Diminished Faculties: A Political Phenomenology of Impairment*. Durham, NC: Duke University Press, 2022.

Sturman, Peter Charles, and Susan Tai, eds. *The Artful Recluse: Painting, Poetry, and Politics in Seventeenth-Century China*. Santa Barbara, CA: Santa Barbara Museum of Art, 2012.

Summers, William. *Félix d'Herelle and the Origins of Molecular Biology*. New Haven, CT: Yale University Press, 1999.

Suzuki, Akihito. "Public Health, Laboratory Experiment, and Asymptomatic Carriers in Japan, ca. 1920–1950." *East Asian Science, Technology, and Society: An International Journal* 13 (2019): 39–55.

Takio, Eiji 滝尾英二. *Chōsen Hansenbyōshi: Nihon shokuminchika no Sorokuto* 朝鮮ハンセン病史：日本植民地下の小鹿島 [History of Hansen's disease in Joseon: Sorok island under the Japanese rule]. Tokyo: Miraisha, 2001.

Takio, Eiji 滝尾英二, ed. *Shinbun kiji ni miru Hansenbyō 1* 新聞記事にみるハンセン病 1 [Hansen's disease through newspaper 1). Vol. 4. 8 vols. Shokuminchika Chōsen ni okeru Hansenbyō shiryō shūsei 植民地下朝鮮におけるハンセン病資料集成 [Collection of material on Hansen's disease in Korea under the Japanese rule]. Tokyo: Fuji Shuppan, 2002.

Takio, Eiji 滝尾英二, ed. *Shinbun kiji ni miru Hansenbyō 2* 新聞記事にみるハンセン病 2 [Hansen's disease through newspaper 2]. Vol. 5. 8 vols. Shokuminchika Chōsen ni okeru Hansenbyō shiryō shūsei 植民地下朝鮮におけるハンセン病資料集成 [Collection of material on Hansen's disease in Korea under the Japanese rule]. Tokyo: Fuji Shuppan, 2002.

Tam, Yee Lok. "Colourful Screens: Water Imaginaries in Documentaries from China and Taiwan." *Interactions: Studies in Communication & Culture* 2, no. 2 (2010): 109–25.

Tamura, Yoshihiko 田村幸彦, Tanaka Toshio 田中敏夫, Ogura Kin'ya 小倉金弥, Ikeda Kazo 池田一夫, Nishimura Masami 西村正美, and Tomiogi Masao 冨尾木正雄. "*Kojima no haru* no zadankai" 「小島の春」の座談会 [Roundtable discussion on *Spring on the Small Island*]. *Eiga to gijutsu* 映画と技術 15, no. 8 (1940): 21–25.

Tanaka, Kathryn M. "Contested Histories and Happiness: Leprosy Literature in Japan." *Health, Culture, and Society* 5, no. 1 (2013): 99–118.

Tanaka, Kathryn M. "For the Purity of the Nation: Ogawa Masako and the Gendered Ethics of *Spring on the Small Island* (*Kojima no haru*)." *U.S.-Japan Women's Journal* 50 (2016): 93–114.

Tanimoto, Kiyoshi 谷本清. *Hiroshima genbaku to Amerikajin: Aru bokushi no heiwa angya* 広島原爆とアメリカ人：ある牧師の平和行脚 [Hiroshima atomic bomb and Americans: A minister's peace pilgrimage]. Tokyo: Nippon hoso shuppan kyokai, 1976.

Taylor, Jeremy E. "From Transnationalism to Nativism? The Rise, Decline and Reinvention of a Regional Hokkien Entertainment Industry." *Inter-Asia Cultural Studies* 9, no. 1 (2008): 62–81.

Taylor, Kim. *Chinese Medicine in Early Communist China, 1945–1963: A Medicine of Revolution*. London: Routledge, 2005.

Taylor, T. L. *Watch Me Play: Twitch and the Rise of Game Live Streaming*. Cambridge, MA: The MIT Press, 2018.

Teaiwa, Teresia K. "bikinis and other s/pacific n/oceans." *The Contemporary Pacific* 6, no. 1 (1994): 87–109.

Teiwes, Frederick C. *Politics and Purges in China: Rectification and the Decline of Party Norms, 1950–1965*. 2nd edition. Armonk, NY: M. E. Sharpe, 1993.

Terranova, Tiziana. "Free Labor: Producing Culture for the Digital Economy." *Social Text* 18.2 (2000): 33–58.

The Committee of Concerned Asian Scholars. *China! Inside the People's Republic*. Toronto: Bantam, 1972.

The Yellow Emperor's Classic of Internal Medicine. Translated and edited by Ilza Veith. Berkeley, CA: University of California Press, 1975.

Theobald, Brianna. *Reproduction on the Reservation: Pregnancy, Childbirth, and Colonialism in the Long Twentieth Century*. Chapel Hill, NC: The University of North Carolina Press, 2019.

This Is Your Life. Season 3, episode 32, "Rev. Kiyoshi Tanimoto." Aired May 11, 1955, on NBC. https://www.dailymotion.com/video/xl3jx5.

"Tottori ken kōshū eisei kacho" 鳥取県公衆衛生課長. Letter to Nagashima Aisei-en Entertainment Committee Chief returning two borrowed films. 25 July 1951. Nagashima Aisei-en Archives. *Iji kankei ippan* 医事関係一般, Showa 26–27.

Tsai, Brian. "U.S. Uninsured Rate Hits Record Low in First Quarter of 2023." Accessed November 15, 2023. https://blogs.cdc.gov/nchs/2023/08/03/7434/#:~:text=Highlights%20from%20the%20report%3A,the%20same%20period%20in%202022.

Tsai, Tsung-lung, Li-ping Yu, and Chin-yuan Ke. "A Glimpse at the Development of the Environmental Documentary in Taiwan." *Concentric: Literary and Cultural Studies* 39, no. 1 (2013): 161–76.

Tu, Jiong. *Health Care Transformation in Contemporary China: Moral Experience in a Socialist Neoliberal Polity*. Dordrecht: Springer, 2019.

Uchida, Jun. *Brokers of Empire: Japanese Settler Colonialism in Korea, 1876–1945*. Cambridge, MA: Harvard University Asia Center, 2011.

Uchida, Morito 内田守人. "Eiga *Kojima no haru* no zakkan" 映画「小島の春」の雑感 [Miscellaneous thoughts on the film *Spring on the Small Island*]. *Nihon dangi* 日本談義 3, no. 10 (1940): 50–51.

Van Dijck, José. *The Culture of Connectivity: A Critical History of Social Media*. Oxford: Oxford University Press, 2013.

Velmet, Aro. *Pasteur's Empire: Bacteriology and Politics in France, Its Colonies, and the World*. Oxford: Oxford University Press, 2020.

Wang, Fangfei. "Narrating China: Reading Li Ziqi and Fangfang from a Nationalist Perspective." Masters thesis, Duke University, 2021.

Wang, Jianxin 汪建新. "Zaidu Mao Zedong 'Qilü ershou songwenshen'" 再讀毛澤東《七律二首•送瘟神》[Revisiting Mao Zedong's "Farewell to the God of Plague"]. February 24, 2020. http://dangshi.people.com.cn/n1/2020/0224/c85037-31601095.html.

Wang, Qiming 王啟明. "Guanyu longya zhenjiu zhiliao qingkuang jieshao" 關於聾啞針灸治療情況介紹 [Results of curing deaf-mutism through acupuncture]. *Zhongyi zazhi*, 中醫雜誌, no. 1 (1956): 36–37.

Wang, Xiajing 汪俠靜. "'Wei' shidaixia zhiyuxi wenhua liuxing xianxiang jiedu" "微"時代下治癒系文化流行現象解讀 [An analysis of the healing culture popular phenomenon in the "micro" era]. *Qingnianjizhe* 青年記者, no. 32 (2018): 30–31.

Wang, Xinyi, François Colbert, and Renaud Legoux. "From Niche Interest to Fashion Trend: *Hanfu* Clothing as a Rising Industry in China." *International Journal of Arts Management* 23.1 (2020): 79–89.

Wang, Yu 王宇. "Yan'an wenxue zhong de yiliaoweisheng xushi" 延安文學中的醫療衛生敘事 [Medical and hygienic narratives in Yan'an literature]. *Xueshu yuekan* 學術月刊 (2017): 132–40.

Watt, John R. *Saving Lives in Wartime China: How Medical Reformers Built Modern Healthcare Systems Amid War and Epidemics, 1928–1945*. Leiden: Brill, 2013.

Wei, Zongdai 魏宗岱. "Zhenci erlong ji shijuezheng zhi jingyan" 針刺耳聾及屍厥症之經驗 [Experience in the acupuncture treatment of deafness and fainting syndromes]. *Yixiue zazhi* 醫學雜誌 35 (1927): 92–94.

Weisgall, Jonathan M. "The Nuclear Nomads of Bikini." *Foreign Policy*, no. 39 (1980): 74–98.

Whitehead, Anne, and Angela Woods. "Introduction." In *The Edinburgh Companion to the Critical Medical Humanities*, edited by Anne Whitehead, Angela Woods, Sarah Atkinson, Jane Macnaughton, and Jennifer Richards, 1–31. Edinburgh: Edinburgh University Press, 2016.

"Wisaenggangyeonhwaldongsajin" [Hygiene lecture and film]. *Maeil Sinbo*, June 18, 1922.

Wŏn, Chu-yŏng. "Ŭishik kaesŏnŭl t'onghan hwan'gyŏng kwalli: 1970-nyŏndae ch'o toshi ŭi hwan'gyŏng munje wa toshi saemaŭl undong" [Urban pollution and the city saemaul movement: An environmental management in the early 1970s]. *Han'guk kwahaksa hakhoeji* 45, no. 1 (2023): 43–69.

Wu, Kang 伍慷. "Qingnian qunti zhiyuxi wenhua liuxing xianxiang touxi" 青年群體治癒系文化流行現象透析 [Close analysis of the healing culture popular phenomenon among youth groups]. *Qingnian tansuo* 青年探索, no. 5 (2017): 94–100.

Wu, Sheng 吳晟. "Zhineng weini xie yishou shi" 只能為你寫一首詩 [Can only write you a poem]. Huanjing zixun zhongxin 環境資訊中心. June 27, 2010. https://e-info.org.tw/node/56856.

Wu, Zhisheng 吳芝昇, and Zhang Zhixue 張知學. "Zhenjiu liaofa zhiliao longya zheng de jige bingan" 針灸療法治療聾啞症的幾個病案 [Several clinical cases on treating deaf-mutism]. *Beijing zhongyi* 北京中醫 3, no. 5 (1953): 20.

Wu, Zhisheng, and Zhang Zhixue. "Shenjingxing longya zhifa chubu jieshao" 神經性聾啞治法初步介紹 [Preliminary introductions on treating neurotic deafness]. *Zhongyi zazhi* 中醫雜誌, no. 1 (1955): 32.

Xiao, Xiong 肖雄. *Xinzhongguo shiqinian zhenjiu tuiguang yudong yanjiu* 新中國十七年針灸推廣運動研究 [A study on the promotion of acupuncture in PRC, 1949–1966]. PhD dissertation. Guangzhou zhongyiyao daxue, 2021.

Xie, Junfeng, et al. "*Shengming de kaige*" 生命的凱歌 [*A Song of Victory for Life*]. *Zhongguo dianying* 中國電影, no. 1 (1959): 53–74.

Xu, Shichang 徐世長. "Zhenci mumang zhi jingyan" 針刺目盲之經驗 [Experience of acupunctural treatment of blindness]. *Yixue zazhi* 醫學雜誌 10 (1922): 101–3.

Xu, Shichang 徐世長. "Banshen busui kouyan woxie cifa" 半身不遂口眼喎斜刺方 [Needling methods for physical and facial paralysis]. *Yixue zazhi* 醫學雜誌 21 (1924): 103.

Yagi, Yasutarō 八木保太郎. "Kyakyuhon *Kojima no haru*" 脚本「小島の春」 [Film script, *Spring on the Small Island*]. *Kinema Junpō bessatsu Nihon eiga daihyō shinario zenshū* キネマ旬報別冊 映画代表シナリオ全集2 (1958): 81–96.

"Yakjin Joseonyeonghwagye munhwayeonghwajejak chaksu" [Rapid progress of Josen film world, initiation of culture film production]. *Chosun ilbo*, February 20, 1940.

Yang, Jie. *Unknotting the Heart: Unemployment and Therapeutic Governance in China*. Ithaca, NY: Cornell University Press, 2015.

Yang, Zongcheng. "Development of Burn Medicine in China." In *Chinese Burn Surgery*, edited by Zongcheng Yang, 1–7. Dordrecht: Springer, 2015.

Yashiro, Naohiro, Reiko Suzuki, and Wataru Suzuki. "Evaluating Japan's Health Care Reform of the 1990s and Its Efforts to Cope with Population Aging." In *Health Care Issues in the United States and Japan*, edited by David A. Wise and Naohiro Yashiro, 17–42. Chicago: The University of Chicago Press, 2006.

Yavenditti, Michael J. "The Hiroshima Maidens and American Benevolence in the 1950s." *Mid-America: An Historical Review* 64, no. 2 (1982): 21–39.

Ye, Zhen. "Streamer-Interface-Viewer Entanglement in Popular Chinese Social Media Apps: An Analysis of the Discursive and Affective Live-Streaming Chatroom Interfaces." *MedieKultur* no. 70 (2020): 131–50.

Yi Bai Qiuen wei guanghui bangyang: Zhongguo yisheng he gongcheng jishu renyuan zai guowai 以白求恩為光輝榜樣：中國醫生和工程技術人員在國外 [Taking Bethune as a shining example—Chinese doctors and engineering technicians abroad]. Shanghai: Shanghai renmin chubanshe, 1970.

Yi, Jun 藝軍. "Gongchanzhuyi sixiang de kaige: kan yingpian *Chunman renjian*" 共產主義思想的凱歌：看影片春滿人間 [A victorious song of the communist spirit: Watching *Spring Reigns Everywhere*]. *Dianying yishu* 電影藝術, no. 2 (1960): 59–61.

Yi, Sŭl-gi. "Nongyak chungsim ŭro pon noksaek hyŏngmyŏng: 1970-nyŏndae chŭngsan kwa konghae e karyŏjin nongyak chungdok" [Pesticide problems in the Korean green revolution: Inequal knowledge production, ignorance, and invisible pesticide poisoning in the 1970s]. *Han'guk kwahaksa hakhoeji* 43, no. 1 (2021): 215–35.

"Yixiang zhongyao de chengjiu" 一項重要的成就 [An Important Achievement]. *Renmin ribao* 人民日報, December 10, 1958, 6.

Yoneyama, Lisa. *Hiroshima Traces: Time, Space, and the Dialectics of Memory*. Berkeley, CA: University of California Press, 1999.

Yoo, Sunyoung. "Sigakgisulloseo hwandeunggwa singminjiui sigakseong" [Magic lantern as a technology of vision and construction of visuality in colonial Korea]. *Eollongwa sahoe* 24, no. 2 (2016): 191–229.

Young, Paul. *The Cinema Dreams of Its Rivals: Media Fantasy Films from Radio to the Internet*. Minneapolis, MN: University of Minnesota Press, 2006.

"YouTube Stats and Analytics for Li Ziqi." *Hypeauditor*. Accessed February 2022. https://hypeauditor.com/youtube/li_zi_qi_liziqi-UCoC47do520os_4DBMEFGg4A/.

Yu, Chang-Min. "Cinema's Turing Test: Consciousness, Digitality, and Operability in *Hardcore Henry*. *NECSUS: European Journal of Media Studies* 6 (2017): 189–207.

Yu, Eun, Chanyong Jung, Hyungkin Kim, and Jaemin Jung. "Impact of Viewer Engagement on Gift-Giving in Live Video Streaming." *Telematics and Informatics* no. 35 (2018): 1450–60.

Yu, He 余賀. "Weishengwu yu jiti" 微生物與機體 [Microbes and organisms]. *Zhexue yanjiu* 哲學研究, no. 3 (1962): 23–28.

Yu, He 余賀. *Xijunxue* 細菌學 [Bacteriology]. Beijing: Renmin weisheng chubanshe, 1956.

Yuan, Mingdong 袁明東 and Chen Xinyuan 陳心園. "Zhenjiu zhiliao longya 153 li de jingyan xiaojie" 針灸治療聾啞153例的經驗小節 [Results of 153 cases on treating deaf-mutism through acupuncture]. *Zhongyi zazhi* 中醫雜誌, no. 12 (1956): 647.

Yun, Che-yon. "Nugu rŭl wihan hwan'gyŏng chŏngch'aek in'ga" [Who are environmental policies for?]. In *Salminya chukŭminya* [Life or death], edited by Chŏng Ho-kyŏng and Kim Chi-ha, 101–5. Seoul: Hyŏngsŏngsa, 1985.

Yurgel, Caio. "Li Ziqi: A Romantic in the Year of the Plague." *Sixth Tone*, December 9, 2021. https://www.sixthtone.com/news/1009177/li-ziqi-a-romantic-in-the-year-of-the-plague.

Zhang, Ge, and Larrisa Hjorth. "Live-Streaming, Games and Politics of Gender Performance: The Case of *Nüzhubo* in China." *Convergence* 25, no. 5–6 (2019): 807–25.

Zhang, Jinfeng 張金鳳. "Zimeiti shiyuxia xiangcun qingnian 'zouhong' xianxiang de chuanboxue tanjiu" 自媒體視野下鄉村青年『走紅』現象的傳播探究 [A communication studies analysis of rural youth's "road to stardom" through the lens of self-media]. *Shiting* 視聽, no. 5 (2020): 210–12.

Zhang, Li. *Anxious China: Inner Revolution and the Politics of Psychotherapy*. Oakland, CA: University of California Press, 2020.

Zhang, Ling. "Foreshadowing the Future of Capitalism: Surveillance Technology and Digital Realism in Xu Bing's *Dragonfly Eyes* (2017)." *Comparative Cinema* 8, no. 14 (2020): 62–81.

Zhang, Wei 張碨. "Rang yaba shuohua de ren" 讓啞巴說話的人 [The person who makes the mute talk]. *Renmin ribao* 人民日報, December 10, 1958, 6.

Zhang, Wei 張碨. "Yang Fuzhi fazhan le zuguo zhenjiu xue" 楊輔之發展了祖國針灸學 [Yang Fuzhi has developed the acupuncture of the motherland]. *Renmin ribao* 人民日報, December 10, 1958, 6.

Zhang, Zijun 張子駿. "Shidaorujin, cai zhenzheng kandongle Li Ziqi de shipin" 事到如今，才真正看懂了李子柒的視頻 [Only when our situation has come to this, do we truly understand Li Ziqi's videos]. *Elle China*, February 19, 2020. https://www.ellechina.com/celeb/gossip/a30991715/liziqi-20220219/.

Zhao, Puyu 趙普羽. "Wuxian zhongyu Mao zhuxi chuangzao qiji" 無限忠於毛主席創造奇蹟 [Unlimited loyalty to Chairman Mao creates miracle]. *Remin ribao* 人民日報, May 19, 1969, 5.

Zhao, Puyu 趙普羽. "Kao Mao Zedong sixiang dakai longya jinqu" 靠毛澤東思想打開聾啞禁區 [Relying on Mao Zedong thought to open the forbidden zone of deaf-mutism]. *Renmin Ribao* 人民日報, October 24, 1969, 4.

Zhao, Zhifang 趙志方. "Zhenjiu zhi longya" 針灸治聾啞 [Curing deaf-mutism with acupuncture]. *Renmin Ribao* 人民日報, August 27, 1958, 7.

"Zhenjiu zhi longya." 針灸治聾啞 [Curing deaf-mutism with acupuncture]. *Shangying huabao* 上影畫報, no. 8 (1959): 23.

Zhonggong zhongyang wenxianshi 中共中央文獻室. *Mao Zedong nianpu* 毛澤東年譜 [Chronology of Mao Zedong]. Beijing: Zhongyang wenxian chubanshe, 1993.

Zhongguo gongchandang Shanghai dier yixueyuan weiyuanhui 中國共產黨上海第二醫院委員會. "Guanyu qiangjiu tangshang gongren Qiu Caikang tongzhi de gongzuo zongjie" 關於搶救燙傷工人邱財康同志的工作總結 [Work summary of rescuing the burned worker comrade Qiu Caikang]. *Shangyi xuebao* 上醫學報, no. 2 (1958): 83–89.

Zhongguo renmin jiefangjun no. 1806 budui zhengzhibu 中國人民解放軍1806部隊政治部. "Beijingshi Disan Longern Xuexiao shisheng huansong Zong Jinguang ruwu" 北京市第三聾啞學校師生歡送宗金廣入伍 [Teachers and students of Beijing No. 3 Deaf-mute School see Zong Jinguang off to join the army]. *Renmin Huabao* 人民畫報, June (1971): 44.

Zhongguo yiliao dui 中國醫療隊. "Zhongguo yisheng ba ta de bing zhihao le: Zhongguo yiliaodui zai Yemen zhiliao longya bingren de shiji" 中國醫生把他的病治好了：中國醫療隊在也門治療聾啞病人的事蹟 [Chinese doctors cured his disease: Chinese medical team treats deaf-mute patients in Yemen]. *Renmin Ribao* 人民日報, November 15, 1969, 5.

Zhu, Lian 朱璉. *Xin zhenjiu xue* 新針灸學 [New acupuncture]. Beijing: Renmin weisheng chubanshe, 1954.

Zuo, Hua 左華. "Women weishenme meiyou baodao hao Qiu Caikang" 我們為什麼沒有報導好邱財康 [Why did we not do well in reporting Qiu Caikang]. *Chuanmei pinglun* 傳媒評論, no. 10 (1958): 17 and 23.

Zuppello, Suzanne. "Slow Food's Elitism Only Fueled My Cravings for McDonald's." *Eater*, October 18, 2018. https://www.eater.com/2018/10/18/17943358/slow-food-manifesto-elitist-fast-food.

Index

Note: Page locators in italics denote endnotes and locators in bold denote photographs or illustrations.

www.ingramcontent.com/pod-product-compliance
Ingram Content Group UK Ltd.
Pitfield, Milton Keynes, MK11 3LW, UK
UKHW021836100926
8556IPUK00004B/385

9 789888 876815